OSCE in Critical Care Medicine-I

OSCE in Critical Care Medicine-I

Editors

Atul Prabhakar Kulkarni
MD FISCCM PGDHHM FICCM

Editor-in-Chief, Indian Journal of Critical Care Medicine
Past President, Indian Society of Critical Care Medicine
Past Chancellor, Indian College of Critical Care Medicine
Past President, Association of SAARC Critical Care Societies
Secretary General, Asia Pacific Association of Critical Care Medicine
Professor and Head, Division of Critical Care Medicine
Department of Anesthesiology, Critical Care and Pain
Tata Memorial Hospital, Homi Bhabha National Institute
Mumbai, Maharashtra India

Shilpushp Jagannath Bhosale
MD DM (Critical Care Medicine)

Associate Professor
Consultant Intensivist, Division of Critical Care
Department of Anesthesiology, Critical Care and Pain
Tata Memorial Hospital, Homi Bhabha National Institute
Mumbai, Maharashtra India

Jacob George Pulinilkunnathil
MD (Respiratory Medicine) DM (Critical Care) IDCCM IFCCM EDIC FCCP

Consultant Pulmonologist and Intensivist
Department of Critical Care Medicine
Mar Sleeva Medicity Palai
Cherpunkal, Kerala, India

JAYPEE

JAYPEE BROTHERS MEDICAL PUBLISHERS
The Health Sciences Publisher
New Delhi | London

Jaypee Brothers Medical Publishers (P) Ltd

Headquarters

Jaypee Brothers Medical Publishers (P) Ltd
4838/24, Ansari Road, Daryaganj
New Delhi 110 002, India
Phone: +91-11-43574357
Fax: +91-11-43574314
Email: jaypee@jaypeebrothers.com

Overseas Office

J.P. Medical Ltd
83 Victoria Street, London
SW1H 0HW (UK)
Phone: +44 20 3170 8910
Fax: +44 (0)20 3008 6180
Email: info@jpmedpub.com

Website: www.jaypeebrothers.com
Website: www.jaypeedigital.com

Inquiries for bulk sales may be solicited at: jaypee@jaypeebrothers.com

OSCE in Critical Care Medicine-I

First Edition: **2020**

ISBN 978-93-90020-49-2

Printed at

Dedicated to

The Most Hard Working Residents in Medicine:
The Critical Care Trainees!

CONTRIBUTORS

Carol Dsilva MD FNB EDIC
Assistant Professor
Department of Critical Care Medicine
St Johns Medical College Hospital
Bengaluru, Karnataka, India

Deepthi Madhu MBBS MD
Consultant Clinical Microbiologist
Mar Sleeva Medicity Palai
Cherpunkal, Kerala, India

Harish Mallapura Maheshwarappa
MBBS MD DM (Critical care medicine) DNB IDCCM EDIC (Dublin) MBA (Health Care Management)
Consultant
Department of Critical Care Medicine
Mazumdar Shaw Medical Center
Narayana Hrudayalaya
Bengaluru, Karnataka, India

Kiran Vishnu Narayan
MD DNB DM Diploma in Allergy and Immunology (CMC Vellore) Specialty certificate in Resp Medicine-MRCP UK European Diploma in Adult Respiratory Medicine (EDARM) European Diploma in Intensive Care Medicine (EDIC)
Assistant Professor
Department of Pulmonary Medicine
Government Medical College
Kottayam, Kerala, India

Manu Varma MK MBBS MD DM PDCC
Assistant Professor
Department of Critical Care Medicine
St John's Medical College and Hospital
Bengaluru, Karnataka, India

Natesh Prabu R
MD DNB DM (Critical Care Medicine)
Assistant Professor
Department of Critical Care Medicine
St John's Medical College and Hospital
Bengaluru, Karnataka, India

Reeba George Pulinilkunnathil
DMRD DNB Radiodiagnosis
Associate Professor
Department of Radiodiagnosis
Government Medical College
Thiruvananthapuram, Kerala, India

Ruchira Khasne
MBBS DA DNB IDCCM EDAIC & EDIC
Consultant and Head
Department of Critical Care Medicine
Ashoka Medicover Hospital
Nashik, Maharashtra, India

Shiva Kumar N
MBBS MD DNB DM (Critical Care) EDIC
Assistant Professor
Department of Critical Care Medicines
St John's Medical College
Bengaluru, Karnataka, India

Suhail Sarwar Siddiqui MD DM EDIC
Assistant Professor
Department of Critical Care Medicine
King George's Medical University (KGMU)
Lucknow, Uttar Pradesh, India

PREFACE

It gives us great pleasure to present the *OSCE in Critical Care Medicine-I.* Objective Structured Clinical Examination (OSCE) was first described by Harden RM and Gleeson FA in 1975. OSCE dramatically changed the assessment of professional competence because it used actors and choreographed scenarios to evaluate the performance of professional behaviors. An OSCE usually comprises a circuit of short (the usual is 5–10 minutes, although some use up to 15 minute) stations. The examination pattern has now changed and the examinee is expected to answer briefly the questions given at each station. These questions may include the results of tests or investigations or laboratory results. Since each question has a standard answer there is no risk of bias of the examiners influencing the marks obtained by the students. It is therefore more credible way to examine the knowledge and ability of the examinee to apply it to clinical problem solving. The OSCEs have become a part of most examinations in Critical Care Medicine, and rightly so. There is no way anyone can predict the questions that the examinee is likely to face in various examinations. But we all know Practice makes Perfect! (this is actually grammatically incorrect and should have been Practice makes Perfection!). This idiom is very old, dates back to 1550, when it was first said "Use makes Perfect" by John Adams, and then in Latin is "Uses promptos facit". Though it is old, it still makes sense, and therefore this book for all our future examinees. As the title suggests, this is but the first book in a series of books on OSCEs in Critical Care Medicine. A word about the origin of the idea. Jacob George, my friend (still!) and a colleague till last year, suggested that such a book will be of great help to the examinees. I am grateful to him for the idea and for the hard work he has put into making this book possible, and hopefully he will still be enthusiastic about the future books in the series. The last but not least, thanks are due to the Contributors who helped in making the book what it is. Their untiring support (of course with some nagging from Shil, Jacob, and me) was invaluable and we hope for their contributions in the future as well.

We wish all of you happy reading and the best for your examinations!

Atul Prabhakar Kulkarni
Shilpushp Jagannath Bhosale
Jacob George Pulinilkunnathil

ACKNOWLEDGMENTS

We would like to acknowledge the support of all our colleagues in the department who worked hard and spared us from our clinical duties so we could work on the book and our sincere thanks to them. Acknowledgments are due to Dr Jigeeshu Divatia, our head, whose support and backing make all our academic endeavors possible. Ms Chetna Malhotra (Associate Director—Content Strategy), an old friend from Jaypee Brothers Medical Publishers (P) Ltd. who always helps in our publication ventures. Our families have been particularly supportive (no fights, at least about this book), while we labored for the sake of the book.

CONTENTS

QUESTIONS

ANSWERS

QUESTIONS

RESPIRATORY MEDICINE

1. You are called in to see a postoperative patient who is becoming difficult to ventilate and desaturating despite providing 100% FiO_2.
   - What is the diagnosis?
   - How will you manage the case?

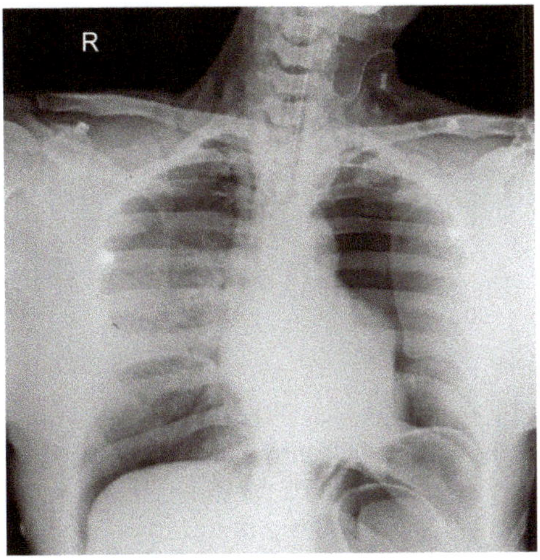

2. Comment on the chest X-ray of a patient who is being electively ventilated for breathlessness.

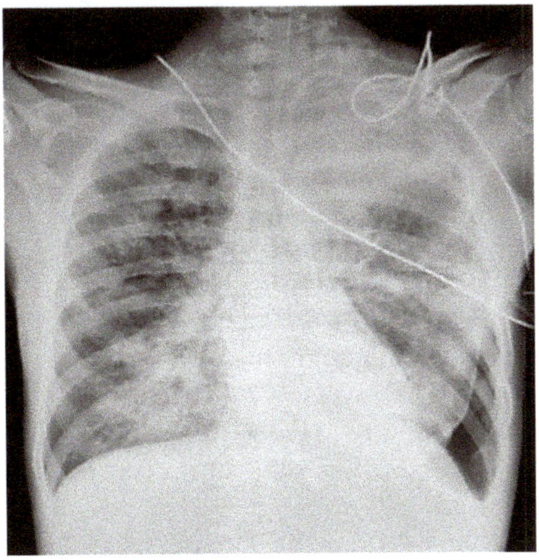

3. This patient was shifted to ICU from OR as a postoperative case for elective ventilation overnight. The patient's saturations are persistently low at 88% despite FiO_2 of 80%.
   - What is the classic radiologic sign in the picture?

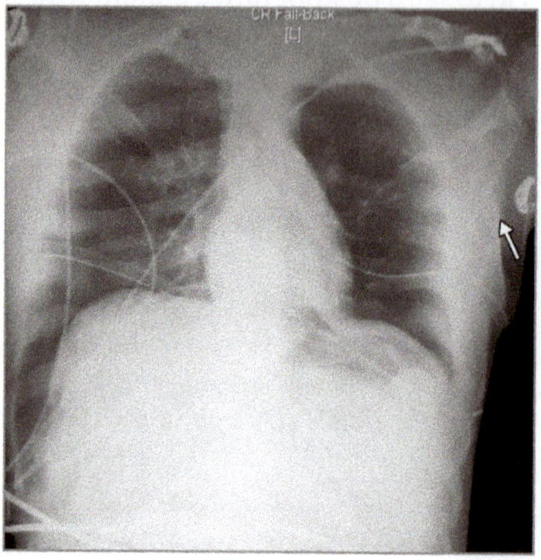

4. A 72-year-old man with past history of hypertension and diabetes mellitus presented to the ER with the sudden onset of intense chest pain radiating to right arm and back for the past half an hour. A contrast CT was taken as chest X-ray showed mediastinal widening.
   - What is the diagnosis and management?

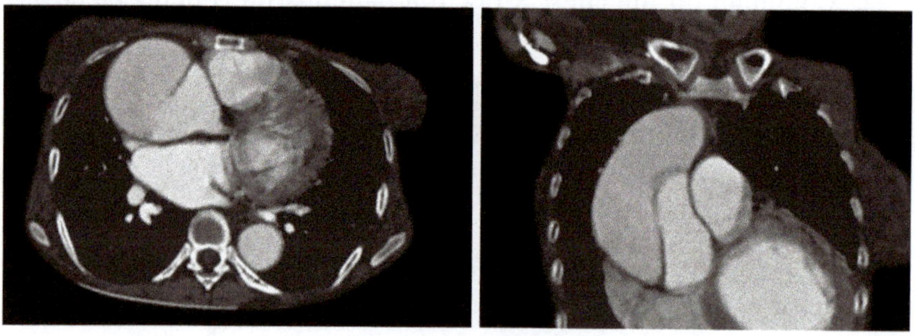

5. A 46-year-old male underwent an upper GI endoscopy for evaluation of esophageal malignancy and dysphagia. Post procedure, he complains of severe chest pain and is admitted to ICU. ECG is normal; HR 115 beats/min; sinus; BP 110/86 mm Hg; RR 26 breaths/min; and saturation 98% on room air. A CT thorax was taken which is shown in image below.
   What is the diagnosis and management?

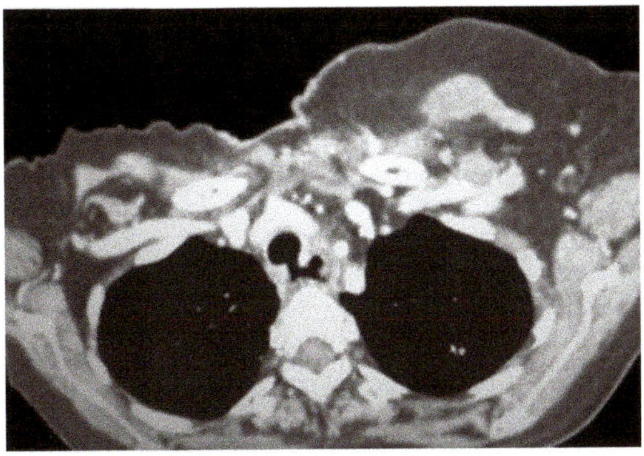

6. A 26-year-old male, a known case of metastatic choriocarcinoma testes, presents with breathing difficulty of 1-week duration. In view of respiratory distress, he is started on noninvasive ventilation (NIV) with a PEEP of 7 cm H_2O, and FiO_2 70%. An ABG showed a PF ratio 180.
As per the BERLIN definition of ARDS, which category of ARDS does he fall into?

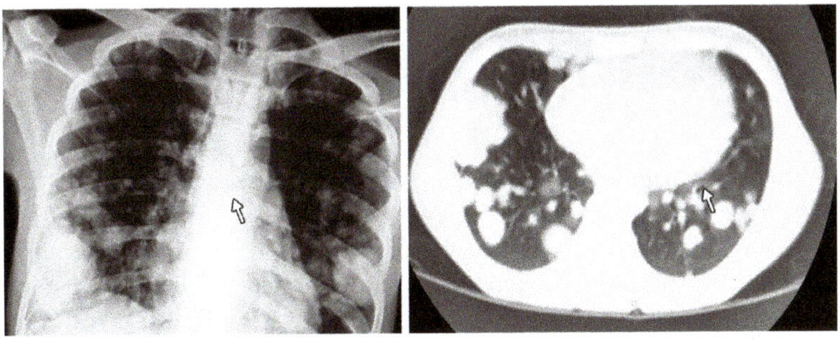

7. An 85-year-old female, known case of HT, DM, and CAD, presented to ER with acute onset fever, chest pain, and breathlessness. What is the possible etiological diagnosis?
   - How will you score the severity of the condition?
   - What is the evidence for HFNC in this condition?

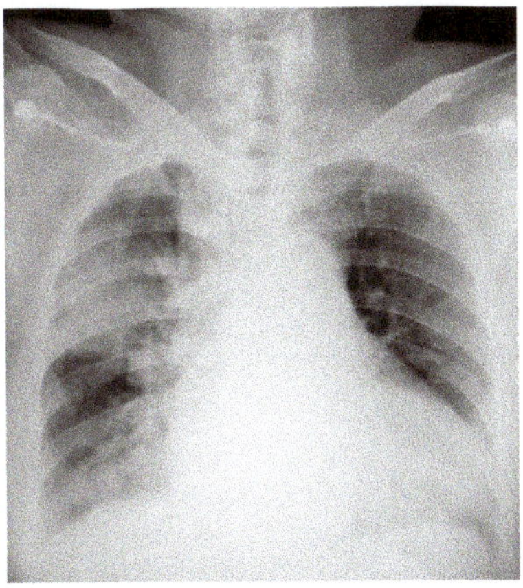

8. A 74-year-old male, a known case of diabetes mellitus, hypertension, and coronary artery disease, is now admitted with breathing difficulty.
   - What is the diagnosis?
   - What are the mechanisms by which noninvasive ventilation will help in managing the patient?

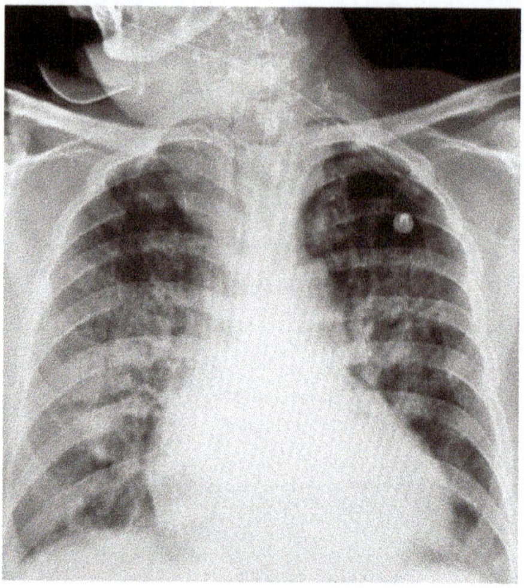

9. This patient is being referred to you with worsening hypoxia, despite being ventilated with 100% FiO_2 and PEEP of 16 cm H_2O. He was apparently normal till last week and the symptoms of cough and breathing difficulty started after a viral prodrome and upper respiratory tract infection. Currently he is being ventilated with 6 mL/kg tidal volume, 16 cm H_2O PEEP and 100% FiO_2 with a respiratory rate of 28. His PaO_2 is 86 mm Hg and PCO_2 is 96 mm Hg with a pH of 7.13. How will you classify the condition?

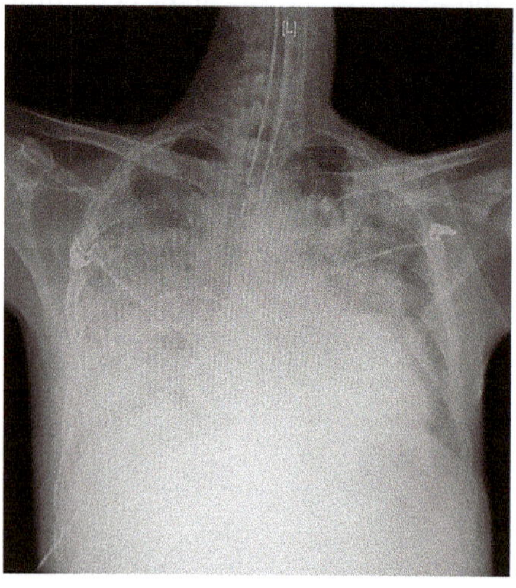

10. Comment on the chest X-ray of a patient, a known case of chronic kidney disease, intubated after being revived from a hyperkalemic cardiac arrest. Post intubation there is a constant alarms of high peak pressures, and the patient is having worsening hypoxia.

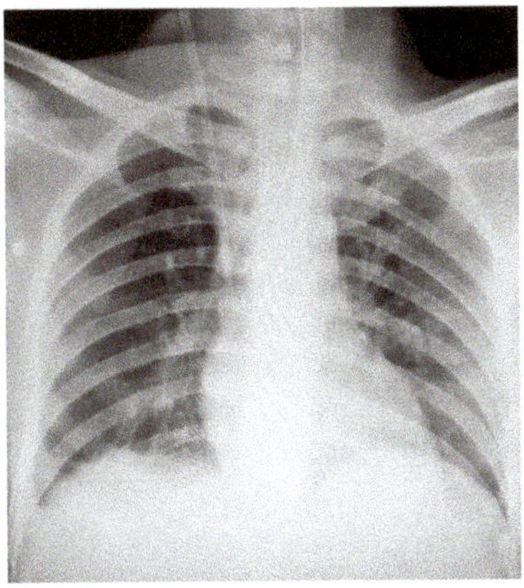

11. Comment on the device seen on chest X-ray.
    What are the class 1 indications for the same?

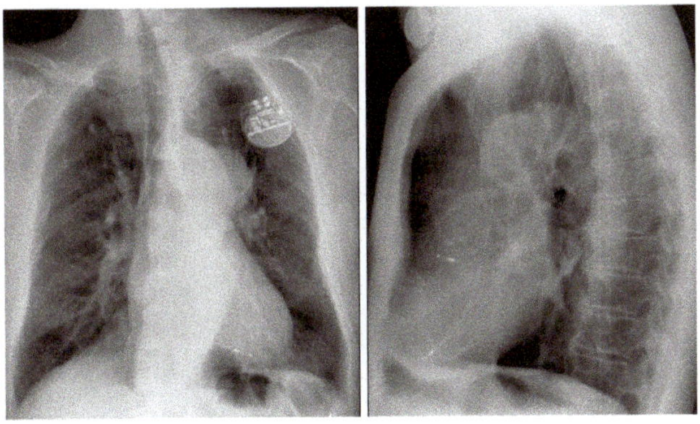

12. Chest X-ray taken after attempt of insertion on right central venous catheter (CVC). Comment on the chest X-ray and what steps needs to be taken?

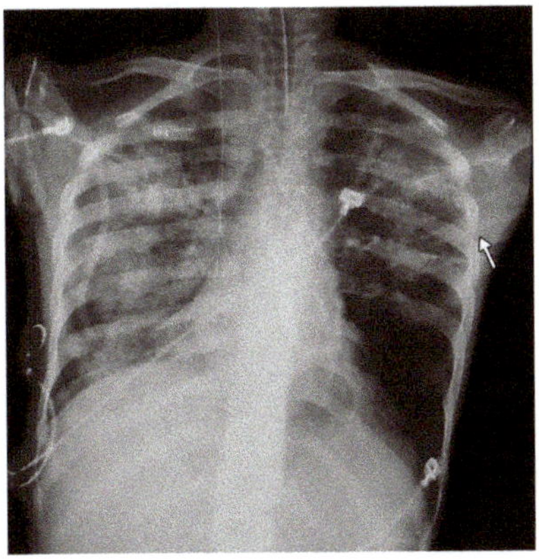

13. A 66-year-old male presented to the ER with chest pain, shortness of breath for 1 week and orthopnea. Ultrasound chest is shown in the image. What is the diagnosis?

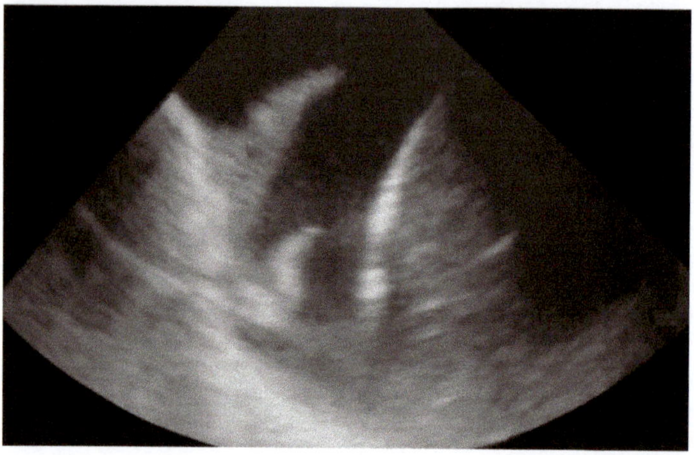

14. This patient is brought to the ER with complaints of giddiness and shortness of breath. After standing for a chest radiograph, the patient felt dizzy and had to be placed on the floor immediately. The resident doctor has placed a cardiac page as he could not feel a pulse. How will you assess the situation?

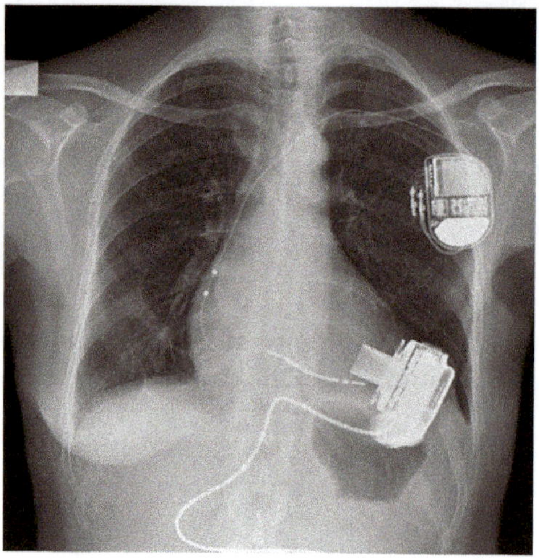

15. Comment on the chest X-ray of the patient admitted with history of trauma.

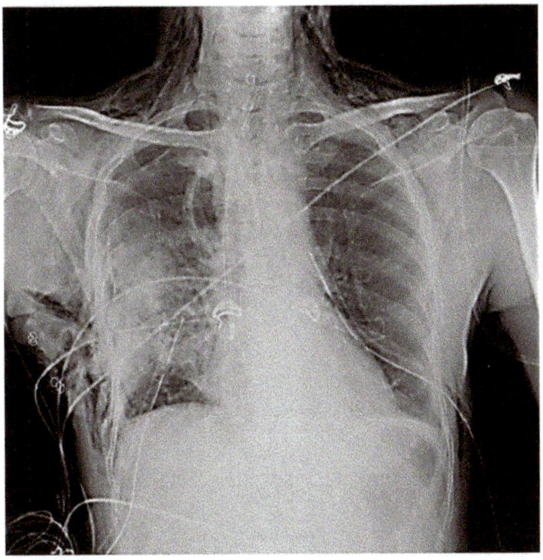

16. A 72-year-old male, a known case of COPD, is currently admitted with complaints of fever, increased expectoration, and breathing difficulty. What are the differential diagnoses and immediate management?

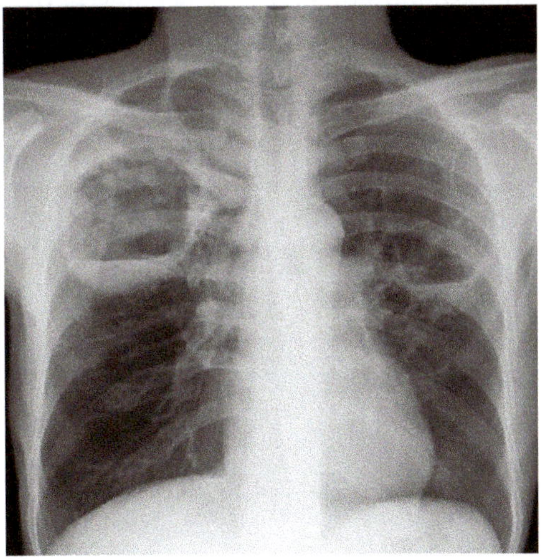

17. What is the Light's criteria for exudative pleural effusion? How will you workup this patient?
What are the diagnostic tests to be done for workup of tuberculosis?

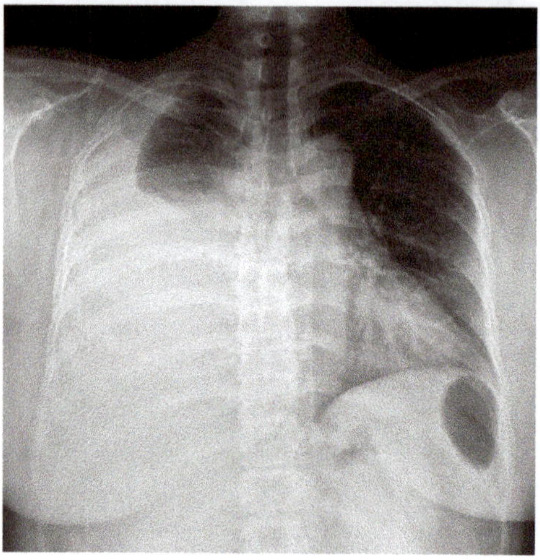

18. A 36-year-old male presented with dyspnea on exertion over 2 weeks. Chest X-ray showed massive pleural effusion and the patient is shifted to ICU for ultrasound-guided thoracocentesis. After draining about 1 liter of pleural fluid, the procedure was stopped as the patient developed cough. Post procedure, the patient is still dyspneic, with heart rate of 105 beats/min and saturation still 90% on room air.
What is the diagnosis and management?

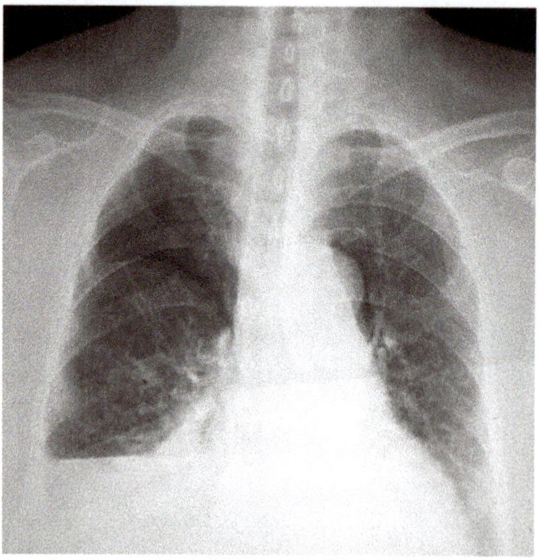

19. A 46-year-old male, a known case of retroviral disease, presented to ICU with breathing difficulty of 3 days duration and dry productive cough. A CT chest obtained is shown in the image below. What are the differential diagnoses? What are the treatment strategies?

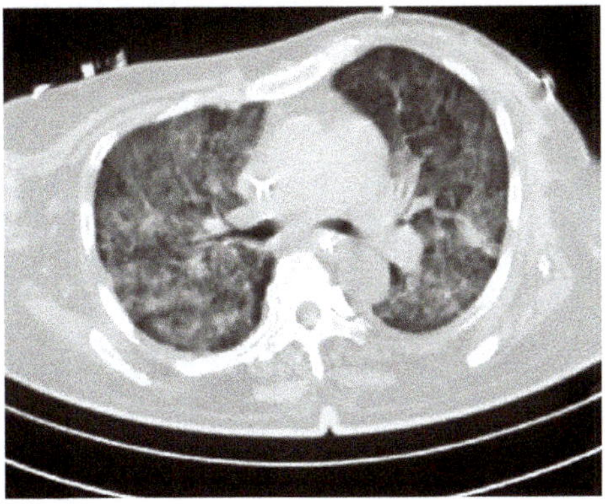

20. A 36-year-old male, with no comorbidities, presented with history of fatigue, weight loss, dry cough, and evening rise of temperature for 3 weeks duration. Sputum for acid fast bacilli, Gram stain, and culture are negative.
What are the differentials for the CT image shown below?

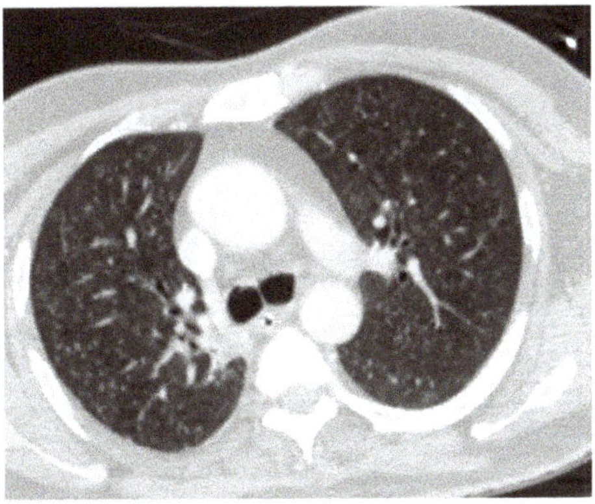

21. A 30-year-old female, software professional while disembarking a 2 hours flight developed acute onset of severe left-sided chest pain and breathlessness and cough and mild blood stain in sputum. In the airport, the documented vitals are—PR: 140/min, BP: 124/70 mm Hg, Chest: B/L clear, RR: 26/min, SpO_2 on room air: 92%, afebrile. Chest X-ray appeared normal and a 12 lead ECG showed sinus tachycardia.
   - CT taken is shown in the image below.

- What are the indications for thrombolysis in this case? What are the approved regimens for thrombolysis? How will you manage anticoagulation if the patient is not a candidate for thrombolysis?

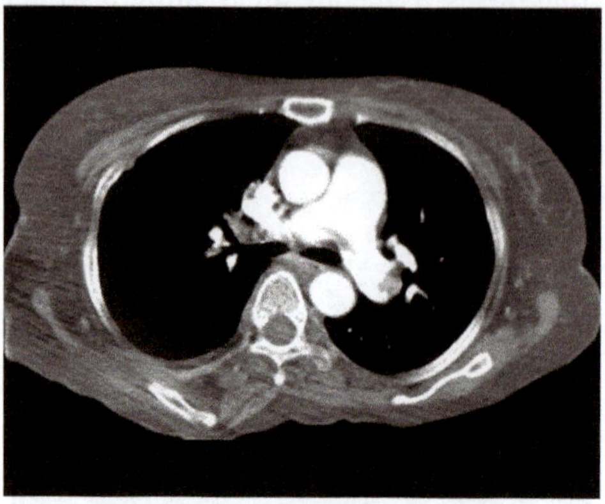

22. Check X-ray after left subclavian line insertion is given below. What is the diagnosis and management?

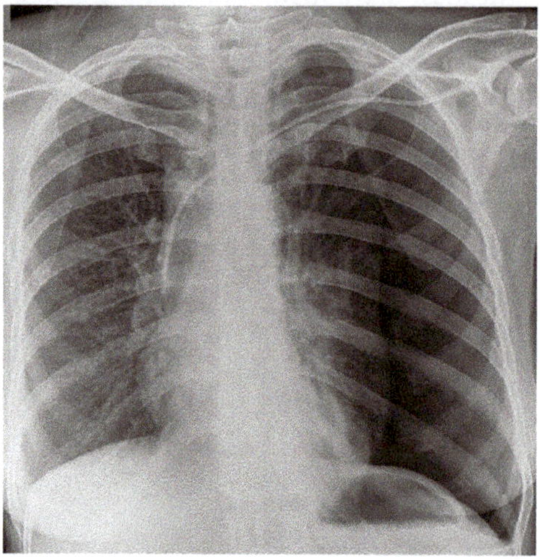

23. Lung ultrasound of a patient presenting to ER with breathing difficulty is shown below. What is the diagnosis?
    - What are the ultrasound features in case of ARDS?

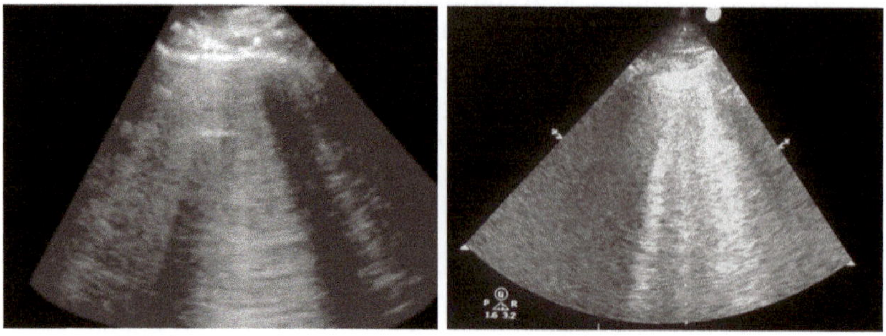

Right lower quadrant   Right upper quadrant

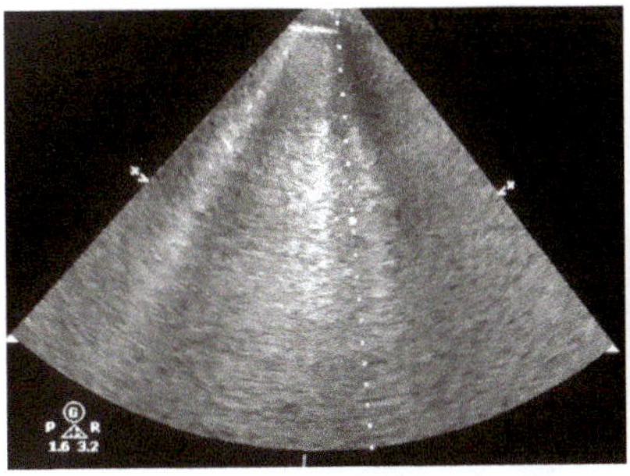

Left upper quadrant

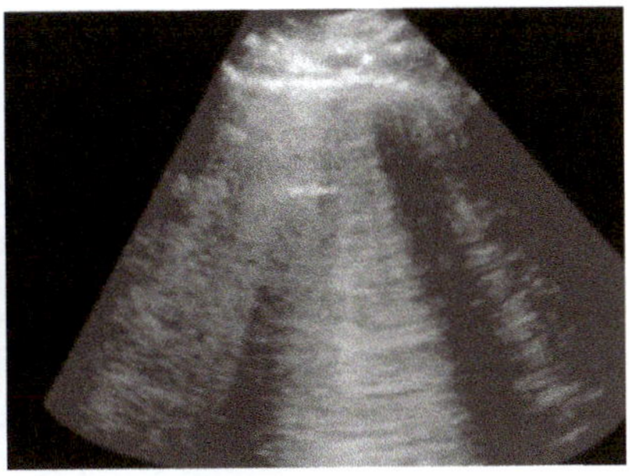

Left lower quadrant

24. Calculate the lung aeration score for each image in this patient.

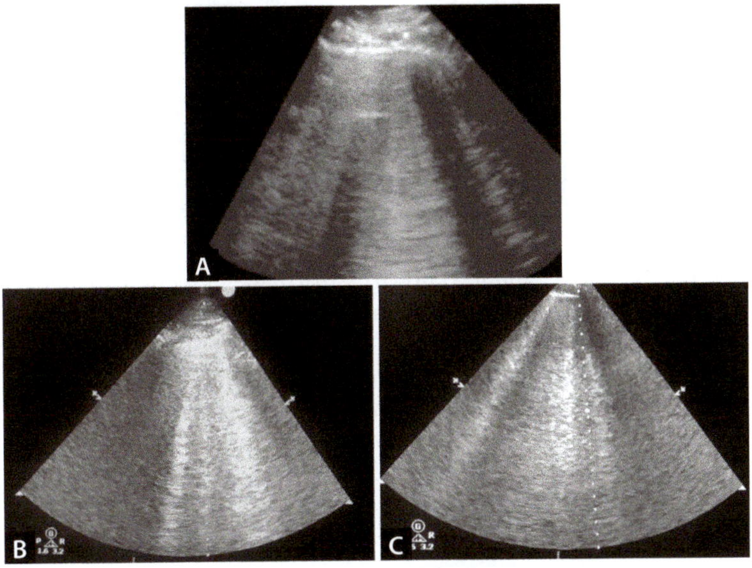

25. This patient is being ventilated with the following settings:
    - Volume control ventilation; TV 380 mL, RR 30/min, 100% FiO_2, and PEEP of 16 cm H_2O.
    - His peak inspiratory pressure is 36, and plateau of 28 cm H_2O.
    - Calculate the oxygenation index if the IE ratio is 1:1.

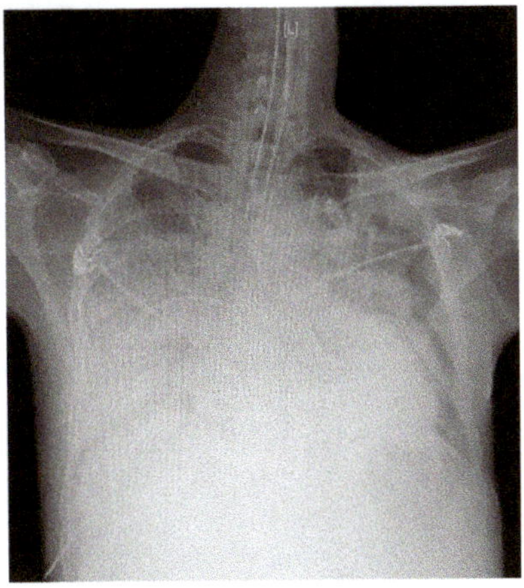

26. Calculate the oxygenation index in this patient being ventilated with the following settings:
    - Pressure control ventilation, PC 28 cm H_2O, RR 30/min, 100% FiO_2, and PEEP of 16 cm H_2O, IE ratio is 1:1.

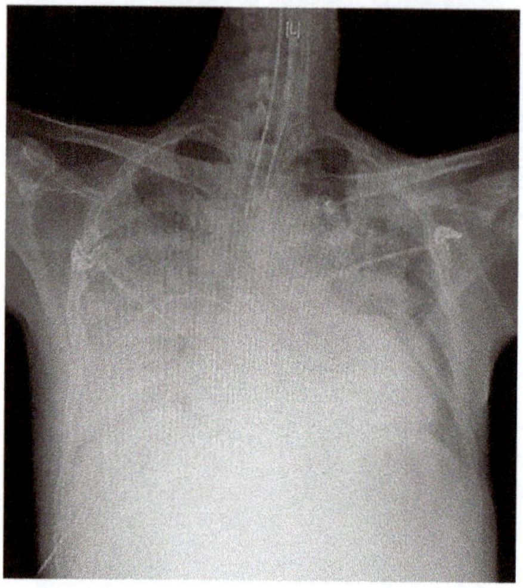

27. This 65-year-old patient, a known case of diabetes mellitus, hypertension, end-stage renal disease, post renal transplant on immunosuppressants now presents with fever, cough, and breathing difficulty that has been progressive over the past 5 days despite antibiotics on an outpatient basis. He was started on meropenem and teicoplanin but without clinical improvement.
    - A CT scan taken is given below. What is the differential diagnosis and and management?

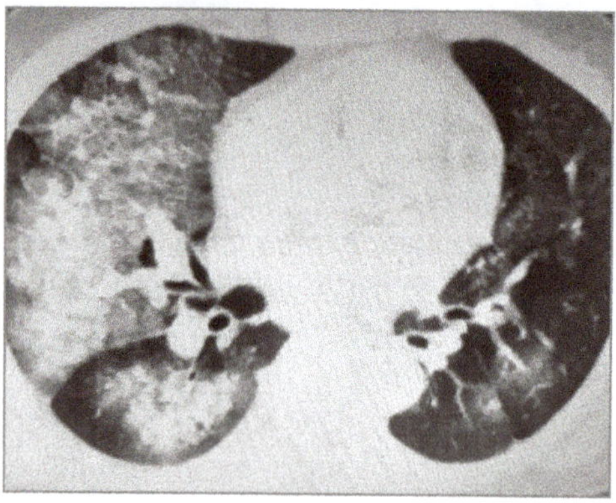

28. Comment on the acceptability criteria of the PFT.

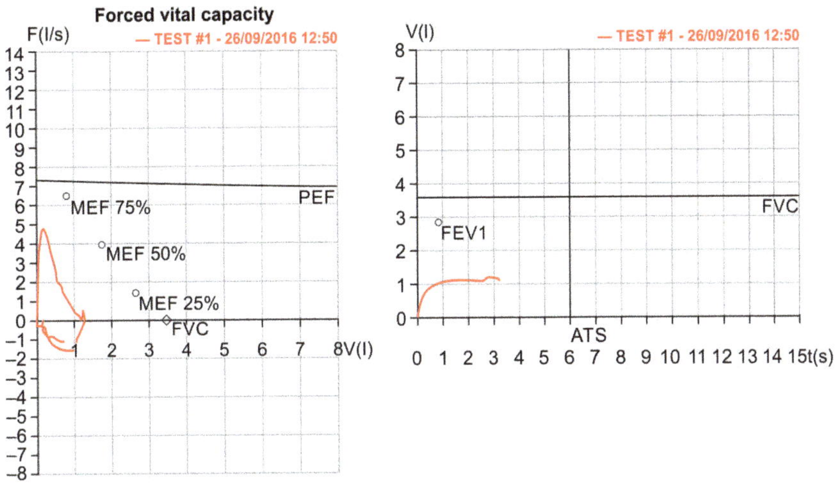

Forced vital capacity				
Parameter	*UM*	*Pred.*	*Test#1*	*% Pred.*
FVC	l (btps)	3.60	1.24	34.5
FEV1	l (btps)	2.90	1.07	37.0
PEF	l/sec	7.25	4.78	65.9
PIF	l/sec		1.55	
FEV1/FVC%	%	77.7	86.3	111.1
FEV1/VC%	%	77.7	94.5	121.6
FEF 25–75%	l/sec	3.23	1.43	44.1
MEF 75%	l/sec	6.35	3.75	59.0
MEF 50%	l/sec	3.89	1.69	43.3
FET 100%	l/sec	1.52	0.60	39.1
FIVC	sec		2.9	
	l (btps)		1.10	

29. Interpret the PFT.

Subject information

ID:	2911	Alternate ID:	
Last Name		First Name	
Population Group:	Indian	Gender:	
Age:		Height:	
BMI:			

Test session information

Test Date:		Device:	Pneumotrac	Serial Number:	25345
No. of Tests:	5	Accuracy Chk:	23/10/2019 02:17	User:	<No user>
Pred. Values:	ERS 93	Pred. Factor:	86%	Posture:	Sitting
Values at BTPS					

Flow/volume graph

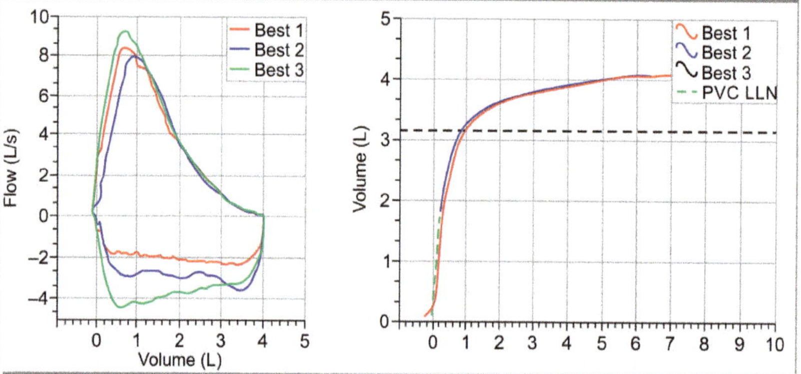

Results

Parameter	Best	Pred	% Pred	Best 1 (Test 2)	Best 2 (Test 4)	Best 3 (Test 5)
Time (hh:mm:ss)				11:17:52	11:18:48	11:19:22
FVC (L)	4.05	3.96	102	4.04	4.05	4.05
FEV1 (L)	3.22	3.19	101	3.22	3.17	3.16
FEV1 Ratio	0.80	0.78	103	0.80	0.78	0.78
PEF (L/min)	661	536	123	509	478	457
FEF 25–75 (L/s)	3.04	4.00	76	3.04	2.82	2.71

30. Patient with history of ARDS ventilation, difficult weaning 20 years back, now comes with progressive difficulty in breathing. Interpret the spirometry image given below

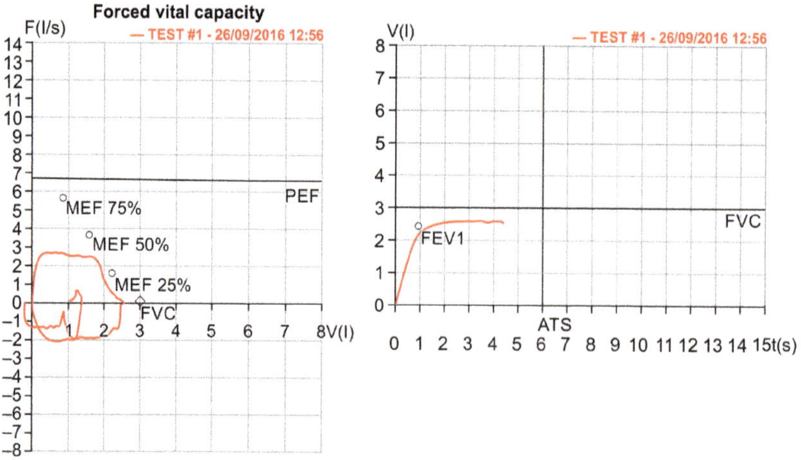

Forced vital capacity				
Parameter	*UM*	*Pred.*	*Test#1*	*% Pred.*
FVC	l (btps)	3.00	2.61	87.0
FEV1	l (btps)	2.47	2.21	89.7
PEF	l/sec	6.64	2.74	41.2
PIF	l/sec		1.91	
FEV1/FVC%	%	78.0	84.7	108.5
FEV1/VC%	%	78.0	97.4	124.8
FEF 25–75%	l/sec	3.09	2.50	80.9
MEF 75%	l/sec	5.79	2.69	46.5
MEF 50%	l/sec	3.52	2.58	73.2
MEF 25%	l/sec	1.28	1.85	144.7
FET 100%	sec		3.2	
FIVC	l (btps)		2.82	

31. A 72-year-old patient, a known case of COPD is admitted to your hospital with a second exacerbation in this year. Pulmonary function test done during admission is as given. If the patient reveals a dyspnea of MMRC grade 3, prior to hospitalization, how will you grade his COPD? What are the options available for reducing frequent exacerbations?

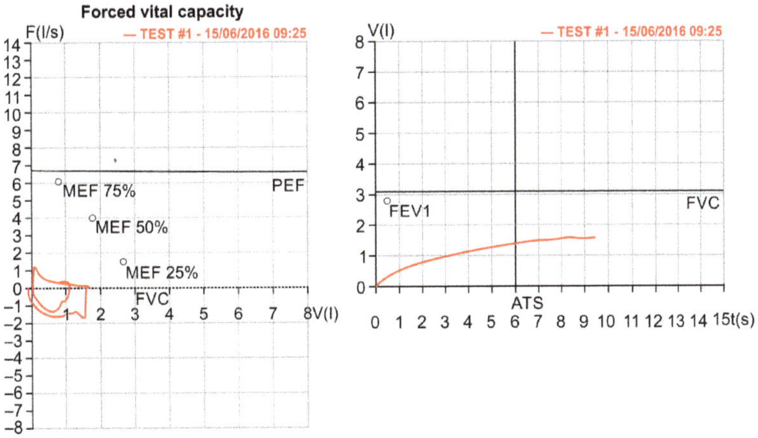

Forced vital capacity				
Parameter	*UM*	*Pred.*	*Test#1*	*% Pred.*
FVC	l (btps)	3.17	1.65	52.1
FEV1	l (btps)	2.60	0.56	21.4
PEF	l/sec	6.83	1.27	18.6
FEV6	l (btps)	3.36	1.49	44.3
PIF	l/sec		1.77	
FEV1/FVC%	%	78.2	33.7	43.1
FEV1/VC%	%	78.2	33.2	42.4
FEV6/FVC%	%		90.1	
FEV1/FEV6%	%		37.4	
FEF 25–75%	l/sec		0.27	8.5
MEF 75%	l/sec	3.18	0.47	7.9
MEF 50%	l/sec	5.96	0.29	8.0
MEF 25%	l/sec	3.65	0.16	11.6
FET 100%	sec	1.37	8.2	
FIVC	l (btps)		1.81	

32. Interpret the PFT with a patient complaining of worsening dyspnea.

Forced vital capacity

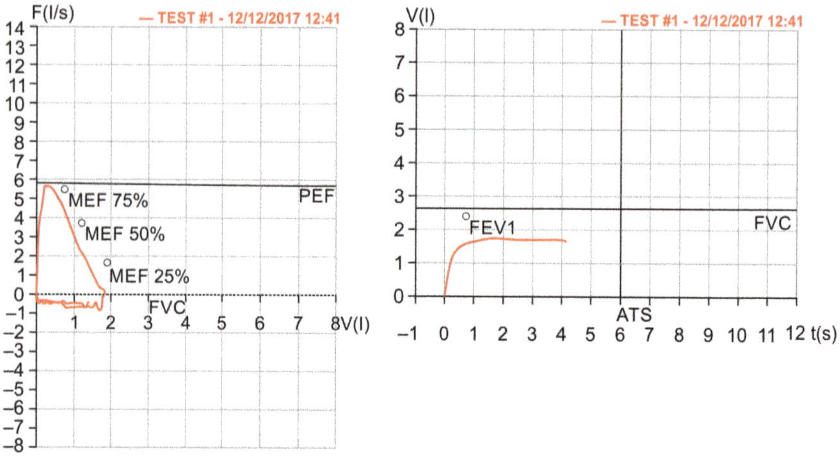

Forced vital capacity					
Parameter	*UM*	*Description*	*Pred.*	*Test#1*	*% Pred.*
Best FVC	l (btps)	Best forced vital capacity	2.57	1.77	69
FVC	l (btps)	Forced vital capacity	2.57	1.77	69
FEV1	l (btps)	Forced exp volume in 1 sec	2.19	1.66	76
PEF	l/sec	Peak expiratory flow	5.77	5.68	98
PIF	l/sec	Peak inspiratory flow		0.77	
FEV1/FVC%	%	FEV 1 as % of FVC	80.7	93.9	116
FEF 25–75%	l/sec	Forced mid-expiratory flow	3.29	2.94	90
MEF 75%	l/sec	Max exp flow @ 25% FVC	5.30	5.38	102
MEF 50%	l/sec	Max exp flow @ 50% FVC	3.71	3.30	89
MEF 25%	l/sec	Max exp flow @ 75% FVC	1.57	1.53	97
FET 100%	sec	Forced expiratory time		2.1	
VEXT	mL	Extrapolated volume		24	
IC	l (btps)	Inspiratory capacity		1.32	

33. A 46-year-old male, known case of hypertension, diabetes, and chronic kidney disease, presented with altered sensorium to the ER.
    - O/E: HR—150 beats/min, BP—100/48 mm Hg, RR—30 breaths/min, and saturation 100% on face mask with 6 L oxygen.
    - Interpret the ABG.
    - Enumerate the differential diagnoses.

Tata Hospital, 2nd Floor ICU

Pat ID

First name

Blood Type Arterial

Blood Gas values (measured at 37. 0C)

pH	6.85	(7.350 - 7.450)
PCO_2	12 mmHg	(35.0 - 45.0)
PO_2	322 mmHg	(80.0 - 100.0)
$cHCO_3$	<3 mmol/L	
BE	_______	
BE(ecf)	_______	
tHb	9.9 g/dl	(11.5 - 17.40)
SO_2	_______	(75.0 - 100)
SO_2 (c)	_______	
Electrolytes		
Na^+	114 mmol/L	(135.0 - 148.0)
K^+	7.3 mmol/L	(3.50 - 4.50)
Cl^-	87 mmol/L	(98.0 - 107.0)
Ca^{++}	0.60 mmol/L	(1.15 - 1.29)
Metabolites		
Glu	> 500 mg/dl	(70 - 110)
Lac	10.6 mmol/L	(0.44 - 2.2)

34. A 46-year-old male, known case of hypertension, diabetes, and chronic kidney disease, presented with altered sensorium to the ER.
    - O/E: HR—150/min, BP—100/48 mm Hg, RR—30/min, and saturation 100% on face mask with 6 L oxygen.
    - What is the corrected sodium if the blood sugar from the laboratory came as 886 mg/dL?

    How will you correct his hyponatremia?

Tata Hospital, 2nd Floor ICU

Pat ID

First name

Blood Type Arterial

Blood Gas values (measured at 37. 0C)

pH	6.85	(7.350 - 7.450)
PCO_2	12 mmHg	(35.0 - 45.0)
PO_2	322 mmHg	(80.0 - 100.0)
$cHCO_3$	<3 mmol/L	
BE	_______	
BE(ecf)	_______	
tHb	9.9 g/dl	(11.5 - 17.40)
SO_2	_______	(75.0 - 100)
SO_2 (c)	_______	
Electrolytes		
Na^+	114 mmol/L	(135.0 - 148.0)
K^+	7.3 mmol/L	(3.50 - 4.50)
Cl^-	87 mmol/L	(98.0 - 107.0)
Ca^{++}	0.60 mmol/L	(1.15 - 1.29)
Metabolites		
Glu	> 500 mg/dl	(70 - 110)
Lac	10.6 mmol/L	(0.44 - 2.2)

35. A 38-year-old male, with no comorbidities, presented to the hospital with complaints of severe fever, prostration, and myalgia of 5 days duration. He has associated nausea, vomiting, and also has severe abdominal pain which has not settled with conservative management. NS1 antigen testing has come positive. How will you classify the condition? How will you resuscitate this patient with dengue and severe symptoms?

Blood Gas Values			
pH	7.090		
pCO_2	40.8	mmHg	[32.0 - 48.0]
pO_2	107	mmHg	[82.0 - 108]
$cHCO_3^-(P)c$	11.8	mmol/L	
cBase(B,ox)c	-20.1	mmol/L	
cBase(Ecf,ox)c	-16.1	mmol/L	
$ctCO_2(P)c$	29.4	Vol%	
Anion Gapc	5.2	mmol/L	
Oximetry Values			
Hctc	68.3	%	
ctHb	22.4	g/dL	
FCOHb	0.3	%	
sO_2	96.3	%	[95.0 - 99.0]
FO_2Hb	95.1	%	[-]
↑ FMetHb	0.9	%	[0.2 - 0.6]
FHHb	3.7	%	
Oxygen Status			
BO_2c	30.8	Vol%	
ctO_2c	30.0	Vol%	
Electrolyte Values			
cK^+	3.9	mmol/L	[3.5 - 5.0]
cNa^+	140	mmol/L	[136 - 146]
↓ cCa^{2+}	1.12	mmol/L	[1.15 - 1.29]
cCl^-	123	mmol/L	[-]
Metabolite Values			
↑ cGlu	334	mg/dL	[70 - 106]
↑ cLac	5.1	mmol/L	[0.5 - 1.6]

VCV mode

FiO_2: 80%

PEEP: 12

RR: 20

TV: 380

36. A 38-year-old male, with no comorbidities, presented to the hospital with complaints of severe fever, prostration, and myalgia of 5 days duration. He has associated nausea, vomiting, and also has severe abdominal pain which has not settled with conservative management. NS1 antigen testing has come positive.

- A chest X-ray showed bilateral haziness with no midline shift.
- Analyze the ABG and calculate the (A-a)O_2 gradient.

Blood Gas Values			
pH	7.090		
pCO_2	40.8	mmHg	
pO_2	107	mmHg	
$cHCO_3^-(P)c$	11.8	mmol/L	
cBase(B,ox)c	-20.1	mmol/L	
cBase(Ecf,ox)c	-16.1	mmol/L	
$ctCO_2(P)c$	29.4	Vol%	
Anion Gapc	5.2	mmol/L	
Oximetry Values			
Hctc	68.3	%	
ctHb	22.4	g/dL	
FCOHb	0.3	%	
sO_2	96.3	%	[95.0 - 99.0]
FO_2Hb	95.1	%	[-]
↑ FMetHb	0.9	%	[0.2 - 0.6]
FHHb	3.7	%	
Oxygen Status			
BO_2c	30.8	Vol%	
ctO_2c	30.0	Vol%	
Electrolyte Values			
cK^+	3.9	mmol/L	[3.5 - 5.0]
cNa^+	140	mmol/L	[136 - 146]
↓ cCa^{2+}	1.12	mmol/L	[1.15 - 1.29]
cCl^-	123	mmol/L	[-]
Metabolite Values			
↑ cGlu	334	mg/dL	[70 - 106]
↑ cLac	5.1	mmol/L	[0.5 - 1.6]

VCV mode

FiO_2: 80%

PEEP: 12

RR: 20

TV: 380

37. A 64-year-old female, known case of diabetes mellitus, peripheral occlusive vascular disease, and coronary artery disease, now presented with altered sensorium and tachypnea of 2 days duration.
    - On examination, she is disoriented, tachycardic, and tachypneic.
    - The right leg is blackish in color and foul smelling.
    - What are the urgent management issues to be undertaken in this patient?

Measurement report

20-10-2019 23:19
Serial number : 11440
Instrument ID : 1
Operator ID :
TATA HOSPITAL 1st Floor ICU

Pat ID	109
Bar	1015.08 mbar
First name	
Location	109
Blood type	Arterial

	Blood gas		
pH	7.064 (--)	[7.350 -	7.450]
PCO_2	33.5 mmHg (-)	[35.0 -	45.0]
PO_2	116.6 mmHg (+)	[80.0 -	100.0]
$cHCO_3^-$	9.4 mmol/L		
BE	-19.6 mmol/L		
BE_{ecf}	-20.9 mmol/L		
Hb	9.29 g/dL (-)	[11.50 -	17.40]
SO_2	97.0 %	[75.0 -	99.0]
SO_2 (c)	95.0 %		
	Electrolytes		
Na^+	126.5 mmol/L (-)	[135.0 -	148.0]
K^+	5.50 mmol/L (+)	[3.50 -	4.50]
Cl^-	96.0 mmol/L (-)	[98.0 -	107.0]
Ca^{2+}	3.46 mg/dL (--)	[4.49 -	5.29]
	Metabolites		
Glu	116.8 mg/dL (+)(!)	[60.0 -	109.9]
Lac	10.06 mmol/L (++)(!)	[0.44 -	2.22]

38. A 46-year-old male, known case of hypertension, diabetes, and chronic kidney disease, presented with altered sensorium to the ER. On examination: HR 150/min, BP 100/48 mm Hg, RR 30/min, and saturation 100% on room air.

- What is the role of bicarbonate in resuscitation of this patient?

Tata Hospital, 2nd Floor ICU

Pat ID

First name

Blood Type Arterial

Blood Gas values (measured at 37. 0C)

pH	6.85	(7.350 - 7.450)
PCO_2	12 mmHg	(35.0 - 45.0)
PO_2	322 mmHg	(80.0 - 100.0)
$cHCO_3$	<3 mmol/L	
BE	________	
BE(ecf)	________	
tHb	9.9 g/dl	(11.5 - 17.40)
SO_2	________	(75.0 - 100)
SO_2 (c)	________	
Electrolytes		
Na^+	114 mmol/L	(135.0 - 148.0)
K^+	7.3 mmol/L	(3.50 - 4.50)
Cl^-	87 mmol/L	(98.0 - 107.0)
Ca^{++}	0.60 mmol/L	(1.15 - 1.29)
Metabolites		
Glu	> 500 mg/dl	(70 - 110)
Lac	10.6 mmol/L	(0.44 - 2.2)

39. A 72-year-old patient, known case of COPD, presented to the emergency department with altered sensorium and breathing difficulty of 1-day duration.
    - Analyze the ABG, given that the albumin levels for this patient are 4.0 g/dL and he is currently on FiO_2 of 40%.

Tata Hospital, 2nd Floor ICU

Pat ID

First name

Blood Type Arterial

Blood Gas values (measured at 37. 0C)

pH	6.96	(7.350 - 7.450)
PCO_2	126.4 mmHg	(35.0 - 45.0)
PO_2	88 mmHg	(80.0 - 100.0)
$cHCO_3$	17.4 mmol/L	
BE	-8.6 mmol/L	
BE(ecf)	-4.5 mmol/L	
tHb	9.9 g/dl	(11.5 - 17.40)
SO_2	87.4	(75.0 - 100)
SO_2 (c)		
Electrolytes		
Na^+	133 mmol/L	(135.0 - 148.0)
K^+	3.47 mmol/L	(3.50 - 4.50)
Cl^-	87 mmol/L	(98.0 - 107.0)
Ca^{++}	0.36 mmol/L	(1.15 - 1.29)
Metabolites		
Glu	138 mg/dl	(70 - 110)
Lac	2.2 mmol/L	(0.44 - 2.2)

40. A 72-year-old patient, known case of COPD, presented to the emergency department with altered sensorium and breathing difficulty of 1-day duration.
    - Analyze the ABG, given that the albumin levels for this patient are 4.0 g/dL and he is currently on FiO_2 of 40%.
    - Calculate the anion gap.
    - What are the causes of negative anion gap?
    - What is normal urinary anion gap and what are its uses?

Tata Hospital, 2nd Floor ICU

Pat ID

First name

Blood Type Arterial

Blood Gas values (measured at 37. 0C)

pH	6.98	(7.350 - 7.450)
PCO_2	88.4 mmHg	(35.0 - 45.0)
PO_2	118 mmHg	(80.0 - 100.0)
$cHCO_3$	20.1 mmol/L	
BE	- 9.8 mmol/L	
BEecf	- 5.5 mmol/L	
tHb	8.7 g/dl	(11.5 - 17.40)
SO_2	97.4	(75.0 - 100)
SO_2 (c)		
Electrolytes		
Na^+	133 mmol/L 92	
K^+	2.74 mmol/L	
Cl^-	106 mmol/L	(98.0 - 107.0)
Ca^{++}	0.86 mmol/L	(1.15 - 1.29)
Metabolites		
Glu	154 mg/dl	(70 - 110)
Lac	1.2 mmol/L	(0.44 - 2.2)

41. What is meant by HCO_3 (std)? What is meant by base excess (B) and base excess (ecf)?

Blood Gas Values			
pH	7.090		VCV mode
pCO_2	40.8	mmHg	FiO_2: 80%
pO_2	107	mmHg	PEEP: 12
$cHCO_3^-$(P)c	11.8	mmol/L	RR: 20
cBase(B,ox)c	-20.1	mmol/L	TV: 380
cBase(Ecf,ox)c	-16.1	mmol/L	
$ctCO_2$(P)c	29.4	Vol%	
Anion Gapc	5.2	mmol/L	
Oximetry Values			
Hctc	68.3	%	
ctHb	22.4	g/dL	
FCOHb	0.3	%	
sO_2	96.3	%	[95.0 - 99.0]
FO_2Hb	95.1	%	[-]
↑ FMetHb	0.9	%	[0.2 - 0.6]
FHHb	3.7	%	
Oxygen Status			
BO_2c	30.8	Vol%	
ctO_2c	30.0	Vol%	
Electrolyte Values			
cK^+	3.9	mmol/L	[3.5 - 5.0]
cNa^+	140	mmol/L	[136 - 146]
↓ cCa^{2+}	1.12	mmol/L	[1.15 - 1.29]
cCl^-	123	mmol/L	[-]
Metabolite Values			
↑ cGlu	334	mg/dL	[70 - 106]
↑ cLac	5.1	mmol/L	[0.5 - 1.6]

42. In Stewart approach of acid–base, what are the independent controllers of acid–base status in body fluids?
    - Albumin is 3.0 g/dL.
    - Calculate the SID and strong ion gap from the ABG.

Measurement report

18-10-2019 11:52
Serial number : 11440
Instrument ID : 1
Operator ID :
TATA HOSPITAL 1st Floor ICU

Pat. ID		A/C ē VC
Barc		TV – 350
First name		RR – 22
Location		Peep – 10
Block type	Arterial	FiO2 – 70%

Blood gas				
pH	7.277 (-)	[	7.350 -	7.450]
PCO_2	37.6 mmHg	[	35.0 -	45.0]
PO_2	67.4 mmHg (-)	[	80.0 -	100.0]
$cHCO_3^-$	17.1 mmol/L			
BE	-8.9 mmol/L			
BE_e	-9.6 mmol/L			
tHb	10.46 g/dL (-)	[	11.50 -	17.40]
SO_2	88.8 %	[	75.0 -	99.0]
SO_2 (c)	89.4 %			
Electrolytes				
Na^+	147.8 mmol/L	[	135.0 -	148.0]
K^+	4.24 mmol/L	[	3.50 -	4.50]
Cl^-	109.3 mmol/L (+)	[	98.0 -	107.0]
Ca^{2+}	4.04 mg/dL (--)	[	4.49 -	5.29]
Metabolites				
Glu	118.9 mg/dL (+)(!)	[	60.0 -	109.9]
Lac	10.48 mmol/L (++)(!)	[	0.44 -	2.22]

Note: Ensure reference ranges match sample type.

43. Comment upon the central venous sample in this patient who presented with meningitis.
    - What are the next measures to be undertaken in this patient?

Status: ACCEPTED
03/12/2019 17:22:56
Sample Type:
Arterial
Sample No.: 27
Operator:
274
Patient:
Name:

Sex:
Instrument:
Model: GEM 3500
S/N: 19081543

Measured (37.0C)

pH	7.29	
pCO2	48	mmHg
pO2	30	mmHg
Na+	128	mmol/L
K+	5.3	mmol/L
Ca++	0.91	mmol/L
Glu	116	mg/dL
Lac	3.1	mmol/L
Hct	38	%

Derived Parameters

Ca++(7.4)	0.87	mmol/L
HCO3-	23.1	mmol/L
HCO3std	20.9	mmol/L
TCO2	24.6	mmol/L
BEecf	-3.5	mmol/L
BE(B)	-3.7	mmol/L
SO2c	49	%
THbc	11.8	g/dL

44. How will you assess adequacy of cardiac output and presence of anaerobic metabolism in this patient with septic shock, hyperlactatemia, and on increasing vasopressor support?

Tata Hospital, 2nd Floor ICU

Pat ID

First name

Blood Type Arterial

Blood Gas values (measured at 37. 0C)

pH	7.277	(7.350 - 7.450)
PCO_2	37.6 mmHg	(35.0 - 45.0)
PO_2	67.4 mmHg	(80.0 - 100.0)
$cHCO_3$	17.1 mmol/L	
BE	-8.9 mmol/L	
BE(ecf)	-9.6 mmol/L	
tHb	10.46 g/dl	(11.5 - 17.40)
SO_2	88.8 %	(75.0 - 100)
SO_2 (c)	89.4 %	
Electrolytes		
Na^+	147.8 mmol/L	(135.0 - 148.0)
K^+	4.24 mmol/L	(3.50 - 4.50)
Cl^-	109.3 mmol/L	(98.0 - 107.0)
Ca^{++}	1.01 mmol/L	(1.15 - 1.29)
Metabolites		
Glu	118.9 mg/dl	(70 - 110)
Lac	10.48 mmol/L	(0.44 - 2.2)

Tata Hospital, 2nd Floor ICU

Pat ID

First name

Blood Type Venous

Blood Gas values (measured at 37. 0C)

pH	7.242	(7.350 - 7.450)
PCO_2	41.3 mmHg	(35.0 - 45.0)
PO_2	38.7 mmHg	(80.0 - 100.0)
$cHCO_3$	17.4 mmol/L	
BE	-9.3 mmol/L	
BE(ecf)	-9.9 mmol/L	
tHb	9.47 g/dl	(11.5 - 17.40)
SO_2	52.7 %	(75.0 - 100)
SO_2 (c)	60.5 %	
Electrolytes		
Na^+	148.0 mmol/L	(135.0 - 148.0)
K^+	3.69 mmol/L	(3.50 - 4.50)
Cl^-	109.9 mmol/L	(98.0 - 107.0)
Ca^{++}	0.93 mmol/L	(1.15 - 1.29)
Metabolites		
Glu	103.5 mg/dl	(70 - 110)
Lac	9.40 mmol/L	(0.44 - 2.2)

45. What are the causes of high anion gap metabolic acidosis and hyperlactatemia in ICU?

Tata Hospital, 2nd Floor ICU

Pat ID

First name

Blood Type Arterial

Blood Gas values (measured at 37. 0C)

pH	7.277	(7.350 - 7.450)
PCO_2	37.6 mmHg	(35.0 - 45.0)
PO_2	67.4 mmHg	(80.0 - 100.0)
$cHCO_3$	17.1 mmol/L	
BE	-8.9 mmol/L	
BE(ecf)	-9.6 mmol/L	
tHb	10.46 g/dl	(11.5 - 17.40)
SO_2	88.8 %	(75.0 - 100)
SO_2 (c)	89.4 %	
Electrolytes		
Na^+	147.8 mmol/L	(135.0 - 148.0)
K^+	4.24 mmol/L	(3.50 - 4.50)
Cl^-	109.3 mmol/L	(98.0 - 107.0)
Ca^{++}	1.01 mmol/L	(1.15 - 1.29)
Metabolites		
Glu	118.9 mg/dl	(70 - 110)
Lac	10.48 mmol/L	(0.44 - 2.2)

46. What are the common causes of metabolic alkalosis in ICU? How will you investigate the patient?

Tata Hospital, 2nd Floor ICU

Pat ID	
First name	
Location	
Blood Type	Arterial
Blood Gas	
pH	7.59
PCO_2	78.4 mmHg
PO_2	119 mmHg
$cHCO_3$	75.2 mmol/L
BE	42.1
BEecf	---
tHb	13.3
SO_2	98.9%
SO_2 (c)	99.4%
Electrolytes	
Na^+	127 mmol/L
K^+	3.39 mmol/L
Cl^-	80 mmol/L
Ca^{++}	0.98 mmol/L
Metabolites	
Glu	146 mg/dl
Lac	1.7 mmol/L

47. Common gap in acid-base balance:
- What is lactate gap?
- What is the importance of saturation gap in ABG?

MEASURED VALUES	
Blood Gas (37°C)	
pH	↑ 7.59
pCO_2	↑ 78.4 mmHg
pO_2	↑ 119 mmHg
Hematocrit	
Hct	41 %
Electrolytes/Metabolites	
cNa^+	↓ 127 mmol/L
cK^+	↓ 3.39 mmol/L
cCa^{2+}	↓ 0.98 mmol/L
cCl^-	↓ 80 mmol/L
cLac	1.7 mmol/L
DERIVED VALUES	
ctHb	13.3 g/dL
$cHCO_3^-$ (P)	75.2 mmol/L
$cHCO_3^-$ (P,st)	73.9 mmol/L
cBase(B)	42.1 mmol/L
cBase(Ecf)	*** mmol/L
cBase(B,ox)	42.0 mmol/L
cBase(Ecf,ox)	*** mmol/L
$ctCO_2$(B)	64.5 mmol/L
$ctCO_2$(P)	77.6 mmol/L
cCa^{2+}(7.40)	1.08 mmol/L
Anion Gap(K^+)	*** mmol/L
Anion Gap	*** mmol/L
pO_2(A)	N/D mmHg
pO_2(A-a)	N/D mmHg
pO_2(a/A)	N/D %
sO_2	98.9 %
ctO_2	18.5 Vol%
RI	N/D %

48. • What are storage lesions?
 • What is the current evidence for use of stored blood versus fresh blood in critically ill patients?

Measurement report
22-12-2019 05 24
Serial number 11444
Instrument ID 2
Operator ID
TATA HOSPITAL 2nd Floor ICU

Pat. ID	rrecovery
First name	
Location	
Blood type	Arterial

	Blood gas		
pH	6.671 (--)	[7.350 -	7.450]
PCO_2	65.5 mmHg (++)	[35.0 -	45.0]
PO_2	76.9 mmHg (-)	[80.0 -	100.0]
$cHCO_3$	7.4 mmol/L		
BE	-30.9 mmol/L		
BE_{ecf}	-29.2 mmol/L		
tHb	16.36 g/dL	[11.50 -	17.40]
SO_2	83.8 %	[75.0 -	99.0]
SO_2(c)	59.9 %		

	Electrolytes		
Na^+	124.5 mmol/L (--)	[135.0 -	148.0]
K^+	17.63 mmol/L (++)	[3.50 -	4.50]
Cl^-	102.8 mmol/L	[98.0 -	107.0]
Ca^{2+}	Out of range (-)	[4.49 -	5.29]

	Metabolites		
Glu	452.6 mg/dL (++)	[60.0 -	109.9]
Lac	16.66 mmol/L (++)	[0.44 -	2.22]

49. • What are the advantages of apneic oxygenation during intubation?
 • What are the measures to reduce hypoxia during intubation attempts?

Measurement report
21-12-2019 11 13
Serial number 11444
Instrument ID 2
Operator ID
TATA HOSPITAL 2nd Floor ICU

Pat ID	Post Intubation
First name	
Location	/28/9/100%
Blood type	Arterial

	Blood gas		
pH	7.177 (--)	[7.350 -	7.450]
PCO_2	15.8 mmHg (--)	[35.0 -	45.0]
PO_2	604.9 mmHg (+)	[80.0 -	100.0]
$cHCO_3$	5.7 mmol/L		
BE	-20.8 mmol/L		
BE_{ecf}	-22.7 mmol/L		
tHb	5.26 g/dL (--)	[11.50 -	17.40]
SO_2	99.2 % (+)	[75.0 -	99.0]
SO_2(c)	100.0 %		

	Electrolytes		
Na^+	128.3 mmol/L (-)	[135.0 -	148.0]
K^+	3.54 mmol/L	[3.50 -	4.50]
Cl^-	95.9 mmol/L (-)	[98.0 -	107.0]
Ca^{2+}	3.97 mg/dL (--)	[4.49 -	5.29]

	Metabolites		
Glu	169.5 mg/dL (++)	[60.0 -	109.9]
Lac	18.89 mmol/L (++)	[0.44 -	2.22]

50. What are the adverse effects of hyperoxia in ICU?

Measurement report

21-12-2019 11:13
Serial number 11444
Instrument ID 2
Operator ID
TATA HOSPITAL 2nd Floor ICU

Pat ID		Post Intubation.
First name		
Location		/28/9/100%.
Blood type	Arterial	

		Blood gas		
pH	7.177	(--)	[7.350 -	7.450]
PCO_2	15.8	mmHg (--)	[35.0 -	45.0]
PO_2	604.9	mmHg (+)	[80.0 -	100.0]
$cHCO_3$	5.7	mmol/L		
BE	-20.8	mmol/L		
BEecf	-22.7	mmol/L		
tHb	5.26	g/dL (--)	[11.50 -	17.40]
SO_2	99.2	% (+)	[75.0 -	99.0]
SO_2(c)	100.0	%		
		Electrolytes		
Na^+	128.3	mmol/L (-)	[135.0 -	148.0]
K^+	3.54	mmol/L	[3.50 -	4.50]
Cl	95.9	mmol/L (-)	[98.0 -	107.0]
Ca^{2+}	3.97	mg/dL (--)	[4.49 -	5.29]
		Metabolites		
Glu	169.5	mg/dL (++)	[60.0 -	109.9]
Lac	18.89	mmol/L (++)	[0.44 -	2.22]

51. A 26-year-old male with no past medical history presented with drowsiness and fatigue of 2 days duration.
   - There is no history of hypertension, or any drug abuse.
   - Comment on the ABG.
   - Mention a few differential diagnoses.

Tata Hospital, 2nd Floor ICU

Pat ID	
First name	
Location	
Blood Type	Arterial
Blood Gas	
pH	7.52
PCO_2	105.3mmHg
PO_2	83mmHg
$cHCO_3$	85.7mmol/L
BE	47
BEecf	-.-
tHb	17.3
SO_2	95.6%
SO_2 (c)	97.2%
Electrolytes	
Na^+	111 mmol/L
K^+	1.80 mmol/L
Cl^-	59 mmol/L
Ca^{++}	0.87 mmol/L
Metabolites	
Glu	214 mg/dl
Lac	0.1 mmol/L

52. What is alpha stat and pH stat in ABG interpretation?
    - What are the clinical implications of the same?

MEASURED VALUES		
Blood Gas (37°C)		
pH	↑	7.52
pCO_2	↑	105.3 mmHg
pO_2		83 mmHg
Hematocrit		
Hct	↑	53 %
Electrolytes/Metabolites		
cNa^+	⇟	111 mmol/L
cK^+	⇟	1.80 mmol/L
cCa^{2+}	↓	0.87 mmol/L
cCl^-	⇟	59 mmol/L
cLac	⇟	0.1 mmol/L

DERIVED VALUES	
ctHb	17.3 g/dL
$cHCO_3^-$(P)	85.7 mmol/L
$cHCO_3^-$(P,st)	83.2 mmol/L
cBase(B)	47.0 mmol/L
cBase(Ecf)	*** mmol/L
cBase(B,ox)	46.9 mmol/L
cBase(Ecf,ox)	*** mmol/L
$ctCO_2$(B)	70.0 mmol/L
$ctCO_2$(P)	88.9 mmol/L
cCa^{2+}(7.40)	0.93 mmol/L
Anion Gap(K^+)	*** mmol/L
Anion Gap	*** mmol/L
pO_2(A)	N/D mmHg
pO_2(A-a)	N/D mmHg
pO_2(a/A)	N/D %
sO_2	95.6 %
ctO_2	23.1 Vol%
RI	N/D %

53. What is the normal calcium level in body?
    - What is the relationship between normal calcium and ionized calcium in body?
    - How will you correct symptomatic hypocalcemia?

Electrolyte Values				
	cK^+	3.9	mmol/L	[3.5 - 5.0]
	cNa^+	140	mmol/L	[136 - 146]
↓	cCa^{2+}	1.12	mmol/L	[1.15 - 1.29]
	cCl^-	123	mmol/L	[-]

Electrolytes			
Na^+	147.8 mmol/L		[135.0 - 148.0]
K^+	4.24 mmol/L		[3.50 - 4.50]
Cl^-	109.3 mmol/L	(+)	[98.0 - 107.0]
Ca^{2+}	4.04 mg/dL	(--)	[4.49 - 5.29]

54. Comment on the CT of a car passenger who was wearing a seat belt and had a high-speed collision.

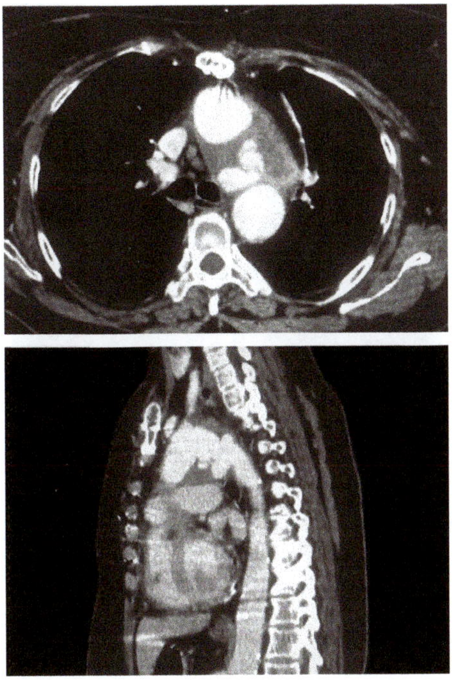

55. What are the different methods of percutaneous tracheostomy at the bedside?

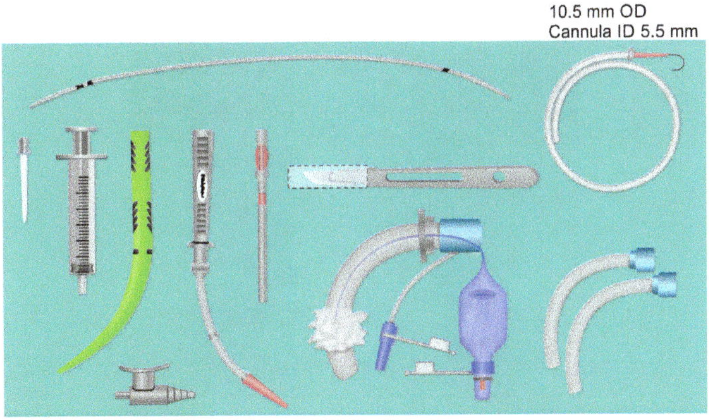

56. A 72-year-old female, a case of well-controlled diabetes mellitus, presents to the ER with fever, cough, and shortness of breath of 1-day duration, while returning from Hajj Pilgrimage. Chest X-ray taken is given below.
   - What is the possible diagnosis?
   - How will you confirm the diagnosis?
   - What is the specific treatment in this case?

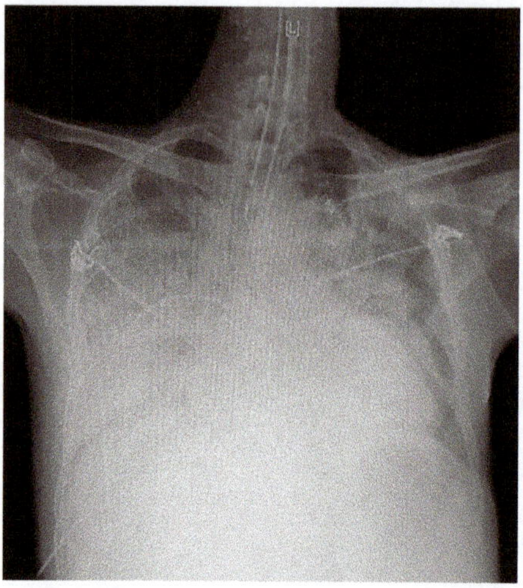

57. X-ray of a COPD patient on NIV. A nasogastric tube was inserted as patient complained of abdominal distention. X-ray taken after nasogastric tube insertion. What is the urgent steps to be taken?

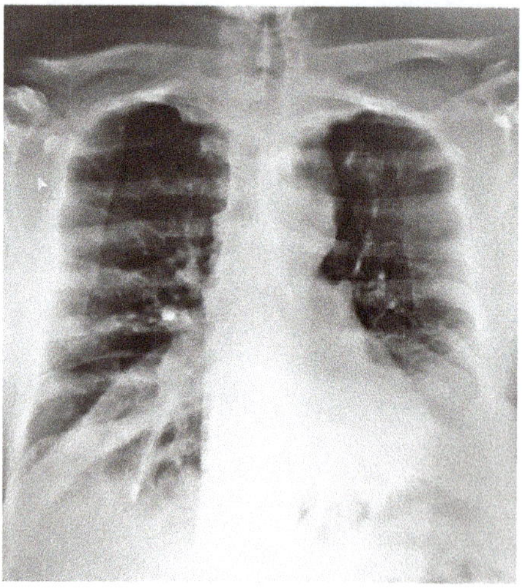

58. A 36-year-old male is admitted to your ICU as a case of road traffic accident. There is diffuse axonal injury and the patient has GCS of only 3. He is electively ventilated. For the past 3 days, he has intermittent fever spikes of 38.4°C, that responds to paracetamol. The nursing staff also reports increased secretions noted from ET, which is mucoid in consistency. Based on the chest X-ray and clinical details, calculate the CPIS score?

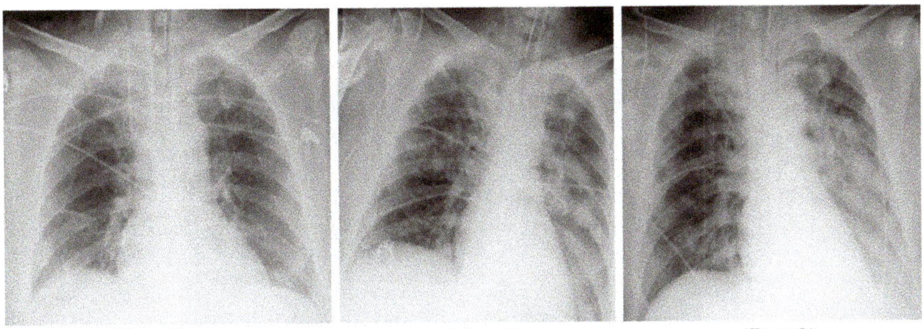

(Day 1)	(Day 2)	(Day 3)
PF ratio 380	PF ratio 260	PF Ratio 200
WBC count 9,800/cm^3	WBC count 8,600/cm^3	WBC count 13,000/cm^3

59. A 36-year-old male, recently detected with retroviral disease, is shifted to the ICU with worsening breathing difficulty and cough, fever, and desaturation.
    - CT taken shows diffuse interstitial and centrilobar nodules with tree in bud appearances and minimal ground glassing.
    - His sputum has come negative for *P. jirovecii* pneumonia (PJP) and pulmonary tuberculosis (PTB) on two occasions.
    - What further tests are recommended for diagnosis of TB in this patient?

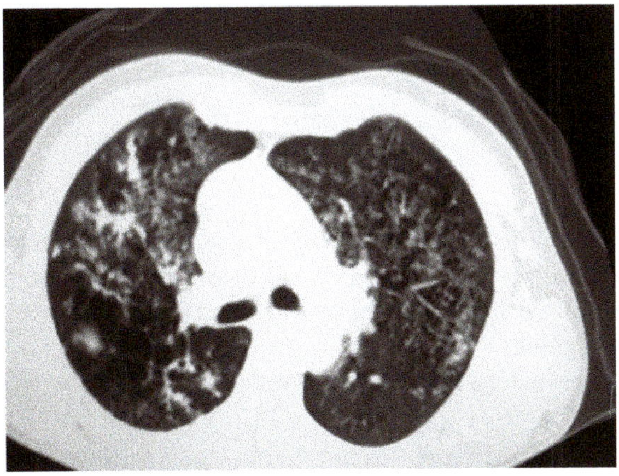

60. A 36-year-old male, recently detected with retroviral disease, is shifted to the ICU with worsening breathing difficulty and cough, fever, and desaturation.
    - CT taken shows diffuse interstitial and centrilobar nodules with tree in bud appearances and minimal ground glassing.
    - Cartridge-based nucleic acid amplification test (CB NAAT) of the sputum has come positive for *Mycobacterium tuberculosis* without detection of rifampicin resistance. How will you start treatment in this case?

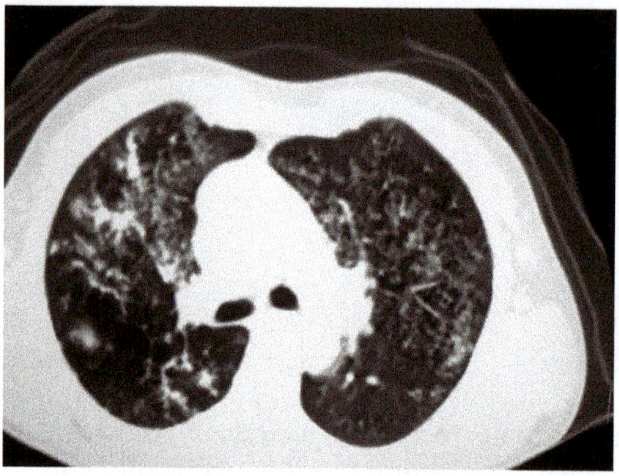

61. A 32-year-old male, recently detected with retroviral disease (CD4 count of 58 cells/μL) and PTB, admitted with respiratory failure due to tuberculosis. 2 weeks after starting antituberculosis treatment, once the respiratory symptoms settled and drug tolerance was acceptable, antiretroviral therapy (ART) was introduced after consultation with an ID specialist. 1 week later, the patient presented with fever, malaise, and worsening breathlessness. Chest imaging revealed development of new parenchymal opacities in both lung fields and mediastinal lymphadenopathy.
    - What is the diagnosis?
    - How will you manage the patient?

NEUROLOGY

62. A 28-year-old male, known case of seizure disorder, is currently admitted with repeated seizures following a week of missed treatment. No history of fever; GCS-E1V1M1. Imaging was done and is as shown below. What is the diagnosis?

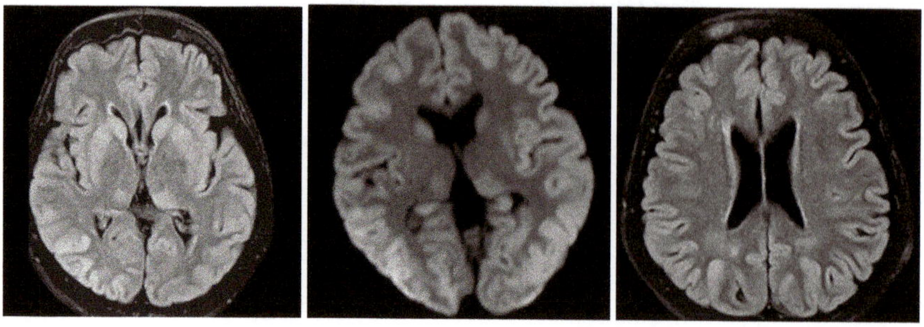

63. A 64-year-old male, chronic alcoholic, was brought to the ER with complaints of seizures.
- On examination, he was hypothermic, bradycardic, and hypotensive.
- Laboratory reports were significant for leukocytosis of 14,000/cm^3, hyponatremia (116 mmol/L), hypokalemia (1.8 mmol/L), and hypochloremia (76 mmol/L).
- He was immediately administered 3% saline 150 mL and as symptoms did not improve, a second bolus was pushed which was followed by potassium correction in normal saline drip. MRI is taken as his sensorium remained dull even after 3 days.
- What is the diagnosis and risk factors?

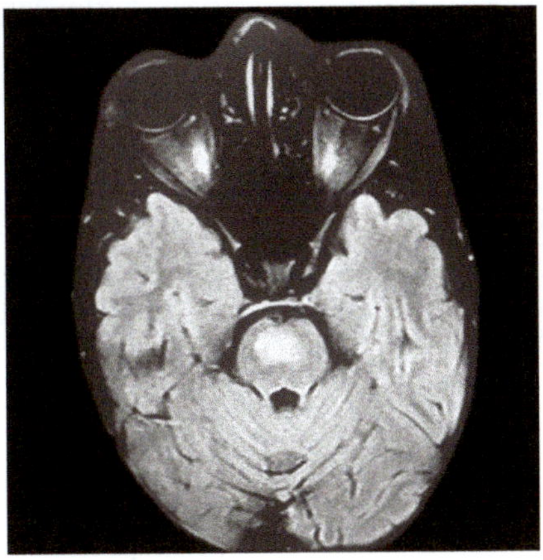

64. A 84-year-old female, with no comorbidities, is brought to ER with complaints of acute onset of focal seizures of lip, loss of consciousness, aphasia, and loss of bowel control.
There is no history of fever. MRI taken is given.
- What is the diagnosis?
- What are the characteristic findings of CSF analysis in herpes encephalitis?
- What is the treatment and treatment duration?

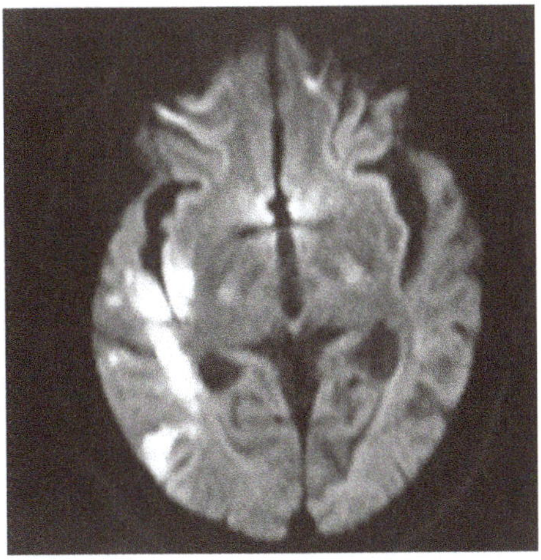

65. Laboratory results of a patient on treatment under neurologist for encephalitis are given below. What are the possible etiologies? How will you manage this patient?

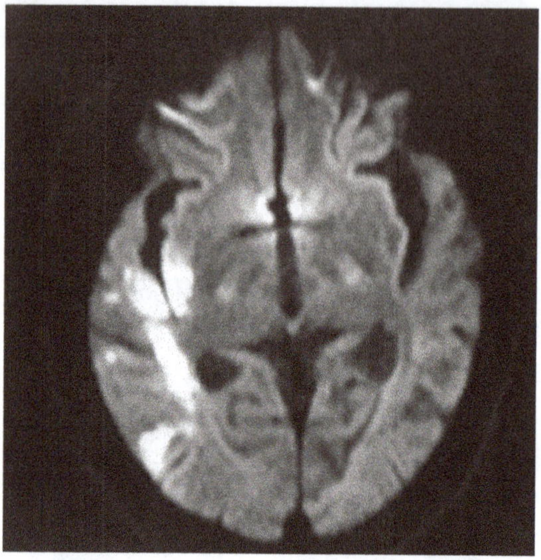

Sodium	143 mmol/L
Potassium	4.2 mmol/L
Chloride	109 mmol/L
Sugar	**246 mg/dL**
Urea	**96 mg/dL**
Creatinine	**2.8 mg/dL**
Hemoglobin	13.6 g/dL
Total count	**14,386**
Platelet	22,600
Urine examination	**Eosinophil cast**
Urine ketone	**1+**
Arterial Blood Gas	
pH	7.38
PCO_2	32 mm Hg
PO_2	64 mm Hg
HCO_3	19 mM
Base excess	–6 mM
Lactate	1.6 mM

66. Patient admitted with acute onset of weakness in right side of the body and loss of consciousness of 6 hours duration. CT angio is given. Comment on the diagnosis and management.

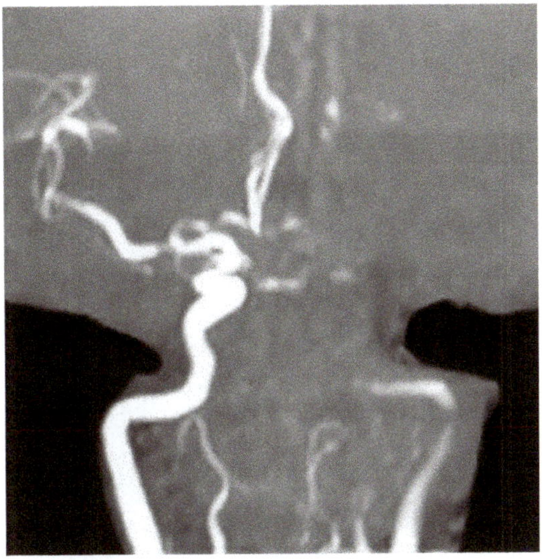

67. Patient presented with headache and seizure of 1-day duration. MRI brain shown in image below.
    - What is the differential diagnosis?

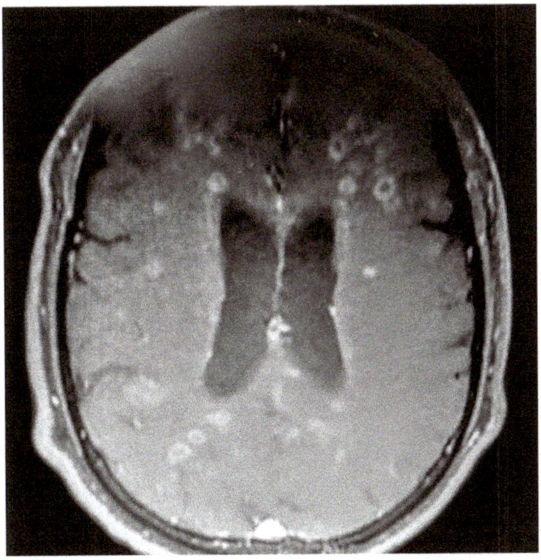

68. A known case of acute leukemia on treatment presented with altered sensorium with a history of falling in bathroom 2 days back.

Laboratory reports:

- Hb: 8.4
- TC: 800/cm^3
- Platelet: 12,000/cm^3
- INR: 1.6

Comment on the diagnosis and management.

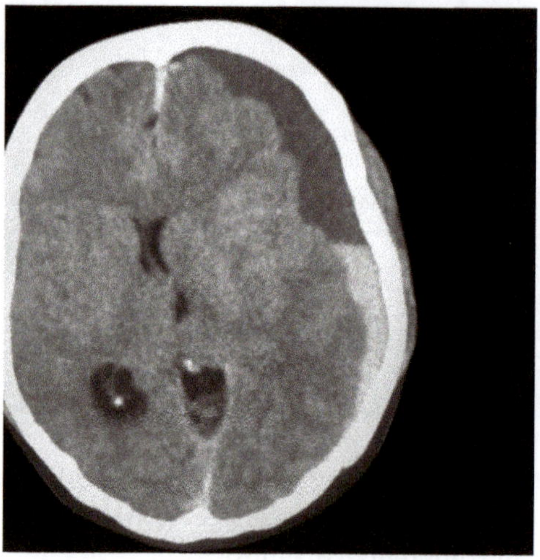

69. CT scan of a patient with history of RTA and altered sensorium is given below.

- Comment on the diagnosis and treatment.

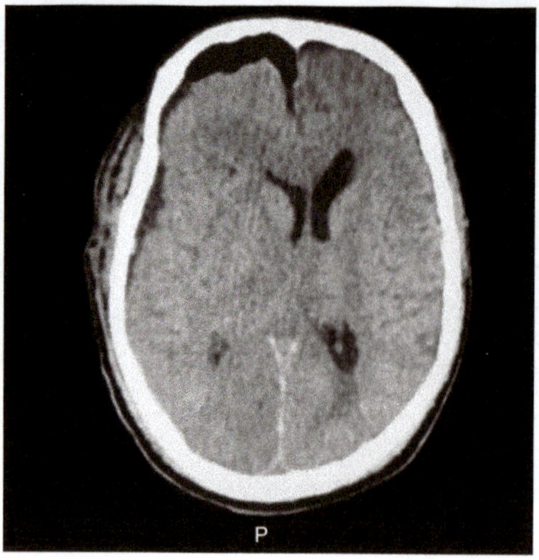

70. The CT scan of a patient with history of RTA is given.
- What is the diagnosis?
- What is Kernohan sign?
- What are the common sites of brain herniation?

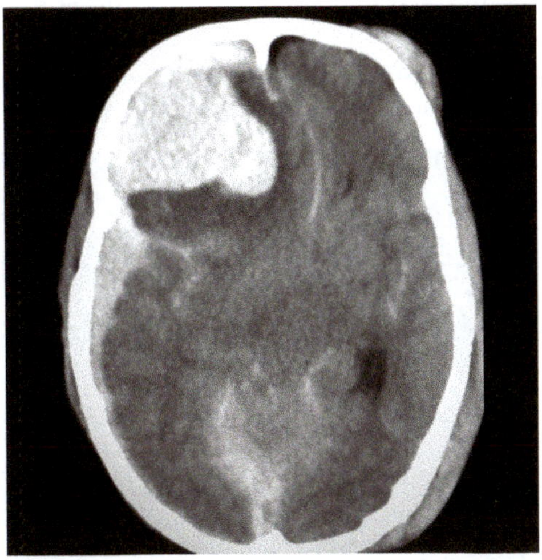

71. A known case of acute leukemia on treatment presented with altered sensorium with a history of falling in bathroom 2 days back.
Laboratory reports:
- Hb: 8.4
- TC: 800/cm^3
- Platelet: 12,000/cm^3
- INR: 1.6

What are the indications of ICP monitoring in TBI?

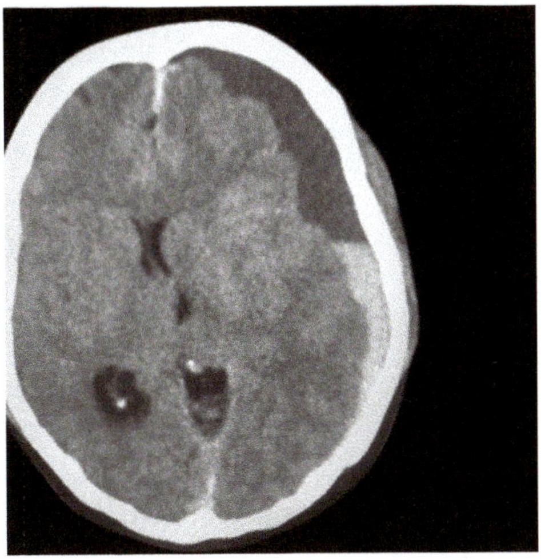

72. A 10-year-old child, with chronic kidney disease stage 5 on hemodialysis, presented to ER with history of seizures half an hour back. Parents give history that the child had refused to take medicines for the past 2 days.
 - On examination, GCS—10/15, PR—110 beats/min, BP—140/100 mm Hg, RR—18 breaths/min, and saturation 86% on room air.
 - MRI taken is as shown below.
 - Comment on the diagnosis and management.

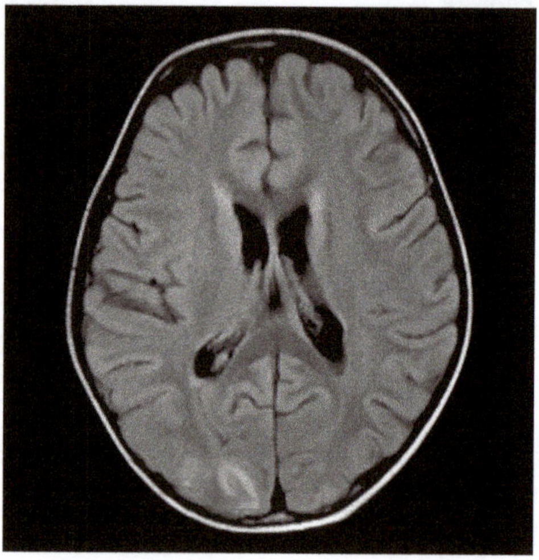

73. CT brain of a 12-year-old child presented with acute onset seizures lasting for more than 2 hours, with child not regaining consciousness in between is as shown in the image below.
 - What is the diagnosis and management?

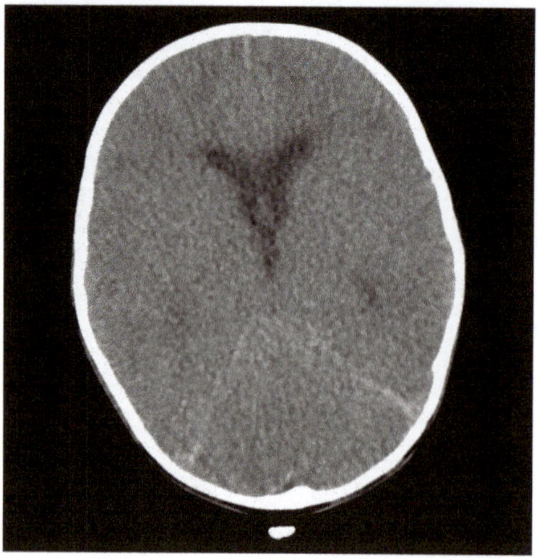

74. A 34-year-old male presented with history of fever of 2 weeks' duration, loss of appetite, and malaise.
Over the past 1 week, he complained of headache and vomiting. He was found to be stuporous for 1 day and had an episode of GTCS at home prior to hospital admission. Clinical evaluation is positive for 6th nerve paralysis and raised ICP.
- MRI taken is as shown below.
- Comment on the diagnosis and management.

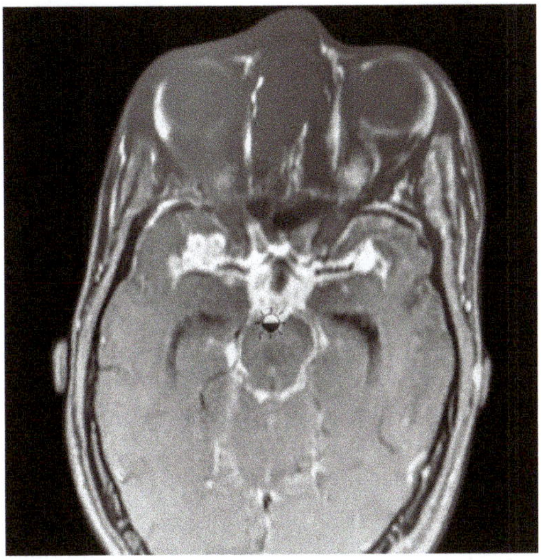

75. CT angiography of a patient with vertigo is given below. Comment on any abnormality noted.

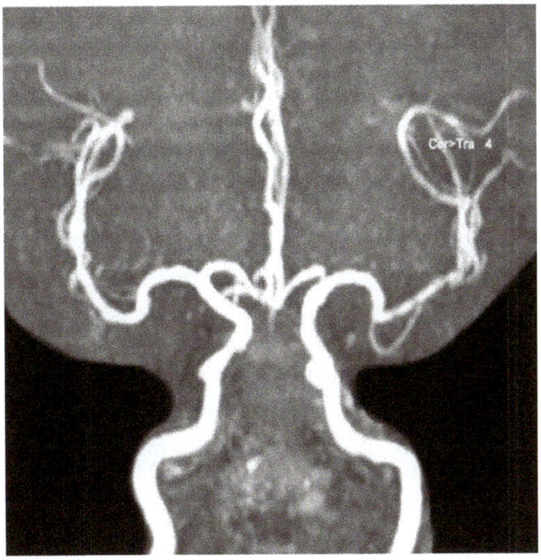

76. A 26-year-old male is brought to ER after being involved in a head-on collision with motor bike and lorry.
    - On arrival, PR—78 beats/min, BP—100/80 mm Hg, RR—12/min irregular, and GCS E2M2V2.
    - CT taken is given in image below. How will you classify the condition?

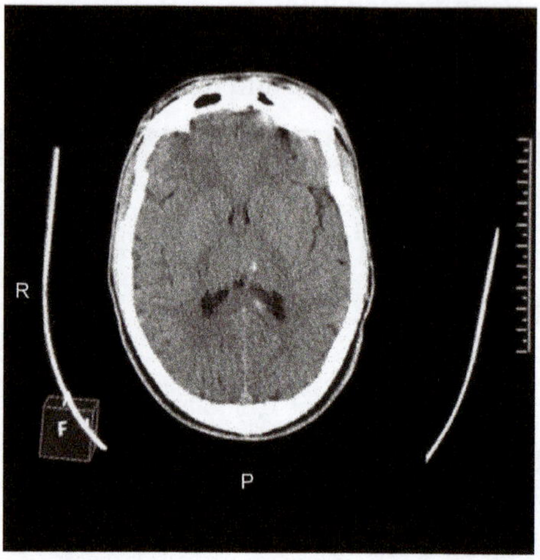

77. A 12-year-old male child, a known case of CNS tumor, is admitted with fever, nausea, vomiting, headache, drop in sensorium, and one episode of seizure.
    - In ICU, GCS—E2M3V3; PR—66 beats/min; BP—110/76 mm Hg; RR—14 breaths/min; saturation 100% on 4-liter face mask; ABG PF ratio of 456; Base excess—7; and Lactate—5.
    - What is the possible differential diagnosis?

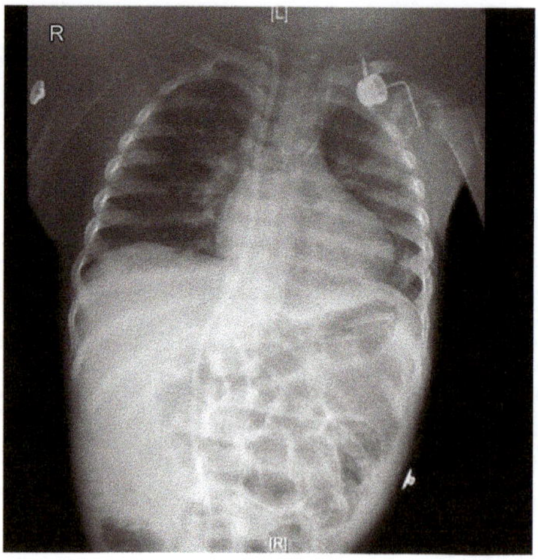

78. A 78-year-old female presented with acute onset loss of consciousness and hemiplegia left side of the body diagnosis.
   - What are the common sites involved?
   - What is the target range for optimal blood pressure control?

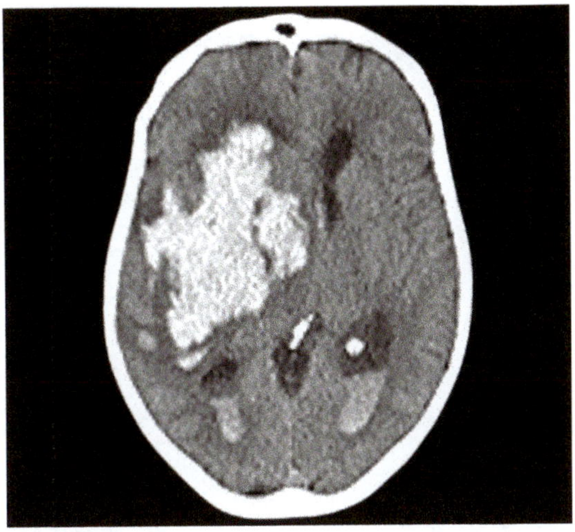

79. A 78-year-old female presented with acute onset loss of consciousness and hemiplegia of left side of the body. What are the prognostic scoring systems to assess outcome in ICH patients?

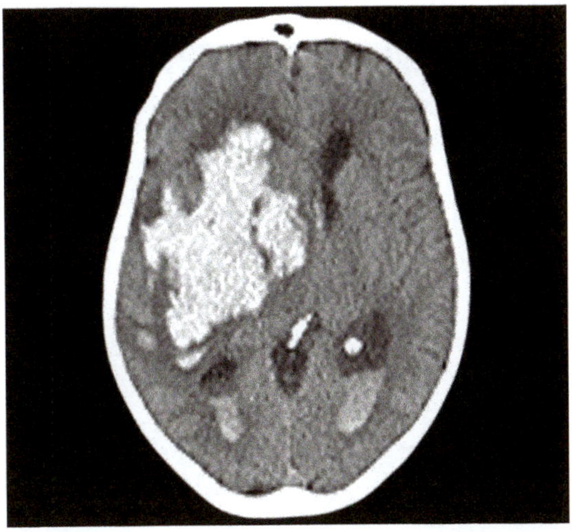

80. A 78-year-old male, with history of hypertension, diabetes mellitus, and chronic atrial fibrillation on warfarin, presents to casualty after sustaining a fall at home. After admission, his GCS has dropped from 13 to 10. A CT scan taken in ER is shown below. What is the diagnosis and what are the urgent measures to be undertaken in managing this patient?

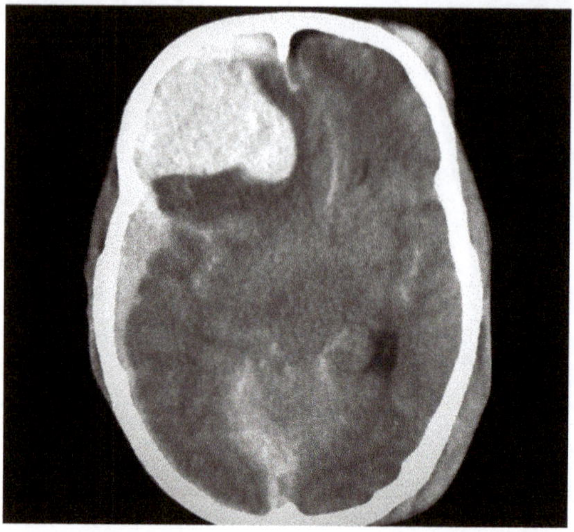

81. A 78-year-old male, with history of hypertension, diabetes mellitus, and chronic atrial fibrillation on warfarin, presents to casualty after sustaining a fall at home. After admission, his GCS has dropped from 13 to 10. A CT scan taken in ER is shown. What are the criteria for surgical evacuation of SDH?

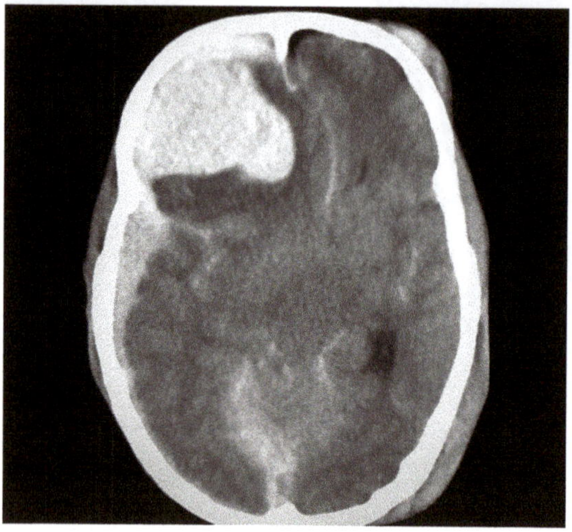

82. A 46-year-old male, a victim of bike colliding on a tree, is brought to the ER. In ER, he is apparently fine except for mild tachycardia of 110/min and chest pain on the left side. He gives a history of loss of consciousness for 5 minutes immediately after the accident, however currently recalls everything.
A whole-body CT scan taken in ER is shown in the image. What is the diagnosis?

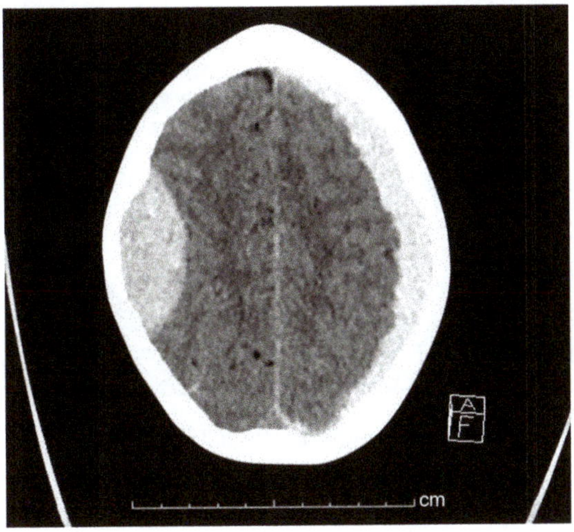

83. What are the indication for neurosurgical intervention for a victim of road traffic accident presenting with the CT given below.

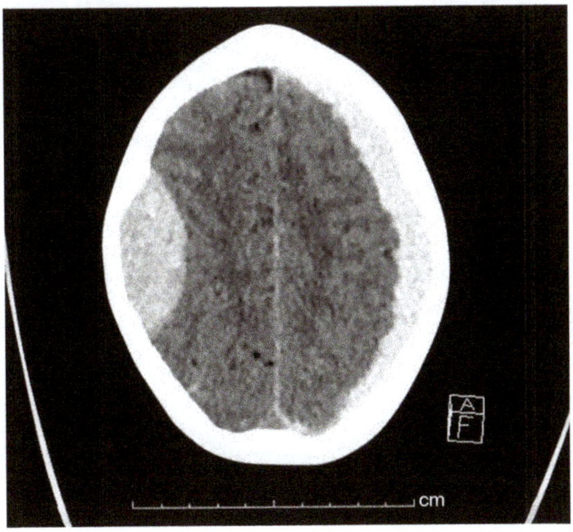

84. The CT brain of a patient admitted to ICU with low GCS is given in the image. What is the diagnosis? What are the indications and complications for craniectomy? Critically appraise the benefit of craniectomy in stroke and trauma.

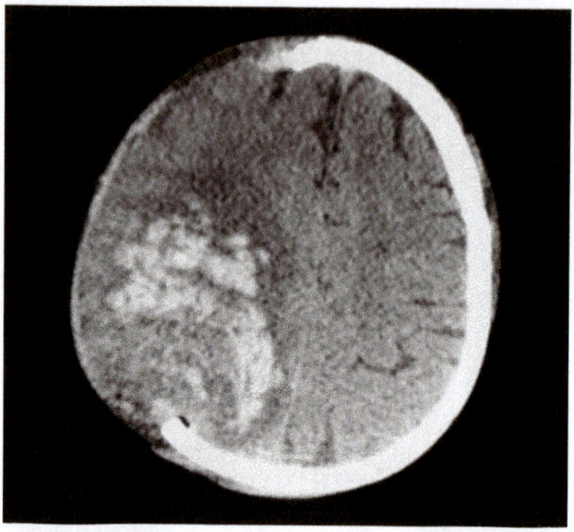

85. A 76-year-old male is brought to the ICU with weakness of right side of the body of 3 hours duaration.
- What is the diagnosis?
- What are the indications/criteria for late thrombectomy after ischemic stroke?

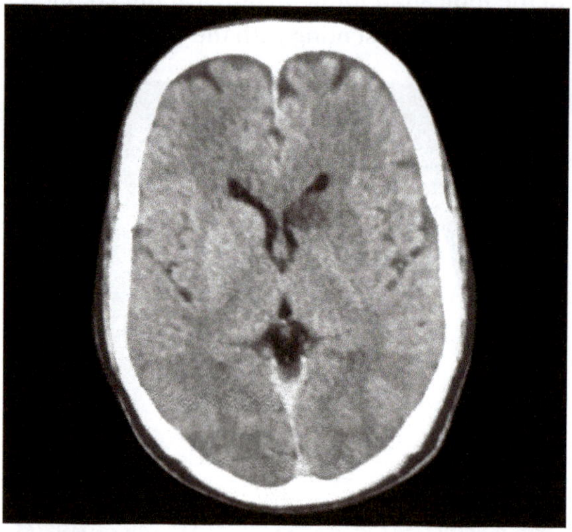

86. For a patient presenting with acute onset weakness of right side of body and CT brain as shown in the image.
- What are the indications for thrombolysis and extended thrombolysis in stroke?
- When is a repeat imaging indicated after thrombolysis in stroke?

- How will you critically evaluate thrombolysis as a therapeutic option for stroke?

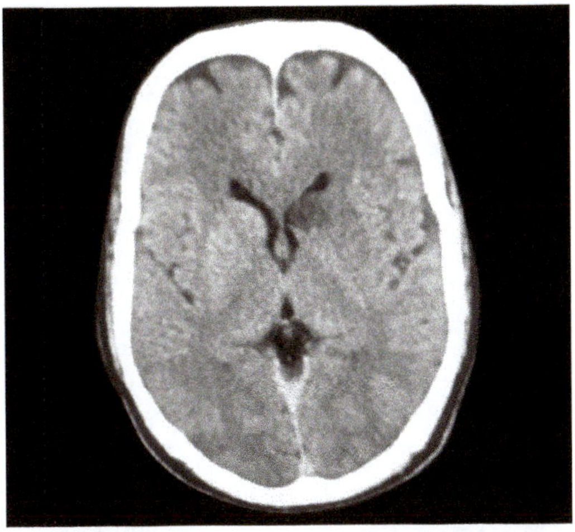

87. CT scan of a patient presenting with right sided weakness of 3 hours duration.
    - What is the immediate medical management in this case?
    - What is the role of heparin?
    - What is the role of dual antiplatelet therapy in these patients?

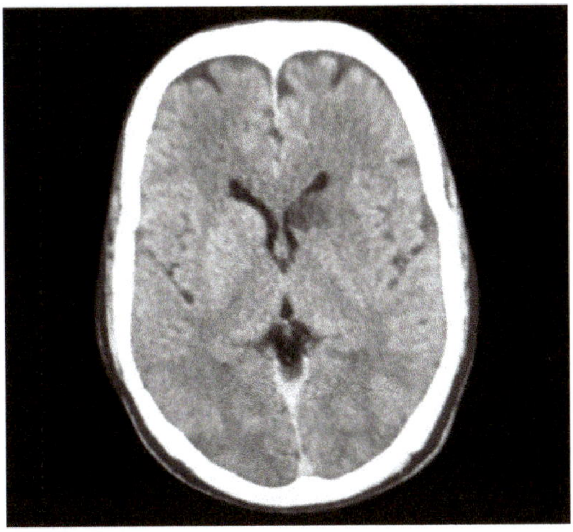

88. A 42-year-old, alcoholic male, presented with altered sensorium. His vitals are normal, except for:
    - Mild tachycardia of 120/min
    - Hypothermia of 96°F
    - Sugars: 56 mg/dL
    - ABG: pH 7.0; HAGMA, Corrected AG—24
    - Lactate—3.5
    - HCO_3—10 mmol/L
    - Urine ketones—positive

He is not improving after correction of hypoglycemia, hypothermia, fluid replacement, and administration of thiamine. MRI taken is shown below. What is the diagnosis in this case?

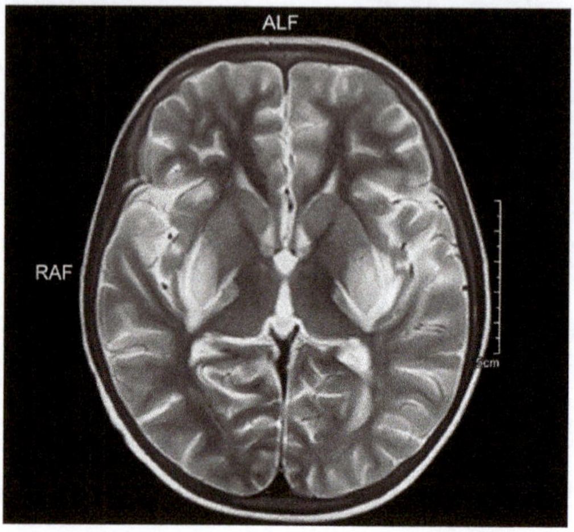

NEPHROLOGY

89. • Identify the renal replacement therapy (RRT) circuits.
    • What are the principles of solute removal in each?

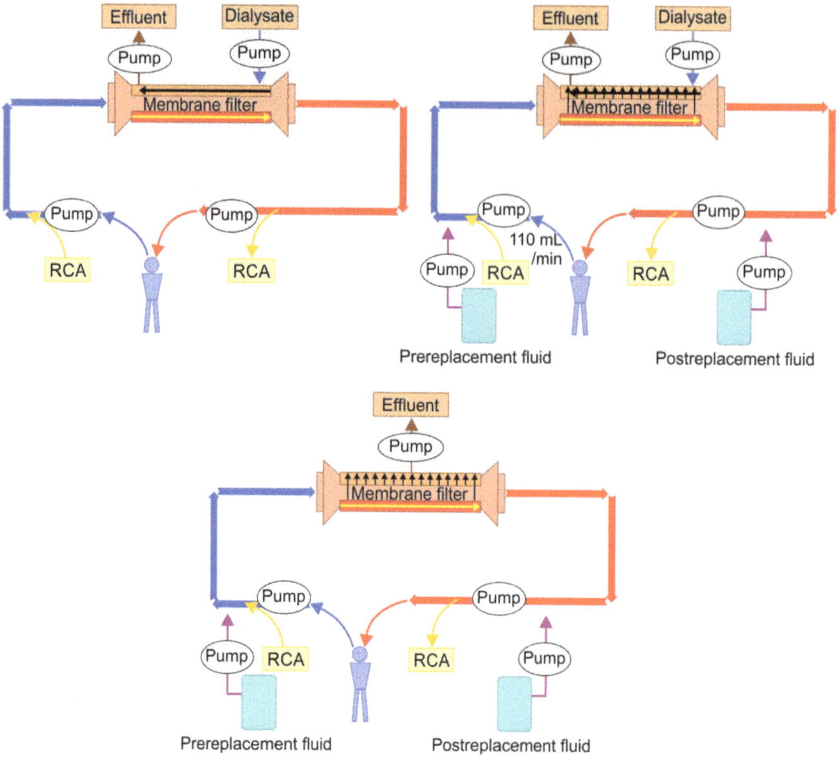

90. What are the maximum rates and commonly prescribed rates of the following?

1. Blood flow in CRRT
2. Rate of fluid replacement
3. Rate of dialysate flow
4. Maximal fluid removal from patient

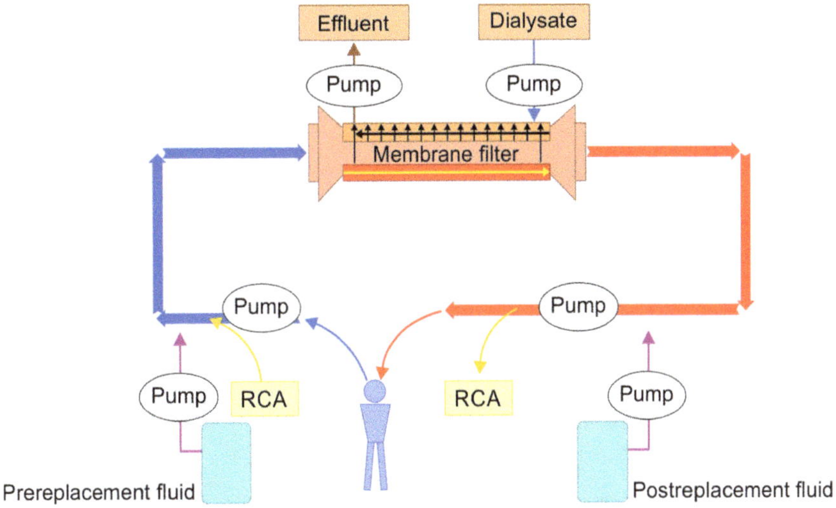

91. • How is the dose of CRRT calculated?
- What is the optimal dose of dialysis that is commonly prescribed?
- What are the interventions to increase the efficiency of dialysis in this circuit?

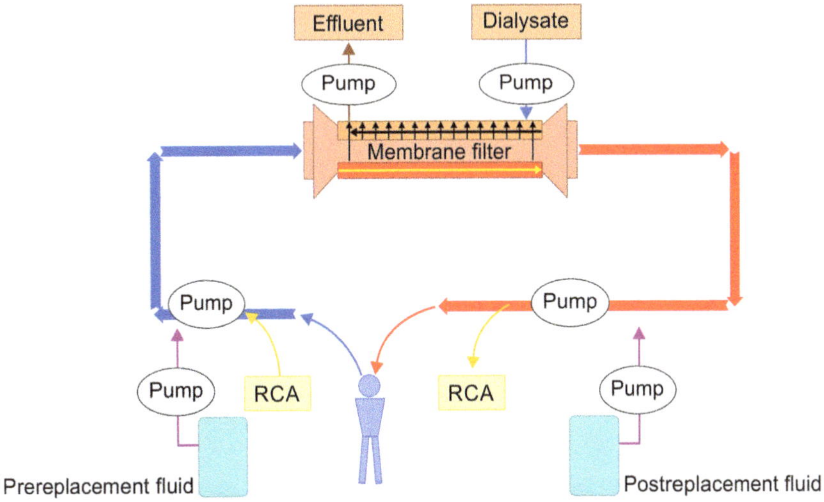

92. • What is drug A and B in regional citrate anticoagulation (RCA)?
• What are the complications of RCA?
• What are the clotting factors inhibited by RCA?

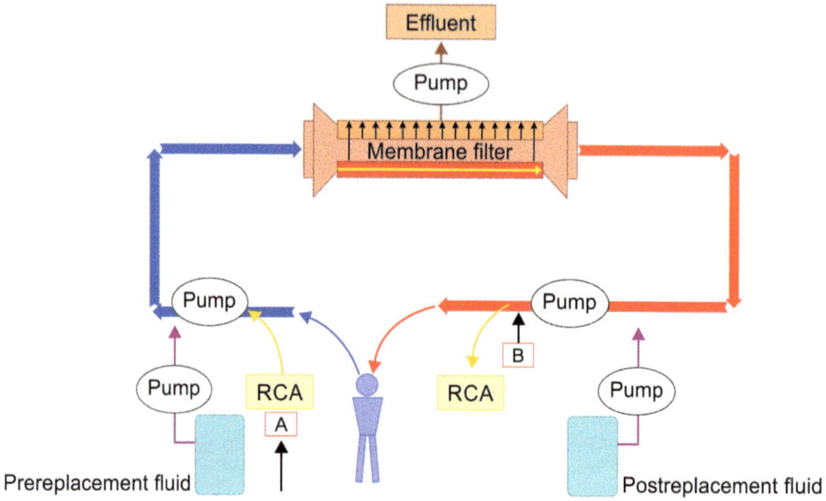

93. What are the strategies to increase filter life?

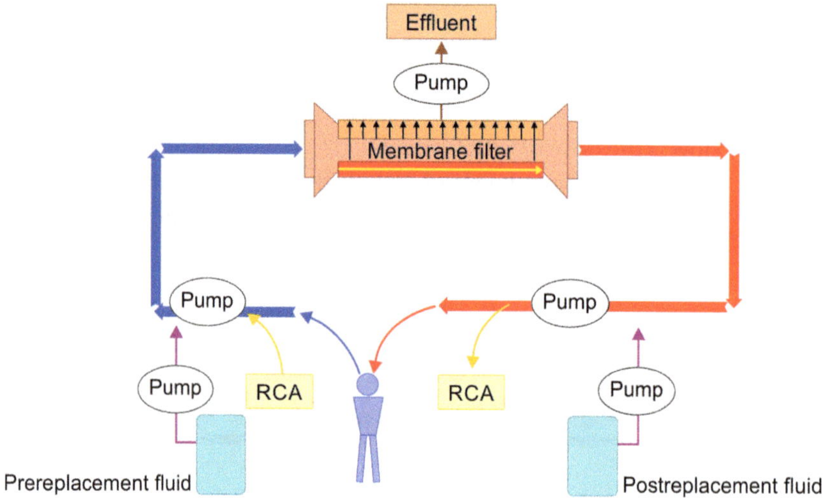

94. How will you troubleshoot a low return pressure?

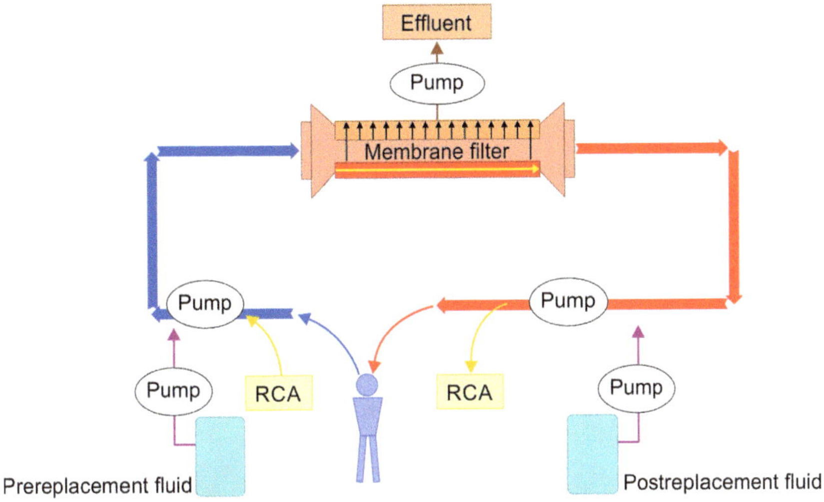

95. • How is transmembrane pressure (TMP) calculated?
- What is filter pressure?
- What are the causes of high TMP alarm?

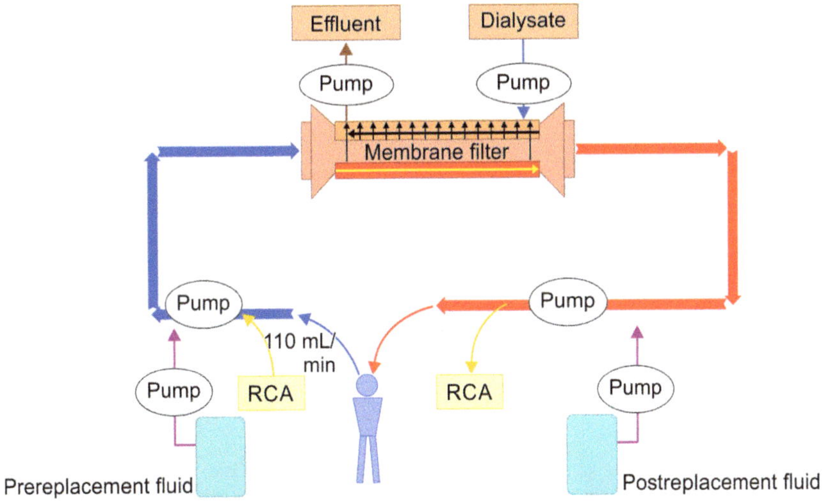

96. • What are the current indications for RRT in ICU?
 • What is the current evidence for the timing of RRT in ICU?

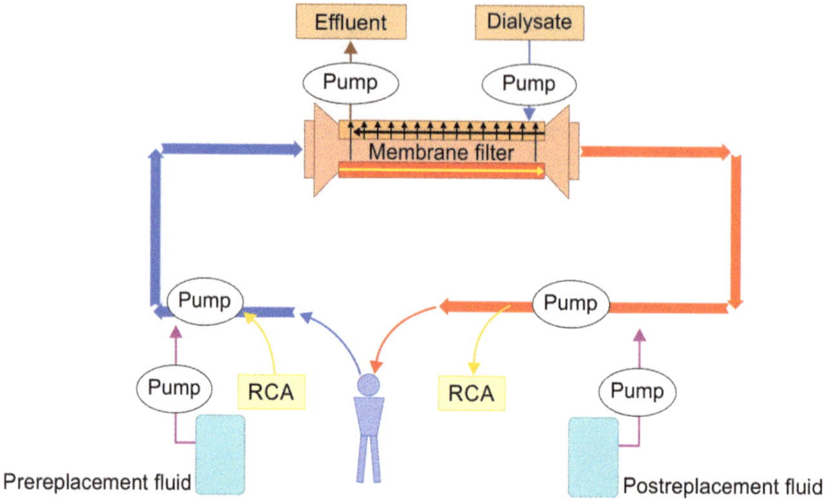

97. What are the factors affecting drug dosing for a patient n CRRT? What are the common dose adjustments required for antibiotics during CRRT?

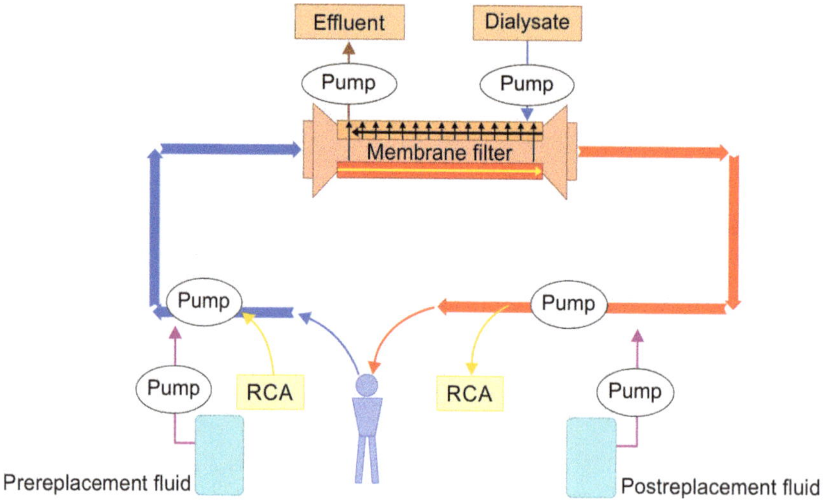

98. What is the typical composition of replacement fluid in CRRT? What are the common electrolyte abnormalities in patients on CRRT?

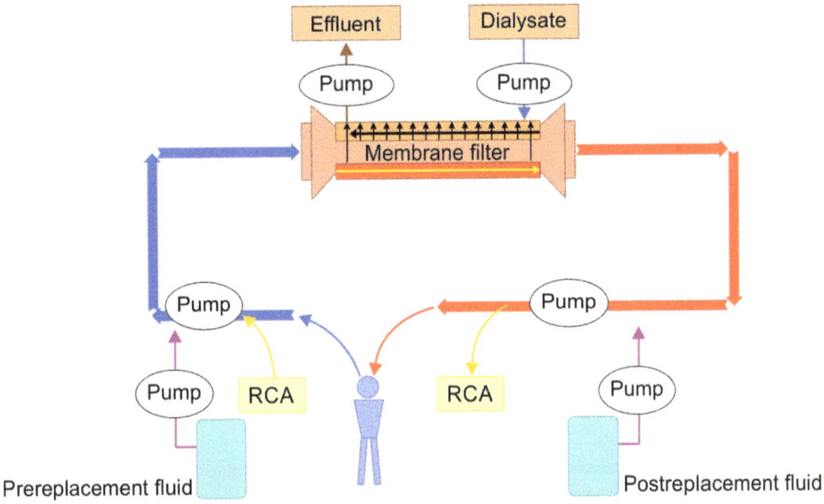

99. Identify the position of the following alarms in circuit.
- Blood leak alarm in circuit.
- Air alarm in circuit.

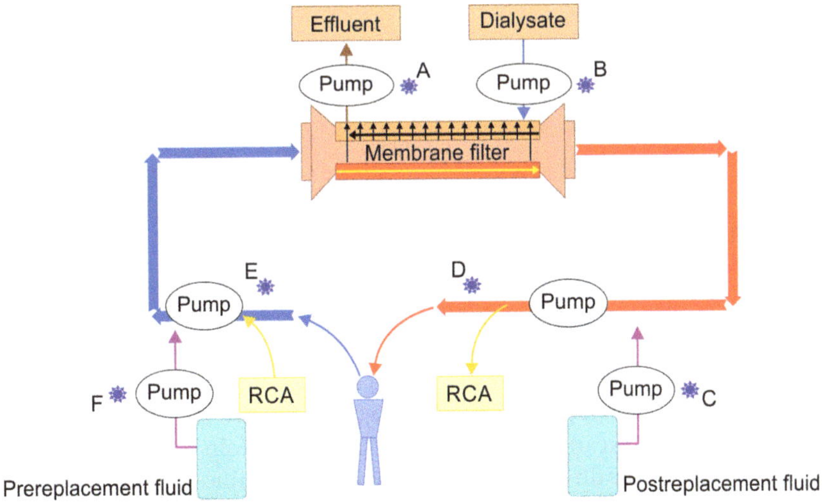

100. A 63-year-old male, a known case of end stage renal dialysis stage 5, who is dialysis naïve, is now admitted with refractory pulmonary edema and breathlessness. His lab values show a urea 246 mg/dL, S Creatine is 14 mg/dL, HCO_3 is 11 mmol/L, Na is 146 mmol/L, K is 6.4 mmol/L, CL is 88 mmol/L as he did not respond to initiation of noninvasive ventilation and a diuretic challenge, it was decided to initiate dialysis via a right jugular catheter. Hemodialysis for 4 hours is initiated in ICU with a planned fluid removal of 2.5 liters. Post-dialysis, the lab values are urea 86 mg/dL, S Cr 4.4 mg/dL, HCO_3 22 mmol/L, Na 140 mmol/L, K 3.3 mmol/L, Cl 100 mmol/L. The patient became drowsy and had one episode of seizure after the dialysis is terminated. What is the probable cause? How could you have prevented it?

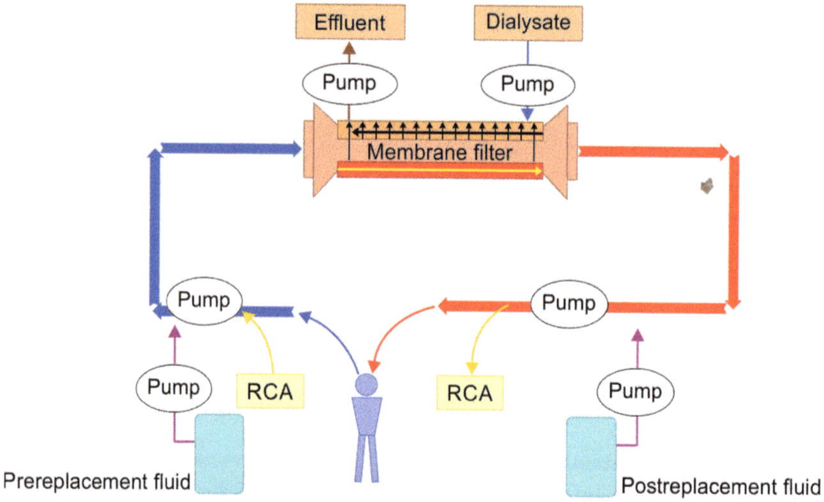

MICROBIOLOGY AND INFECTION CONTROL

101. A 52-year-old farmer presented with fever, retro-orbital headache, chills, myalgia, and decreased urine output of 3 days duration. On examination, the patient is having conjunctival suffusion and calf muscle tenderness. Laboratory investigations sent showed hemoglobin (Hb) 9.2 g/dL, white blood cell (WBC) count of 12,000/cc with 76% neutrophils, and platelet count of 80,000/cumm, serum bilirubin 3.2 mg/dL (direct 0.8 mg/dL, indirect 2.4 mg/dL), aspartate aminotransferase (AST)/serum glutamic oxaloacetic transaminase (SGOT) 39 IU/L, alanine aminotransferase (AST)/serum glutamic pyruvic transaminase (SGPT) 40 IU/L, alkaline phosphatase (ALP) 136 IU/L, blood urea 158 mg/dL, and serum creatine 5.6 mg/dL. Dengue and malaria were reported as negative.

1. What is the presumptive diagnosis?
2. What are the tests you can opt for, to confirm the diagnosis?
3. What is the sample of choice if you choose to do a culture?

102. A 42-year-old alcoholic patient is admitted with complaints of fever, headache, and vomiting of 3 days duration. Clinical examination is positive for photophobia, irritability, and neck stiffness. Laboratory investigation sent has reported the hemoglobin of 9.8 g/dL, WBC count of 14,000/cc, and platelet count of 188,000/cc.
Lumbar puncture revealed hazy cerebrospinal fluid (CSF), and CSF analysis showed 250 cells per cc, 80% polymorphs and 20% lymphocytes, glucose 39.6 mg/dL, protein 78.4 mg/dL, and adenosine deaminase 4.19 U. Serum glucose at the time of lumbar puncture was 112 mg/dL. Gram's stain of CSF showed gram-positive bacilli.
    1. What is the presumptive diagnosis?
    2. What is the suggested empirical therapy for this patient?

103. A 62-year-old social worker is admitted into your intensive care unit (ICU) with altered sensorium, high-grade fever, chills, photophobia, and one episode of seizure. She had a history of fever for the past 5 days and was on treatment for the same. Blood routine was unremarkable except for an erythrocyte sedimentation rate (ESR) of 60 mm/h and C-reactive protein (CRP) of 88 mg/L.
Cerebrospinal fluid studies revealed mildly elevated opening pressure, clear CSF, 14 cells/cumm with 85% lymphocytes, protein 274 mg/dL, and glucose 59 mg/dL. CSF Gram's stain, acid-fast stain, and wet mount showed no bacteria/fungal elements.
    1. What is the diagnosis?
    2. What are the common etiological agents?
    3. What extra investigations need to be called for confirming the diagnosis?

104. A 66-year-old diabetic man admitted into ICU with right upper lobe consolidation. He is confused, mildly tachycardic (heart rate of 110 beats/min), blood pressure (BP) 98/56 mm Hg, respiratory rate of 30 breaths/min, and requiring oxygen of 4 L via face mask to maintain a saturation of 96%.
Arterial blood gases (ABGs) revealed a PaO_2/FiO_2 (partial pressure of oxygen in arterial blood/fraction of inspired oxygen) ratio of 202 and a pH of 7.38. His laboratory analysis is positive for a leukocytosis of 12,400/cc with a neutrophil:lymphocyte ratio of 4, serum albumin of 2.4 g/dL, urea of 66 g/dL, and normal creatinine.
Gram's stain of sputum showed capsulated gram-positive diplococci. The culture is positive and shown in Figure.
    - What is the empirical treatment for community-acquired pneumonia (CAP)?
    - What antibiotic would you chose for the patient not responding to initial therapy?

- Postresolution, what advice would be given to this patient?

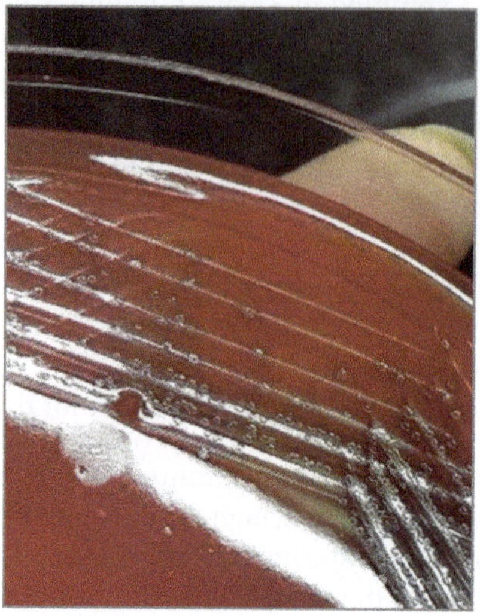

105. A 56-year-old man presents to the emergency room (ER) with fever, myalgia, dry cough, and breathing difficulty of 3 days duration. On admission to ER, pulse rate (PR) was 113 beats/min, BP: 146/90 mm Hg, respiratory rate (RR): 32 breaths/min, and saturation was 85%. Chest X-ray showed bilateral (B/L) lung consolidation. He was admitted to ICU and started high-flow nasal cannula @ 60 L flow and 60% FiO_2 with which he maintained a saturation of 94%. The Labs reveal Hb 11.6 g/dL, pancytopenia with WBC count of 2,900/cc, 58% polymorphs, 11% lymphocytes, and 13% monocytes, and platelet count 110,000/cc. Other results seem to be unremarkable.
Sputum Gram's stain showed gram-positive cocci in clusters.
The relatives give history that his wife was suffering from of H1N1 pneumonia a week ago, and currently recuperating from that.
    1. What would be the investigation of choice?
    2. What is the advantage this test offers, over the other options?

106. A patient got admitted with fever, chills, breathing difficulty, and hacking cough with mild hemoptysis. He was on treatment for CAP for 2 weeks with not much clinical improvement. CT scan taken on admission shows multilobar consolidation, right upper lobe cavity, and scattered nodules in both right and left lungs.
Initial workup for tuberculosis including sputum acid-fast bacilli (AFB) stain and cartridge-based nucleic acid amplification (CB-NAAT) were negative.
Bronchoalveolar lavage taken was negative for malignancy. A modified ZN staining showed filamentous bacteria as shown in the image. What is the empirical therapy?

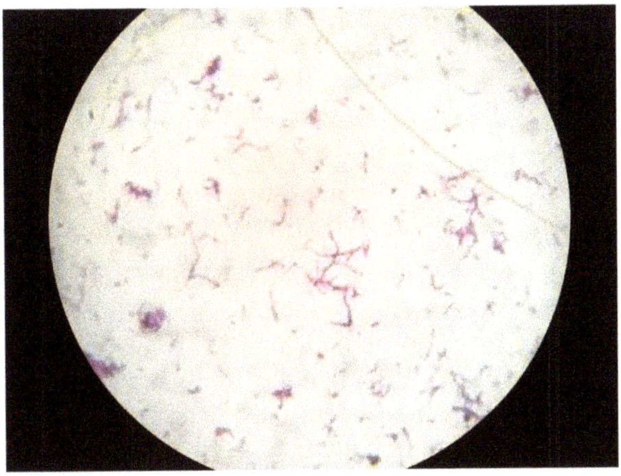

107. A 24-year-old male, recently diagnosed to have acute lymphoid leukemia on chemotherapy, presents with fever, cough, and worsening dyspnea. He was initially started on meropenem, vancomycin, and colistin. Symptomatic and radiologic worsening was noted.
High-resolution computed tomography (HRCT) is shown in the Figure. Bronchoalveolar lavage (BAL) sample on culture yielded this growth.
1. How will you modify the treatment?
2. Name a serologic test that can aid in the presumptive diagnosis of such cases.
3. How will you classify the treatment based on evidence as compared to a treatment based on clinical suspicion?

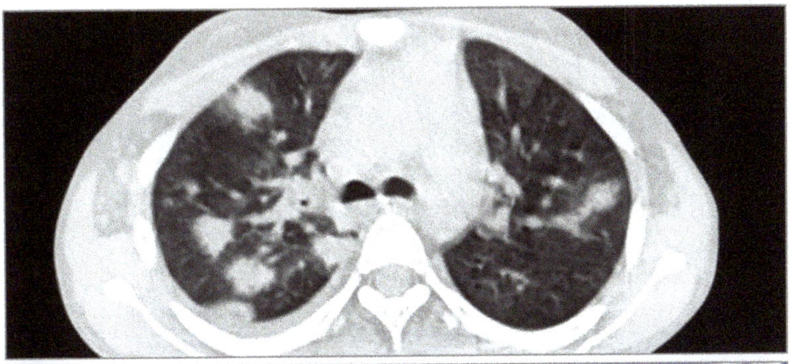

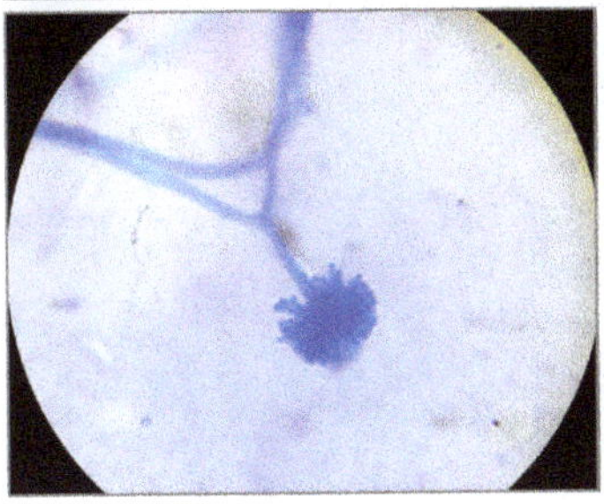

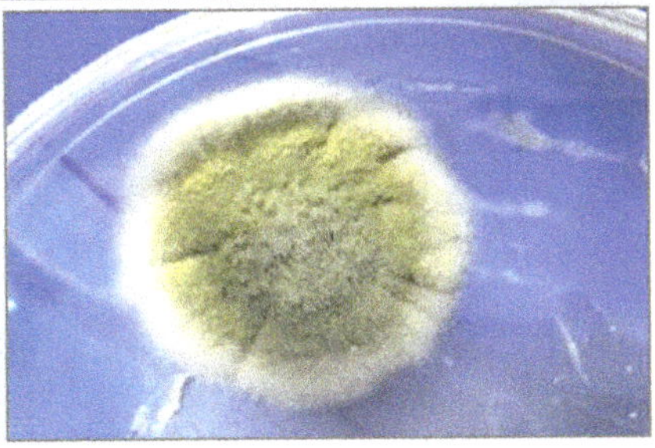

108. A 36-year-old male, recently diagnosed as retroviral disease, is being referred to the ICU with chronic watery diarrhea, mild crampy abdominal pain, and severe dehydration.
He has not responded to initial treatment given on outpatient basis.
1. Which are the probable pathogens?
2. Which are the first-line diagnostic investigations?
3. Apart from fluid resuscitation, what is the empirical therapy?

109. A 36-year-old non-resident Indian (NRI) from California, on visit to his Indian hometown, presented to the hospital with complaints of fever, chills, nausea, dry cough, and malaise of 1 week duration.
Chest CT shows right-sided pleural effusion, right lower lobe infiltrates, and B/L hilar lymphadenopathy. Clinical examination reveals B/L femoral suppurative lymphadenitis.
1. Given the travel history, what are the possible differentials?
2. Which are the investigations of choice?
3. How will you manage this patient in ICU?

110. A 21-year-old man presented with dry cough and dyspnea on exertion over past 3 months. CT showed tissue infiltration into B/L atria, interatrial septum, superior vena cava (SVC) and B/L pulmonary veins.
As bone marrow evaluation did not reveal malignancy and the hemogram was normal, fine needle aspirate of the mass was attempted and sent for histopathology examination and culture. Culture obtained is shown in the image.
1. What are the differentials in this case?
2. Name the molecular method that helps in determination of fungal pathogens.

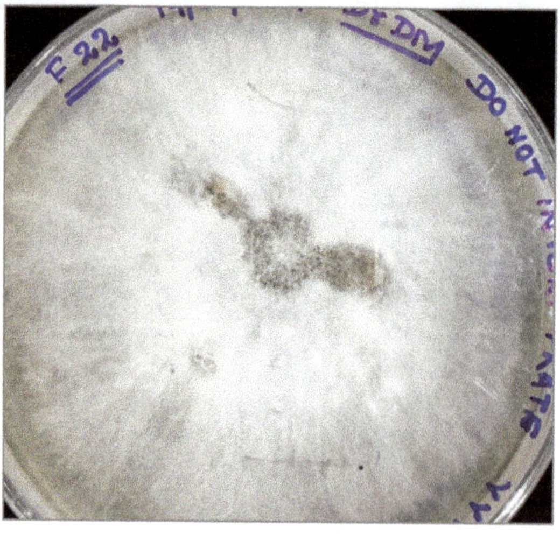

111. A 14-year-old female presented with acute onset of respiratory distress and noisy breathing of 12-hour duration. Her mother gives history of fever and sore throat with difficulty in swallowing over past 1 week. Her

immunization history is unknown and mother says that she might have missed the immunizations.

Direct laryngoscopy showed a swollen epiglottis and a dirty yellow membrane over the tonsil, which bleeds to touch.

1. What is the presumptive diagnosis?
2. How will you confirm the diagnosis?
3. How would you manage the case?

112. The urine culture and sensitivity report of a 26-year-old woman who presented with symptomatic bacteriuria in the third trimester is given in the Figure.
   1. What would your choice for initial antibiotics?
   2. How would the decision be different from a case with similar blood culture isolate?

Organism: *Escherichia coli*
Resistance: Extended spectrum beta-lactamase (ESBL)
Genotype: bla-CTXM

Antimicrobial	*Minimum inhibitory concentration (MIC)*	*Interpretation*
Nitrofurantoin	≤16	S
Amikacin	4	S
Gentamicin	≤1	S
Ciprofloxacin	>2	R
Ampicillin	>16	R
Amoxicillin clavulanate	8	S
Piperacillin tazobactam	8	S
Cefoperazone sulbactam	16	S
Cefuroxime	>32	R
Ceftriaxone	>32	R
Cefepime	>32	R
Imipenem	≤0.25	S
Meropenem	≤25	S

(R: resistant; S: susceptible)

113. A 47-year-old man was admitted into ICU with fever and erythematous rash over chest, hands, back, and legs. This was followed by peeling of skin and later on by dark-brown-colored macules over legs and arms. Gram stain of sample from the lesions showed gram-positive cocci in clusters.
   1. What is the presumptive diagnosis? What would you start the patient on?
   2. What extra tests would you order for the workup of the patient?
   3. How would you modify the treatment if the strain is positive for inducible clindamycin resistance?

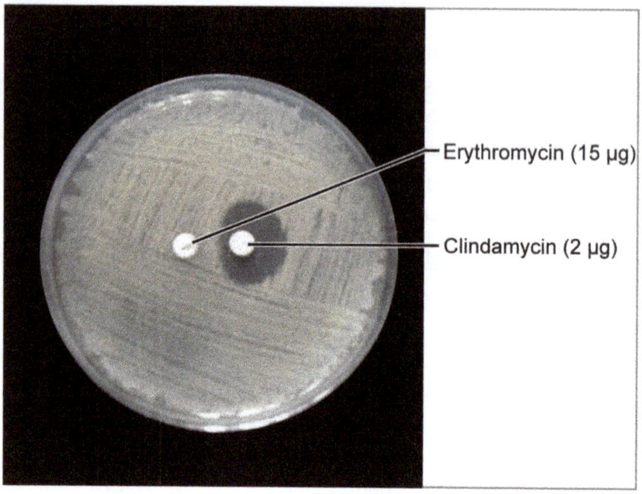

114. A 35-year-old presented to ED with acute onset crampy abdominal pain, profuse watery diarrhea of 15 times/day, and four episodes of vomiting of 1-day duration. He gave history of having consumed raw egg prior to disease onset.
Stool microscopy showed 10–15 polymorphs/hpf and abundant mucus. He was started empirically on ciprofloxacin 500 mg twice a day along with fluid resuscitation.
After 3 days, stool culture yielded *Salmonella typhimurium*.
1. How would you manage the case?
2. What precautions would you instruct your staff to take?

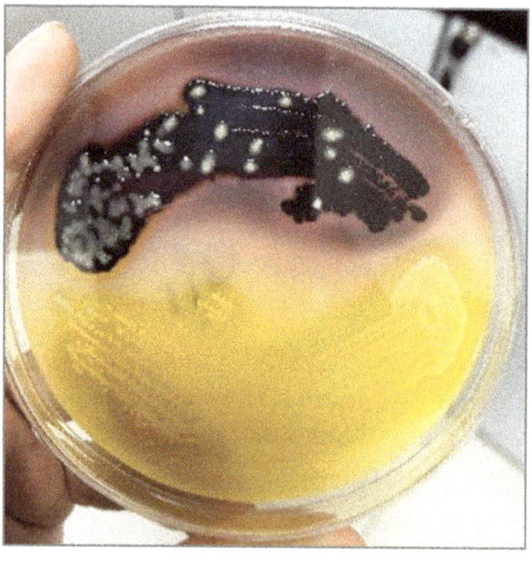

115. A 32-year-old man who returned from a business trip got admitted to hospital with fever, headache, vomiting, and myalgia. Physical examination revealed generalized maculopapular rash. Initial lab

workup for malaria, dengue, and Japanese Encephalitis were negative. He had a rapid worsening of symptoms, with drop in Glasgow Coma Scale (GCS) to 11 and was shifted to ICU after 14 hours of hospital admission.

Laboratory investigations revealed severe thrombocytopenia.

Clinical examination revealed neck stiffness and CSF studies were opted under platelet transfusion. CSF analysis showed a protein of 545 mg/dL and CSF glucose of 40 mg/dL. CSF Gram's stain showed 1,400 cells, 98% polymorphonuclear cells, and gram-negative diplococci.

1. What are the differential diagnoses?
2. What is the empirical treatment in suspected patients?
3. How will you manage the immediate contacts of this case?

116. A 36-year-old male, diagnosed of non-Hodgkin's lymphoma, on chemotherapy for the past 3 months, presented to the ER with fever, hypotension, tachycardia, and oliguria. On examination, he is having cold peripheries, sinus tachycardia of 130 beats/min, and blood pressure of 80/40 mm Hg despite fluid resuscitation. In view of refractory hypotension, he was admitted to ICU, blood cultures were sent, and he was started on meropenem and vancomycin. In view of clinical worsening, caspofungin was added on day 2. On day 3, the blood cultures came positive for *Enterococcus gallinarum*.
    1. What will your empirical therapy be?
    2. How will you modify the treatment if Film array of positive blood culture shows species to be *E. gallinarum*.

117. A 45-year-old male was admitted into the coronary care unit after an inferior wall myocardial infarction (MI) and cardiac arrest. After angioplasty, the patient required high vasopressor supports and intra-aortic balloon pump (IABP) support. A central line was inserted for inotropic agents, which are being tapered according to the target mean arterial pressure (MAP). After 2 days, he developed a high-grade fever spike of 102°F, associated with hypotension.
    A paired blood culture was sent and the sample sent from the central line grew *Staphylococcus epidermidis*.
    1. How would you confirm the diagnosis of central-line-associated blood stream infection (CLABSI)?
    2. How would you manage the patient?

118. A 68-year-old female is being treated for a chest infection that she developed after a surgery for joint replacement. She is on amoxicillin-clavulanate and clindamycin for 10 days and has remained afebrile for 3 days. On the day of the scheduled discharge, she developed acute watery diarrhea that did not respond to changing the nutrition formula and antisecretory agents.
    1. What is the differential diagnosis?
    2. How will you manage the case?

119. A 59-year-old known case of myasthenia gravis is admitted to the ICU following a cardiac arrest and successful resuscitation. He is currently intubated and on day 3, developed fever and dyspnea with increased secretions from endotracheal tube. Tracheal aspirate yielded the organism in culture.
    1. Identify the organism.
    2. What is the main risk factor for ventilator-associated pneumonia (VAP) by this organism?

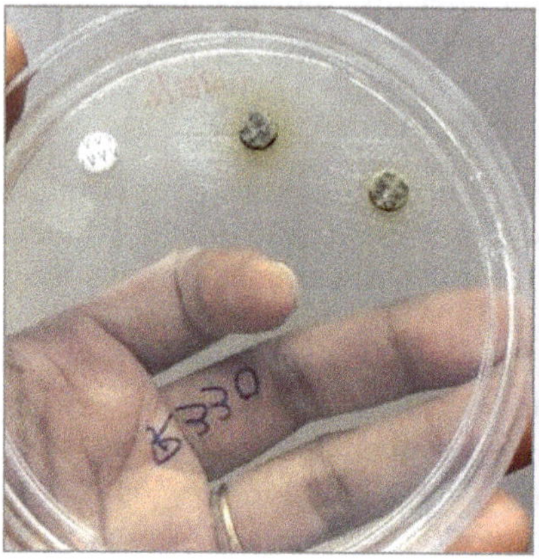
Fig. 1A

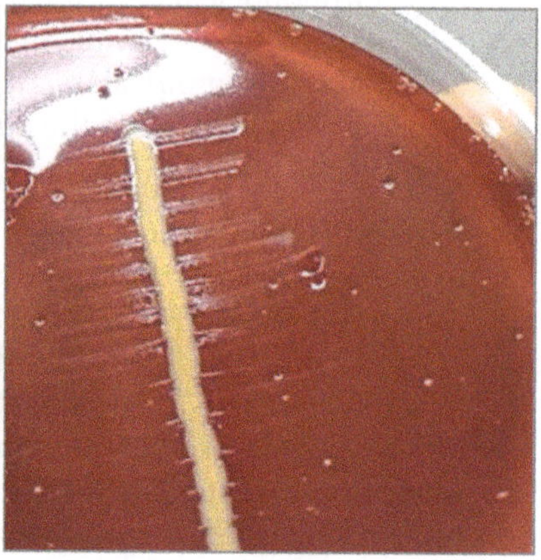
Fig. 1B

120. In a 22-bedded ICU, over a period of 5 days, three patients developed *Burkholderia cepacia* septicemia and another two were found to have their indwelling devices asymptomatically colonized.
    1. What makes this a dreaded organism in the ICU?
    2. How will you track the cause of the outbreak?

121. A 72-year-old immunocompetent, otherwise healthy man, presented with intermittent fever, malaise, weight loss (nearly 7 kg), and abdominal distension over the past 4–5 weeks. As he has not responded to initial treatment, the treating physician suspects brucellosis.
    1. What serologic tests can aid in the diagnosis of Brucellosis?
    2. What is the treatment for this?

122. A 45-year-old man admitted into your ICU was diagnosed to be hepatitis B positive during routine viral serology screening, done as a part of ICU admission policy.
    1. What tests would you do next?
    2. What precautionary measures would you take?

123. A 63-year-old male known case of retroviral disease on antiretroviral therapy (ART), presented with fever, chills, dry cough, and dyspnea on exertion. Auscultation revealed dry crackles in all areas. TLC is 4300/cc and Hb is 10 g/dL. Latest CD4 count is 300/L.

1. What is the organism you would like to confirm/rule out?
2. What is the ideal sample? What tests can be opted?
3. What are HIV indicator infections?

124. Following ileocecal anastomosis for perforation peritonitis, patient was admitted into surgical ICU with central line and urinary catheter *in situ*. On day 5 of ICU stay, while on broad-spectrum antibiotic coverage, a new onset high grade fever with chills was documented. Urine routine showed abundant yeast cells.
    1. What is the use of 1,3-beta D glucan in this case?
    2. What is *Candida* score?
    3. What is colonization index?

125. A 41-year-old otherwise healthy, farmer presented with fever severe headache and altered sensorium of 14-day duration. His blood workup revealed hemoglobin 13.3 g/dL and WBC count was 5,890/cumm. Cerebrospinal fluid showed 290 polymorphs and protein 79 mg/dL and low sugar. Negative staining done is shown in Figure.
    1. Name a test that will aid to confirm the diagnosis at the earliest.
    2. What additional workup would you do?
    3. What would be your preferred initial treatment for this patient?

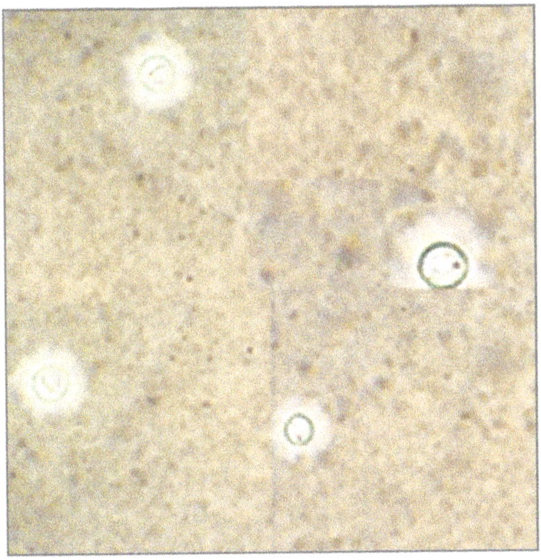

126. The peripheral blood culture sample of a patient in ICU has grown Candida glabrata after 24 hours of inoculation, although the central line culture is still negative. The laboratory has informed the same to you. Antifungal susceptibility report will be available only in another 24 hours.
    1. What would be your empirical antifungal?

127. A 43-year-old hypertensive male presents to the ICU with complaints of worsening dyspnea over the past 3 days which has been gradually increasing over the past 3 months. He was previously admitted for evaluation in the medical ward and was under evaluation for the same complaint. He has history of dry cough for the past 3 months and has an unintentional weight loss of 12 kg. In ICU, the vitals are pulse rate of 108 beats/min, regular, respiratory rate 28 breaths/min, blood pressure 130/86 mm Hg, and temperature of 99.8°F. Clinical examination is positive for diffuse crepitations and scattered wheezing across the chest.

- *Laboratory studies*: Hemoglobin 9.3 g/dL, WBC count 3,000/cumm, and a platelet count of 54,000 per mm^3, and ESR 65 mm/hour; other investigations were normal, and blood cultures reports are awaited.
- Chest X-ray taken is as shown in Figure. Based on the history of pets at home (doves), the infectious disease (ID) consultant suspects histoplasmosis.

1. What are the investigations of choice to confirm/rule out pulmonary histoplasmosis?
2. How would you manage the case?

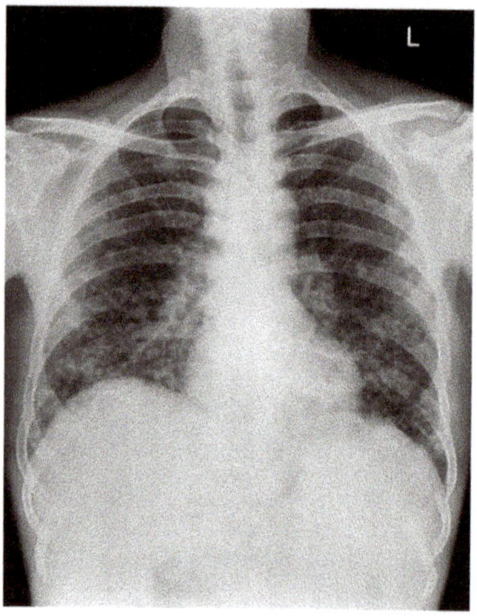

128. A 38-year-old female is admitted to the ICU with history of fever, difficulty in swallowing, hypersalivation, photophobia, dyspnea, and one episode of seizure of 1-day duration. There is history of a stray dog bite 5 weeks prior to onset of symptoms, which was ignored at that time.

1. What is your presumptive diagnosis? How will you confirm it in this case?
2. What is the recommended prophylaxis for the tending staff?
3. What is Milwaukee protocol?

129. Given is the sensitivity report of *Acinetobacter baumannii* isolated from urine of a patient in ICU.
Suggest three injectable antibiotics you will like to treat this patient with.

Organism: A. *baumannii*
Resistance mechanism: OXA-48

Antimicrobial	*Minimum inhibitory concentration (MIC)*	*Interpretation*
Gentamicin	>8	R
Ciprofloxacin	>2	R
Levofloxacin	>4	R
Ticarcillin clavulanate	>64	R
Piperacillin tazobactam	>64	R
Cefoperazone sulbactam	>32	R
Ceftazidime	>32	R
Cefepime	>32	R
Imipenem	>8	R
Meropenem	>8	R
Polymyxin B	≤0.5	S

(R: resistant; S: susceptible)

130. A 24-week-pregnant nurse working in ICU is caring for a sick patient in ICU. On examination, the patient is found to have lesions as in the image. After her duty shift, she has now reported to you for advice. What will be your advice for her?

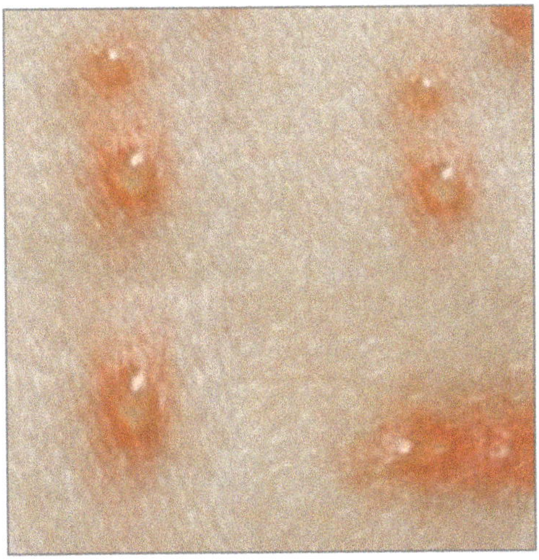

131. Attached is the sensitivity report of *Serratia marcescens* isolated from the sputum of a patient who presented with hemoptysis.
Name a few bacteria which are intrinsically resistant to colistin.

Sample Sputum
Organism: *S. marcescens*

Antimicrobial	*Interpretation*
Nitrofurantoin	S
Amikacin	S
Gentamicin	S
Ciprofloxacin	R
Ampicillin	R
Amoxicillin clavulanate	R
Piperacillin tazobactam	S
Cefoperazone sulbactam	S
Cefuroxime	R
Ceftriaxone	R
Cefepime	R
Imipenem	S
Meropenem	S
Colistin	R

(R: resistant; S: susceptible)

132. A resident doctor in the ICU sustains an accidental needlestick injury to his finger while trying to secure a central venous access. As the head of the ICU, what will be your advice to him as the immediate action? What are the indications for antiviral medications?

133. A 20-year-old male presented to the ICU in septic shock while on being treatment for an abscess in his leg that was reported as MRSA.
   1. What are the antibiotics with anti-MRSA activity?
   2. How would you manage this case?

134. A 23-year-old male presented to the ICU with high-grade fever and altered sensorium of 2-day duration. On admission into ICU, he was disoriented, hemodynamically stable, and had a fever of 40°C. Laboratory results show Hb 9.2 g/dL, TLC 4500/cc, CRP of 127, and lactate dehydrogenase of 278 U/L. Peripheral smear showed *Plasmodium falciparum* infected erythrocytes.
   1. How will you classify malaria?
   2. What are the methods of confirming the diagnosis of malaria?
   3. What is the treatment for severe malaria in ICU?

135. An 18-year-old boy was admitted into ICU with history of fever, headache, and one episode of seizure. Clinical examination revealed altered sensorium and neck stiffness. A lumbar puncture was done and the CSF showed WBC count of 1,120/cumm. Gram's stain and India ink stain were negative. Despite starting steroids, meningitis dose of meropenem and vancomycin, the boy continued to worsen in sensorium and fever. The family members gave history of the boy having gone for swimming lessons at a local pond a week earlier.
   1. What will the differential diagnosis be now?
   2. What test would you specifically ask for, to aid the diagnosis?

136. A 35-year-old female presented with fever, headache, muscular pain, and extensive petechial rash of 2 days duration. On examination, the system examinations were unrewarding. Laboratories revealed a total count of 10,000/cumm and 70% polymorphs, Hb of 14 mg/dL, and platelets of 80000/cc. Peripheral smear for malaria was negative.
   1. What could be the possible diagnosis?
   2. What are the differentials?

137. A 22-year-old man, presented with fever, headache, and loss of appetite of 4 days duration. At the time of presentation to ICU, he was found to be delirious with a temperature of 101°F, BP 88/46 mm Hg, and heart rate 82 beats/min. His friends gave history having gone on a trekking trip 2 weeks prior to onset of symptoms. Clinical examination of the extremities revealed a lesion as shown in Figure.
   1. Which test would you choose to confirm the clinical diagnosis?

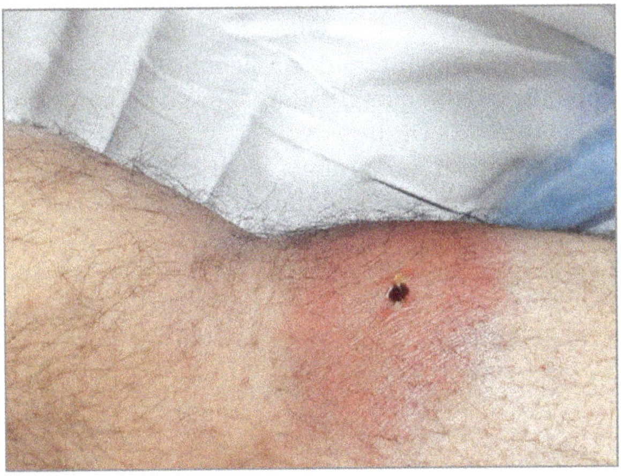

138. A 36-year-old male, admitted to the ICU as a case of trauma with diffuse axonal injury currently is running high-grade fever, increased secretions via tracheostomy tube which have changed in consistency, and also has increased oxygen requirements. Blood culture sent on the day of initial fever spike has grown *P. aeruginosa*.
   Enumerate the beta-lactams that have anti-*Pseudomonas* action.

139. A 45-year-old male, a known case of hypertensive, end-stage renal failure, postrenal transplant 3 months prior is now admitted to the ICU with severe, abdominal pain, nausea, vomiting, diarrhea, and breathing difficulty. He was admitted with pneumonia for the past 10 days in the hospital but has not responded to empiric treatment. A CT scan taken shows diffuse ground glassing in both lungs. The nephrologist is concerned for CMV infection as the kidney donor was seropositive for CMV.
    1. What are the methods of diagnosing/ruling out CMV in this situation?
    2. Give the treatment strategy.

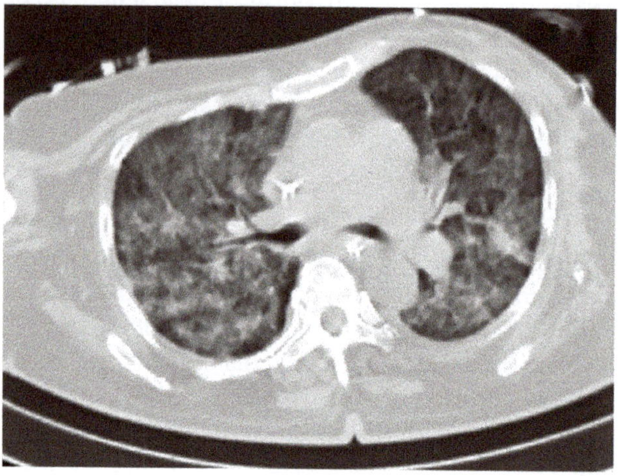

140. A 36-year-old male patient with short bowel syndrome, on total parenteral nutrition with lipid supplements, developed septic shock during his hospital stay. Blood culture showed budding yeast cells, which grew on Sabouraud's Dextrose Agar.
    1. What is the probable causative agent?
    2. What will your empiric antifungal be?

141. • How will you classify beta-lactamases?
    • How will you test for synergistic effect versus additive effect in the microbiology lab?

142. Blood culture of a patient admitted with VAP and CRBSI is given in image. What are the various resistance mechanism for gram negative bacteria?
Organism: *Acinetobacter baumanii*
Resistance mechanism: OXA-48

Antimicrobial	*MIC*	*Interpretation*
Gentamicin	>8	R
Ciprofloxacin	>2	R
Levofloxacin	>4	R
Ticarcillin clavulanate	>64	R
Piperacillin tazobactam	>64	R
Cefoperazone sulbactam	>32	R
Ceftazidime	>32	R
Cefepime	>32	R
Imipenem	>8	R
Meropenem	>8	R
Polymyxin B	≤0.5	S

143. • What are the precautions healthcare personnel should take for needle stick injury? How will you dispose needles after usage?
• What are the mandatory vaccination for healthcare professionals to avoid infections?

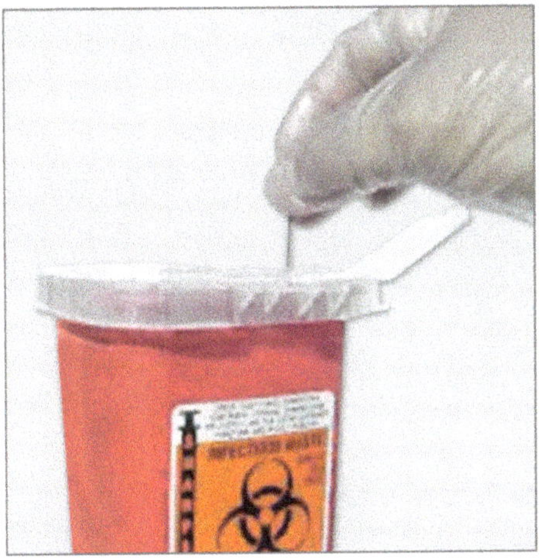

144. A patient in day 7 of ICU has developed diarrhea. Clinical features are suggestive *of C. difficile* bacteria.
   1. Which agent should be used for washing hands after care for this patient?
   2. Define an outbreak of Clostridium infection in ICU.

145. Hand washing is an important precaution to prevent hospital-acquired infections.
   1. What are the common antimicrobial agents used for hand washing?

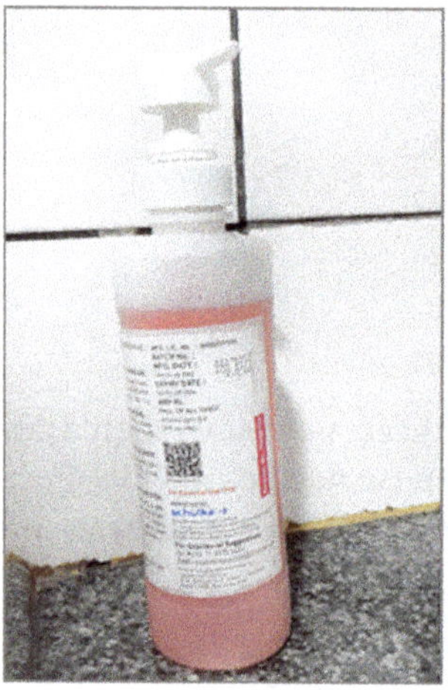

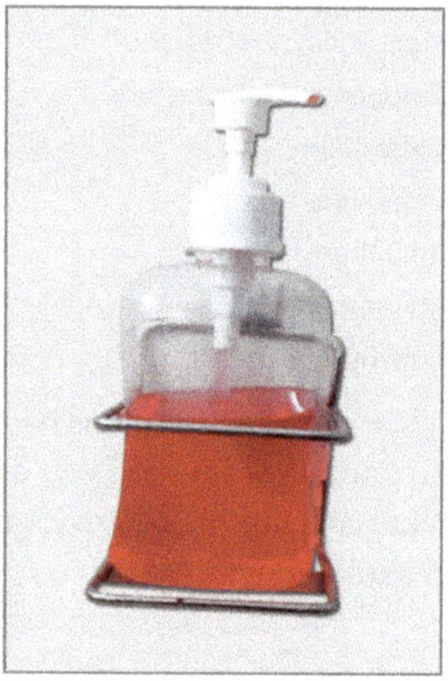

146. 1. Identify the device.
   2. Describe various types of isolation.

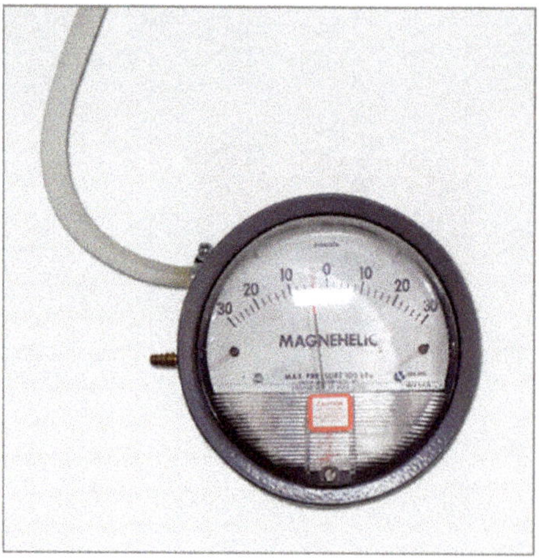

147. 1. Identify the device.
  2. What are the initial steps taken if encountered with eye splash injury at ICU?

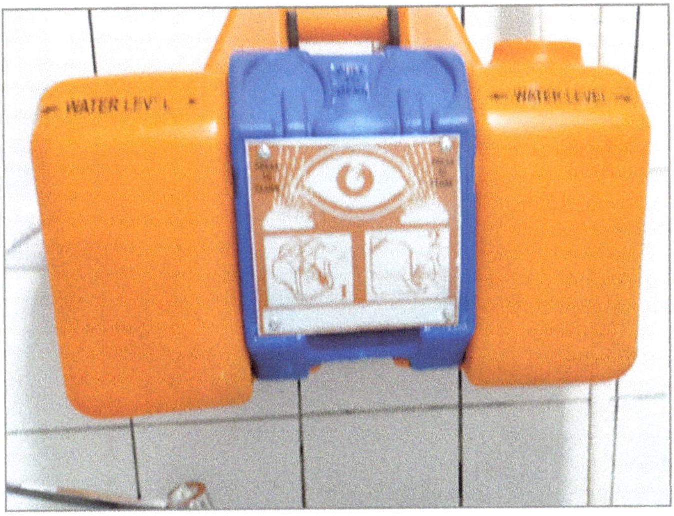

148. 1. What is a biomedical waste (BMW)?
  2. What are the principles of good BMW management?\

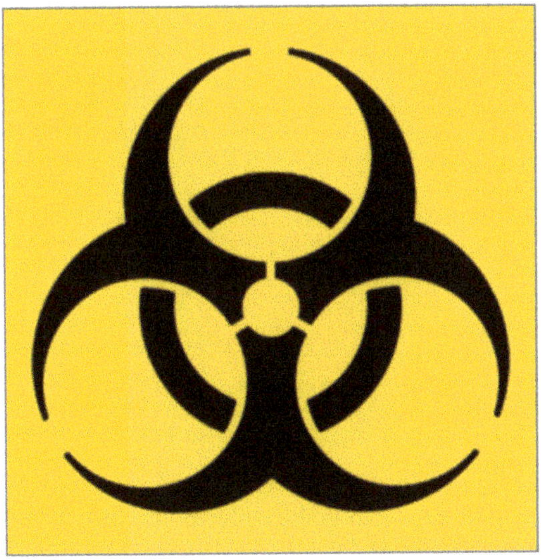

149. 1. Which is the most common scenario in which sodium hypochlorite 1% solution is used?
   2. How long should we wait after this solution is used, before proceeding to next step?

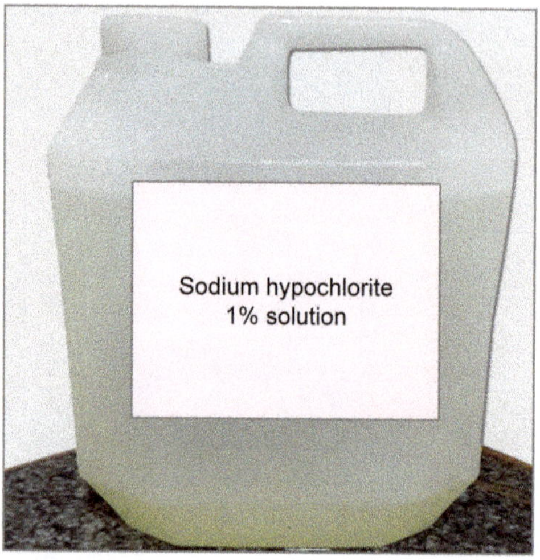

150. 1. Discuss the five moments of hand wash.
   2. Define disinfectant and describe their types.

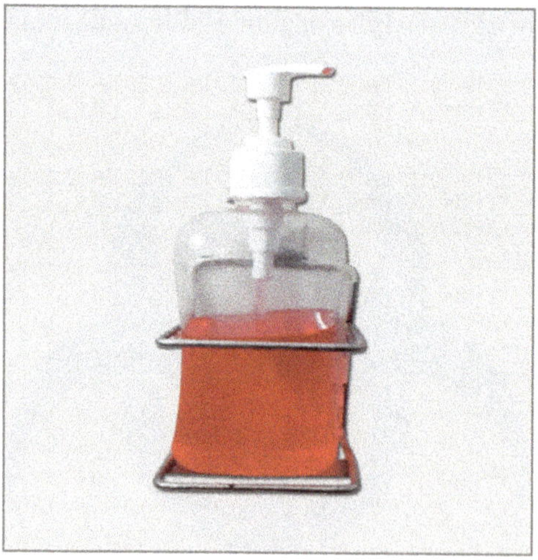

151. What is the sensitivity of blood culture for bacteremia and candidemia?
   - How much blood should be collected for blood culture in a patient with suspected blood stream infection?
   - What is the rate of culture positivity with one-paired sample, two-paired samples, and three-paired samples?

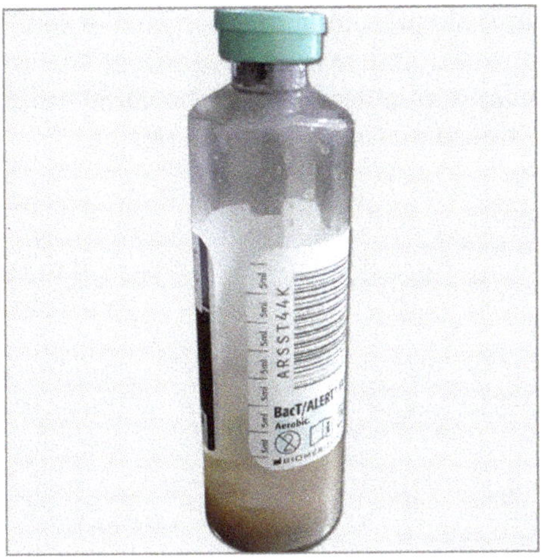

152. A 72-year-old female, a case of well-controlled diabetes mellitus, presents to the ER with fever, cough, and shortness of breath of 1-day duration, while returning from Hajj pilgrimage. A diagnosis of MERS CoV ARDS is made and patient is intubated and ventilated.
   - What type of isolation precaution needs to be taken for this patient?
   - In what order does the PPE need to be removed?

HEMODYNAMICS

153. A 74-year-old male presented to emergency room (ER) with syncope. Patient is confused and sweating is present. His pulse rate (PR) was 55 beats/min and irregular, and BP was 80/60 mm Hg. ECG is shown. What is the diagnosis and management?

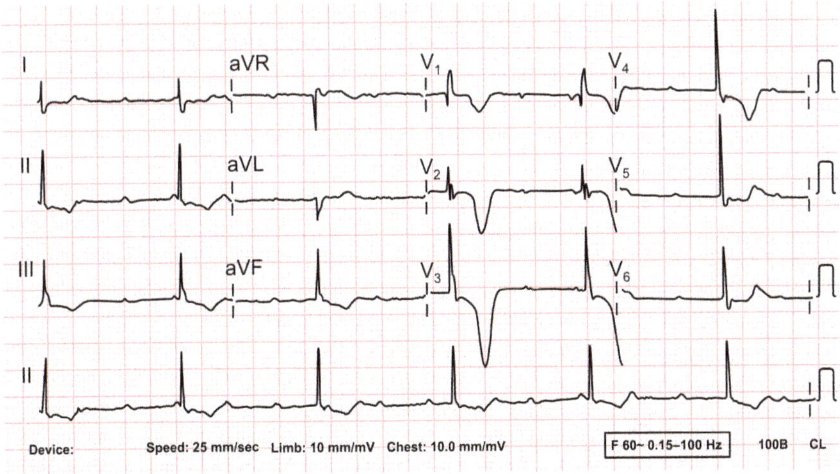

154. A 74-year-old male presented to emergency room (ER) with syncope. Patient is confused and sweating is present. His pulse rate (PR) was 55 beats/min and irregular, and BP was 80/60 mm Hg. ECG is shown. Name a few indications for permanent pacing.

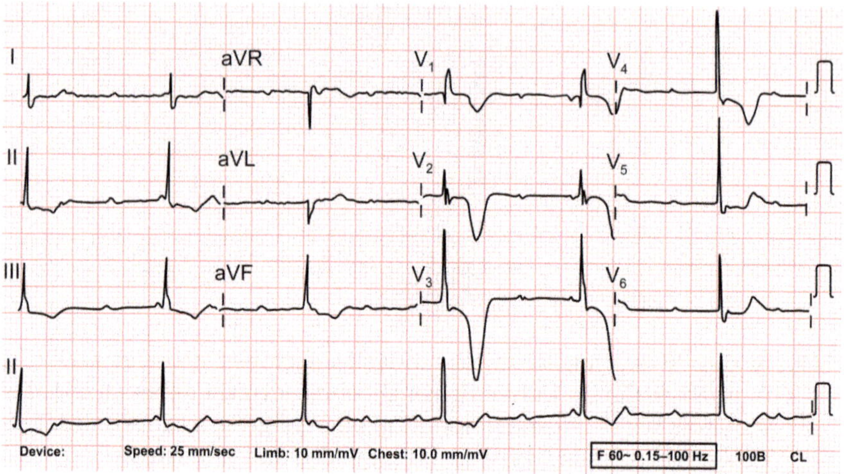

155. A 65-year-old male with diabetes mellitus (DM), hypertension (HTN), atrial fibrillation (A. fib) on digoxin, and chronic kidney disease is admitted to the ICU with nausea, vomiting and and giddiness.
   1. Comment on the ECG.

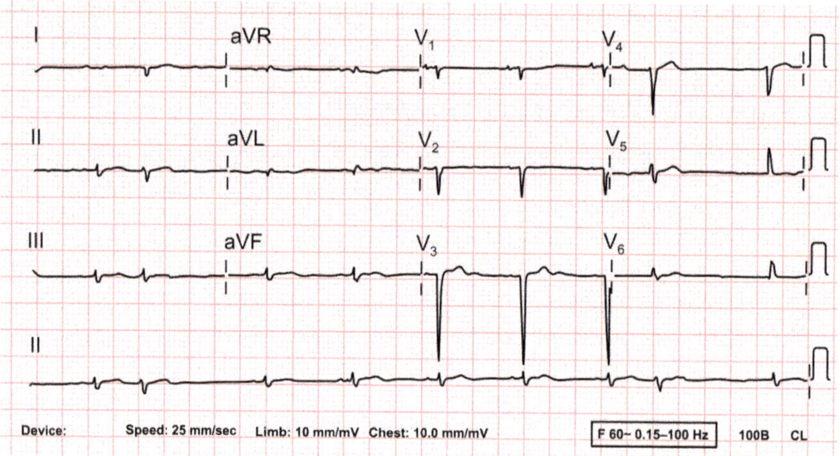

156. A 76-year-old female presented with acute onset chest pain of 4 hours duration. ECG is shown.
    1. Comment on the possible culprit artery

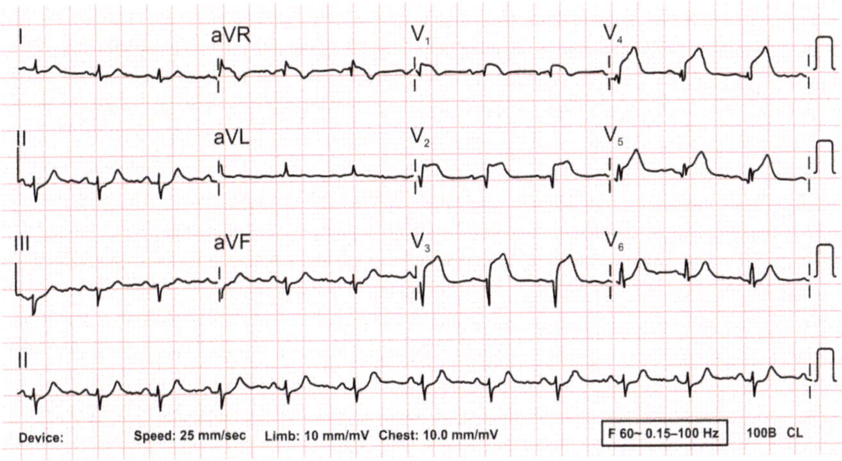

157. A 76-year-old female, diabetic (on treatment) presented with acute onset chest pain of 24 hours duration. ECG is shown. She is hemodynamically stable.
    1. How will you manage the patient?

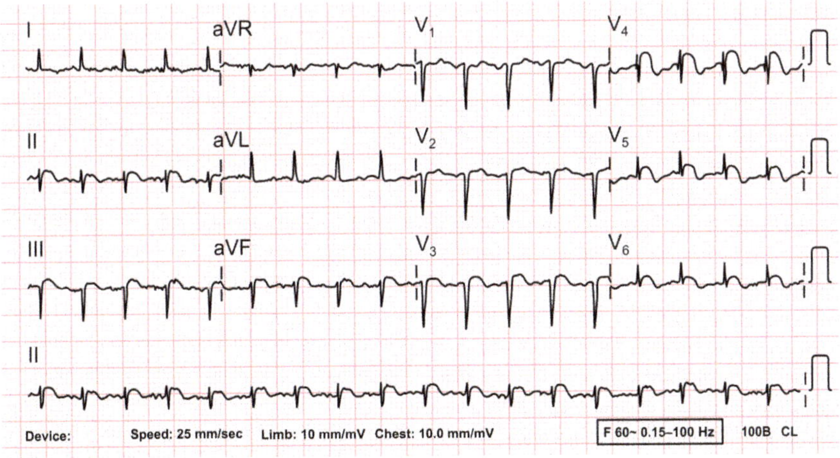

158. A 76-year-old female presented with acute onset chest pain of 4 hours duration. ECG taken is as shown.
    1. How will you manage the patient?

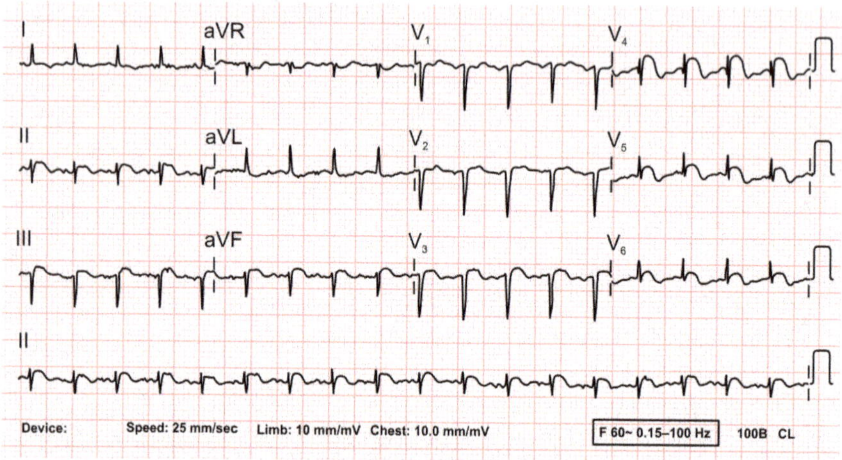

159. ECG of a patient presented with persisting chest pain 6 hours after thrombolysis with streptokinase.
    1. What are the indications for PCI after thrombolysis?

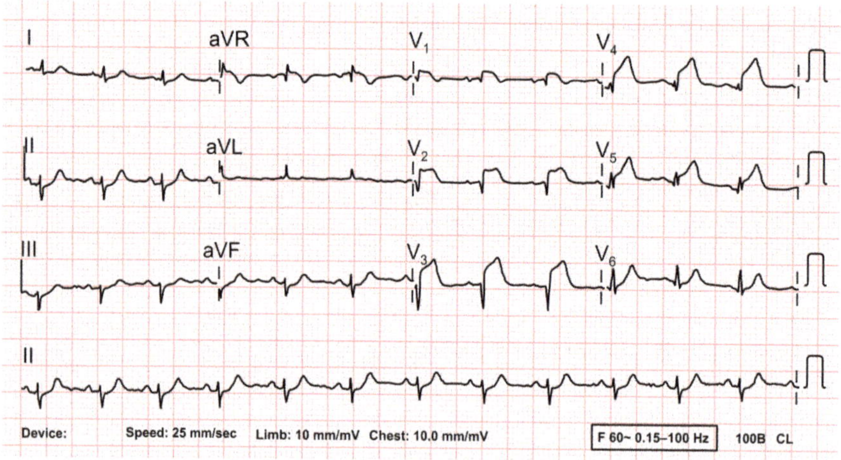

160. Comment on the ECG given in image below. What are the causes of right bundle branch block in ECG?

1. What are the causes of right bundle branch block (RBBB) in ECG?

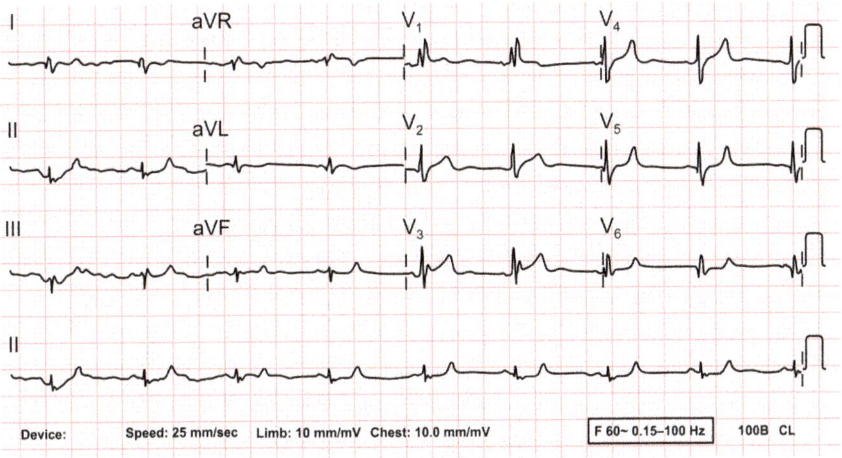

161. How will you determine axis of the heart on ECG.

1. How will you determine axis of the heart on ECG?

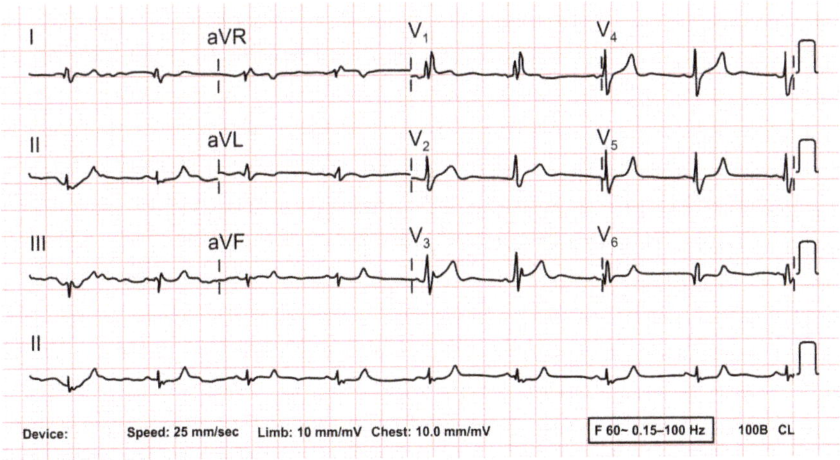

162. 1. What are the acute measures to be undertaken for a patient presenting to the ER and having an ECG as shown in image?
2. How will you manage the patient if he is on digoxin?

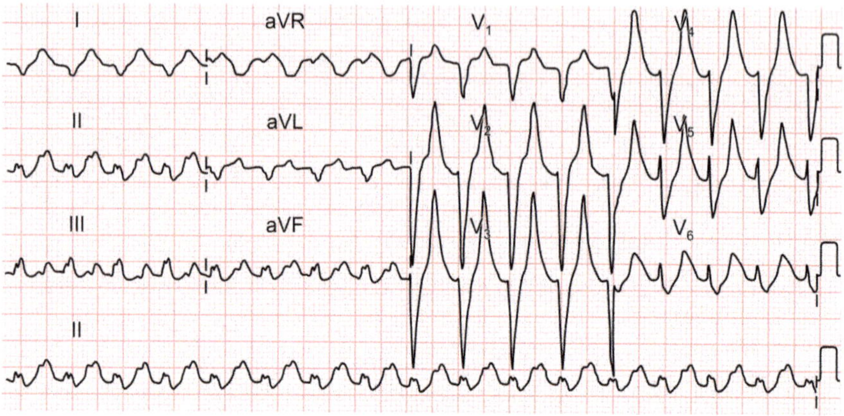

163. What are the ECG changes seen in hypokalemia and hyperkalemia?

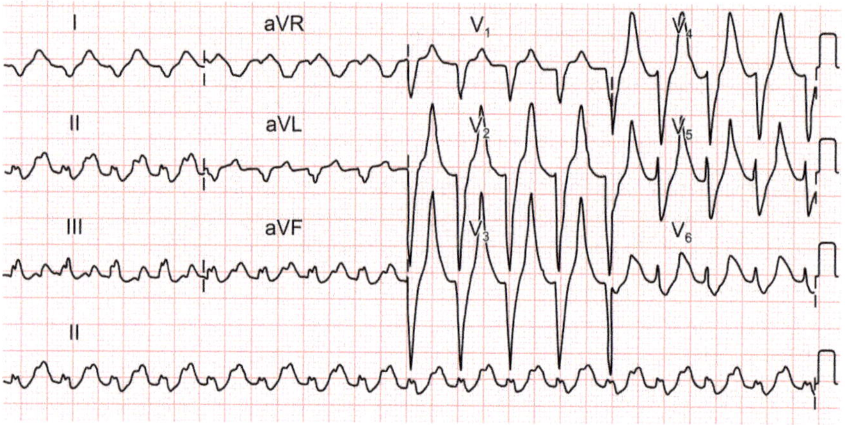

164. What is the diagnosis and management of a patient presenting with palpitations to ER.

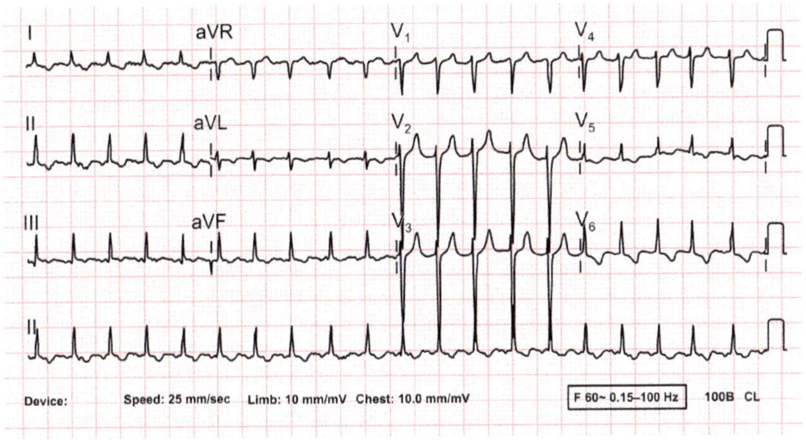

165. Describe the types of supraventricular tachycardia.

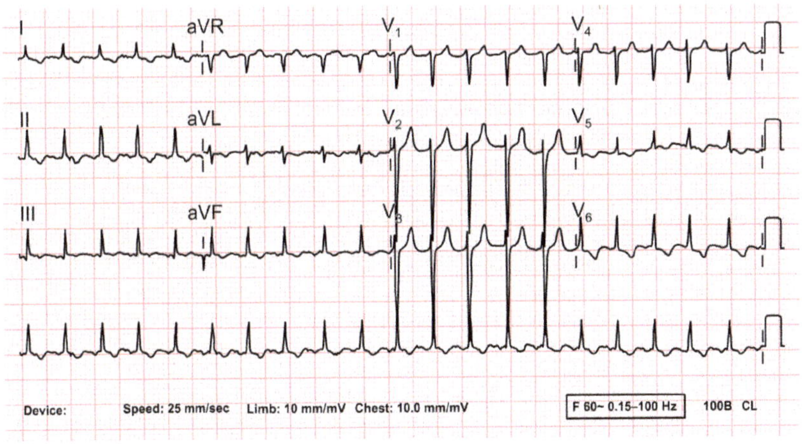

166. Name a few drugs causing this condition.

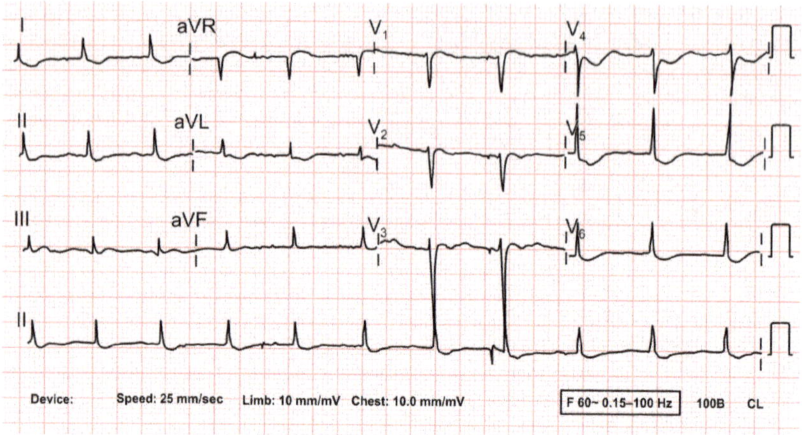

167. What are the causes of broad complex QRS and management?

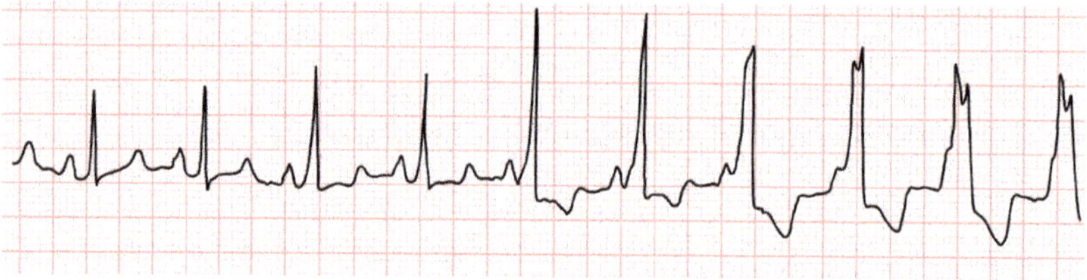

168. A 76-year-old female who was hypertensive and on nebivolol presented to ER with giddiness and one episode of syncope.

1. What are the diagnosis and management?

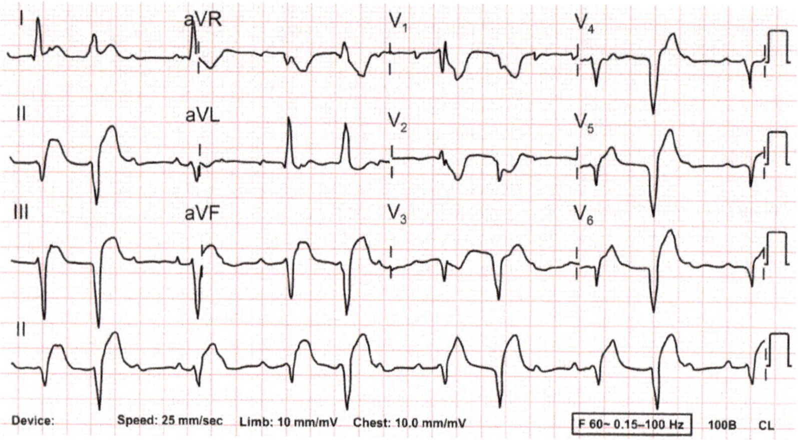

169. 1. Comment on the given ECG.
2. Identify the type of pacing applied.

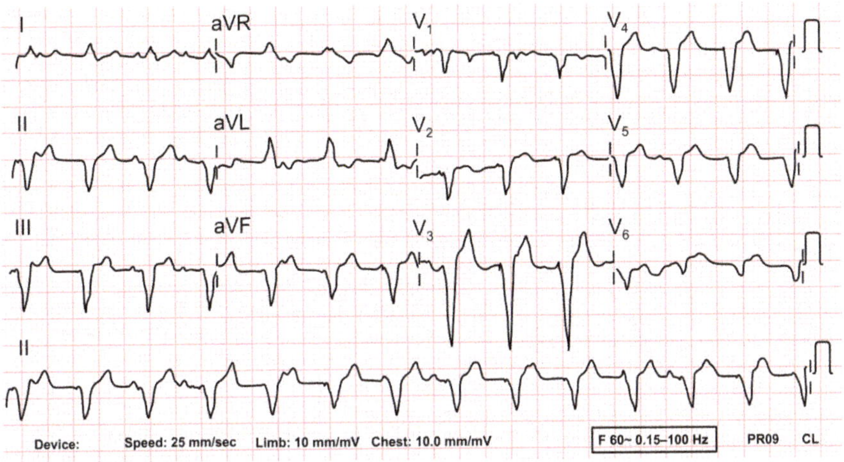

170. A 65-year-old male presented to ER with complaints of giddiness. His pulse rate was 156 beats/min and BP was 70/40 mm Hg and appears confused. ECG is shown.
1. How will you manage the patient?

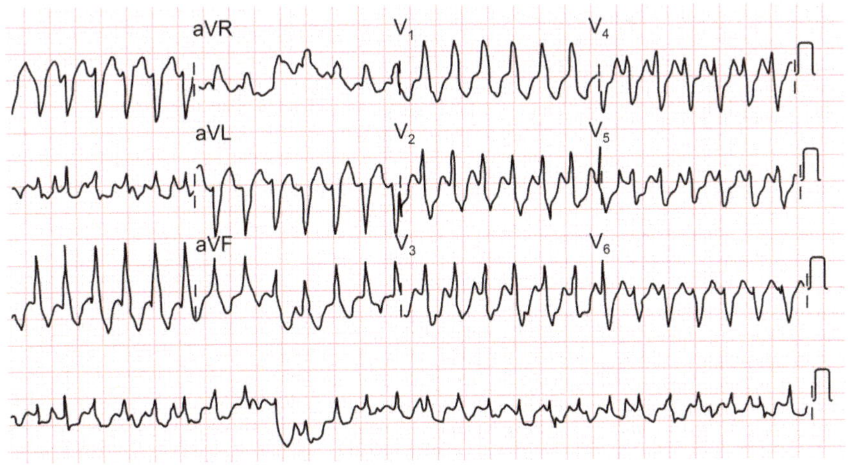

171. A 65-year-old male, known case of coronary artery disease (CAD) presented to emergency room (ER) and collapsed shortly. Vitals are not recordable. ECG is shown.

1. How will you manage the patient?

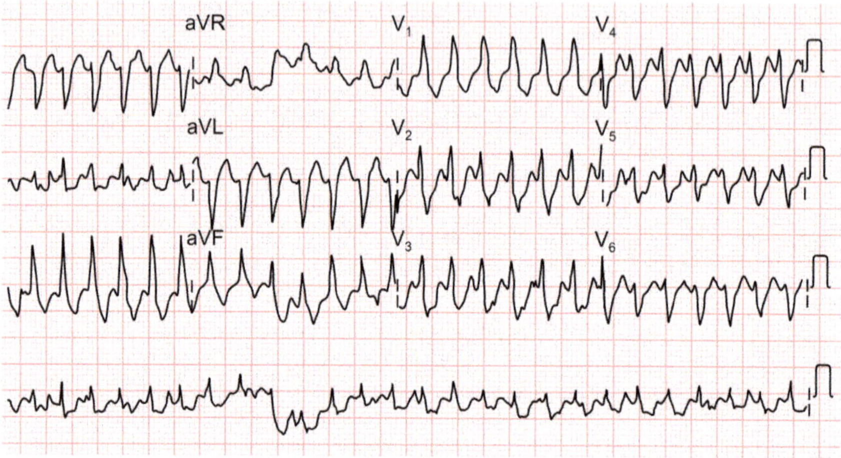

172. What is the diagnosis based on ECG?

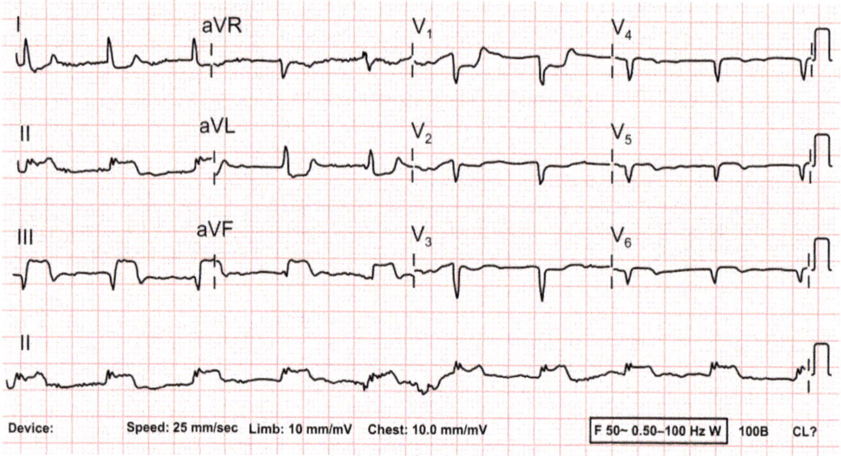

173. What is the diagnosis based on ECG?

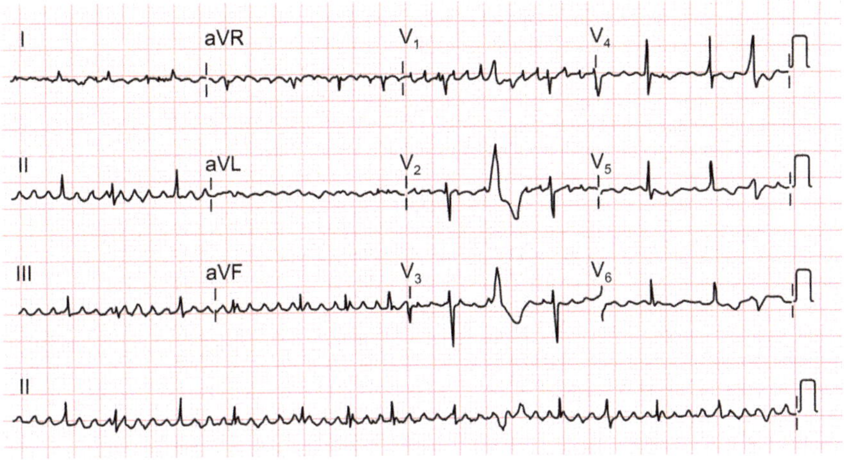

174. What is the ECG abnormality and enumerate a few conditions causing this?

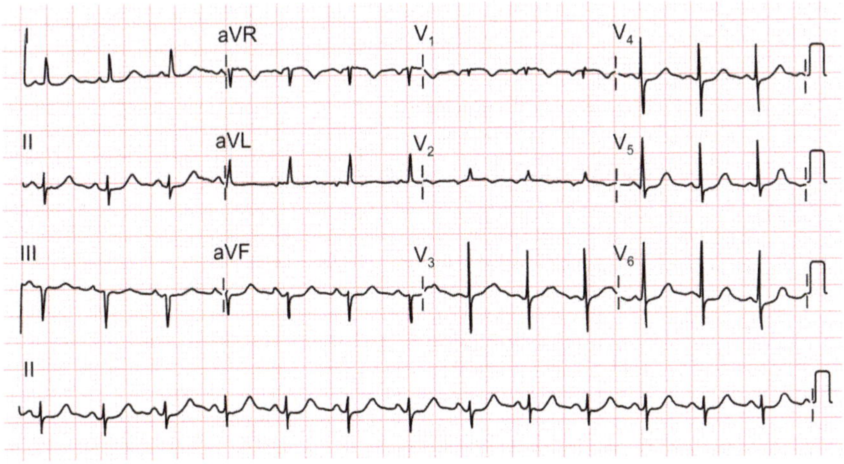

175. 1. Describe the catheter and its parts.
2. What is the principle of cardiac output monitoring with pulmonary artery (PA) catheter?
3. What are the values obtained from this?

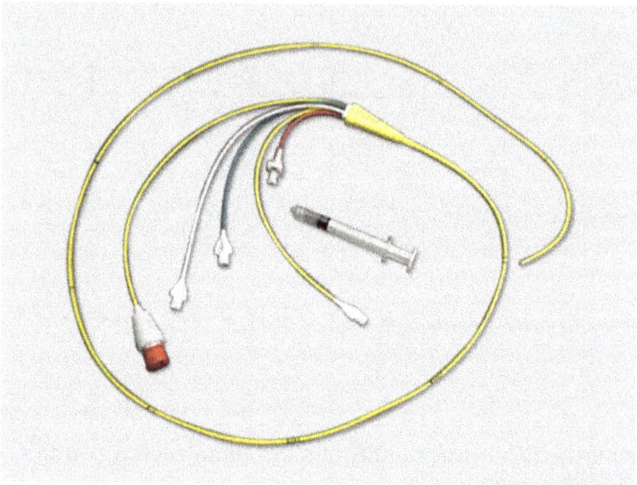

176. 1. What is the relation between central venous oxygen saturation ($ScVO_2$) and mixed venous oxygen saturation (SVO_2) in normal and disease states?
2. What is the normal relation between pulmonary artery diastolic pressure (PADP) and pulmonary artery occlusion pressure (PAOP)?
3. How is cardiac output measured with this?

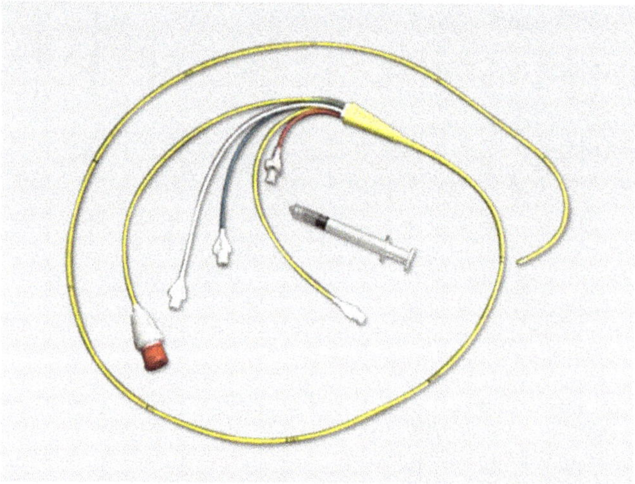

177. 1. What is the current evidence regarding use of PA catheter in intensive care unit (ICU)?
2. Enumerate the complications associated with PA catheter.

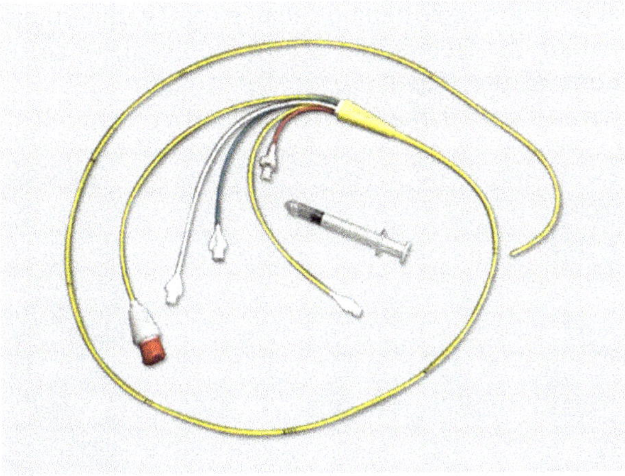

178. 1. What are the zones of west?
2. How will you identify a correctly wedged PA catheter?

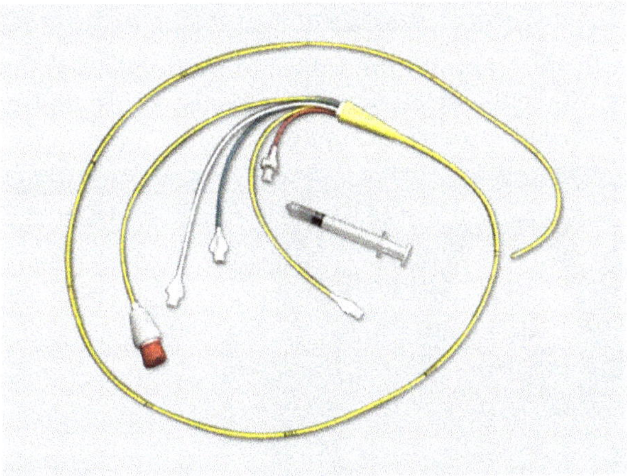

179. List a few absolute indications for PA catheter in ICU.

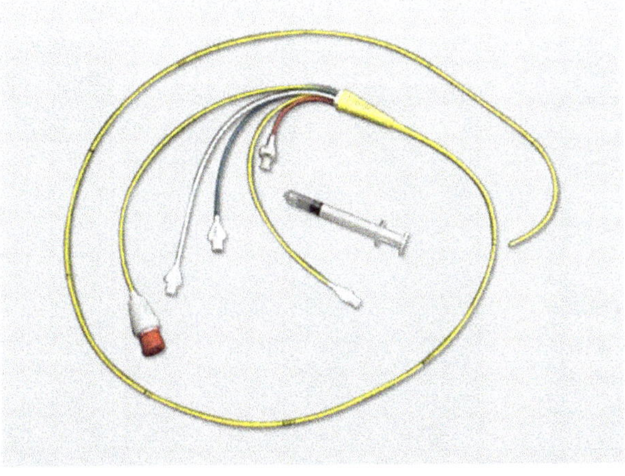

180. 1. What is the principle behind calculation of cardiac output?
  2. What are the factors that determine the slope and shape of the thermodilution curve?
  3. What are the limitations of transpulmonary thermodilution (TPTD)?

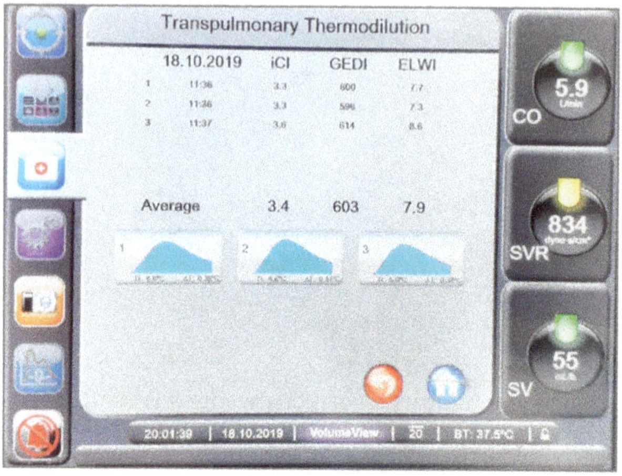

181. How will you interpret the values of thermodilution obtained in a patient with septic shock, increasing fraction of inspired oxygen (FiO_2), and increasing vasopressor supports?

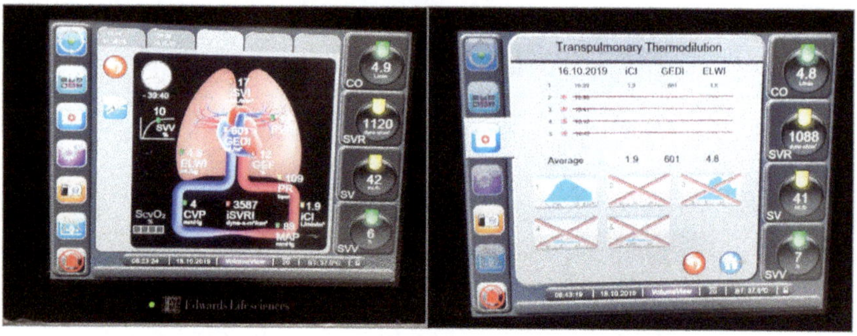

182. How will you explain the mechanism of pulmonary edema in the patient whose transpulmonary thermodilution data is shown?

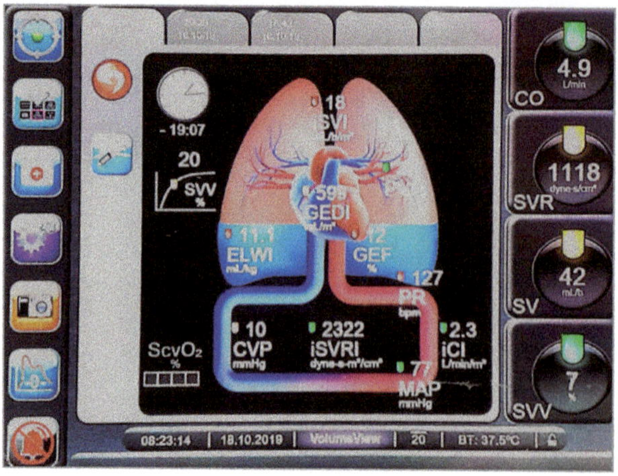

183. • What is the principle behind calculation of cardiac output?
- How will you assess fluid responsiveness using this monitor?
- Compare this with thermodilution-based cardiac output monitors. Mention the limitation of shown monitor.

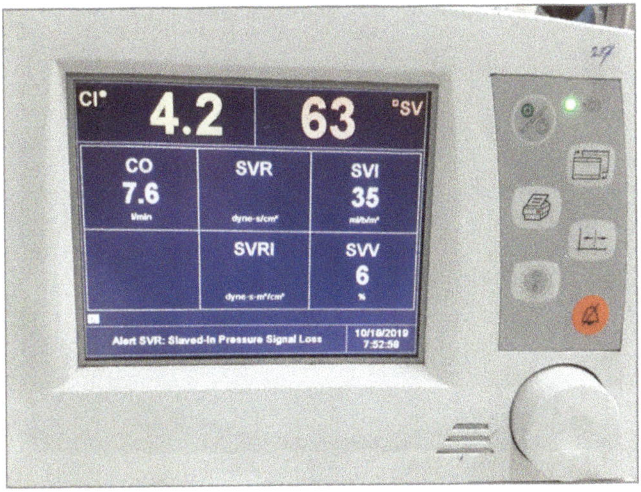

184. Explain the change in SVV 20 to 7. Give the possible explanations.

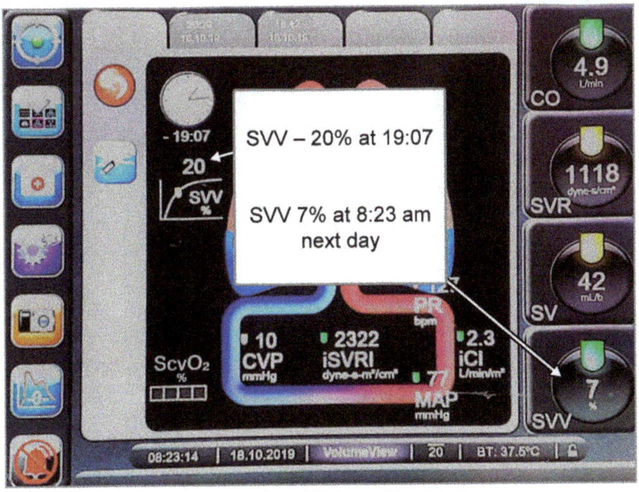

185. A 68-year-old male, diabetic, hypertensive, atrial fibrillation on treatment and coronary artery disease, presented with right-sided weakness of 12-hour duration and hypotension. Comment on the subcoastal view shown in the image.

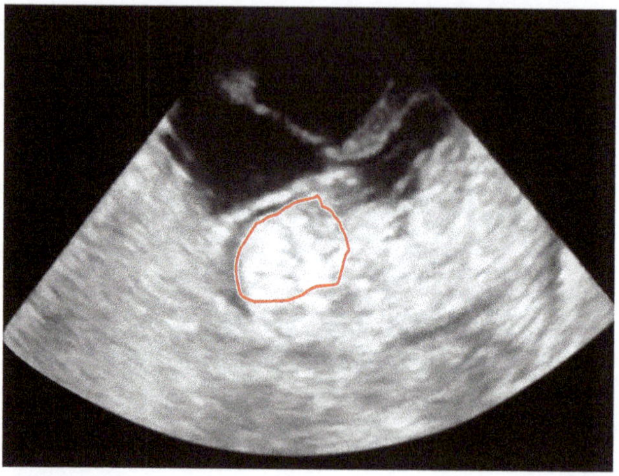

186. 1. Identify the view.
2. Identify the abnormalities seen.

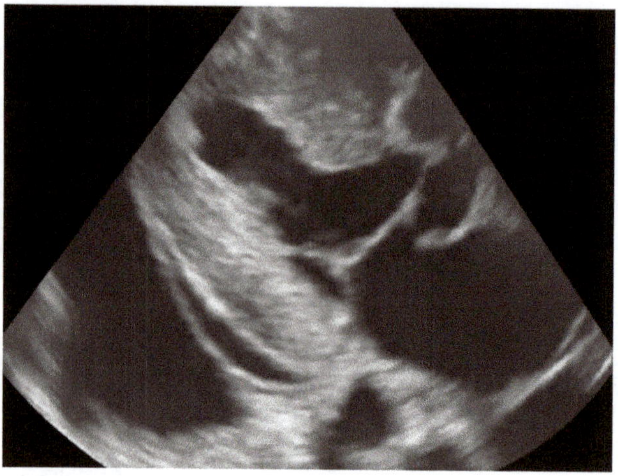

187. A 36-year-old female, presented to ER in cardiac arrest.
    1. Identify the view and abnormalities seen.

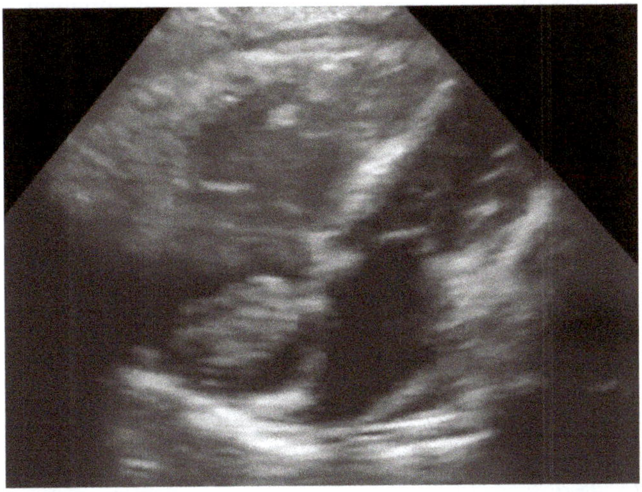

188. What is the management of a patient presenting with cardiac arrest due to pulmonary embolism?

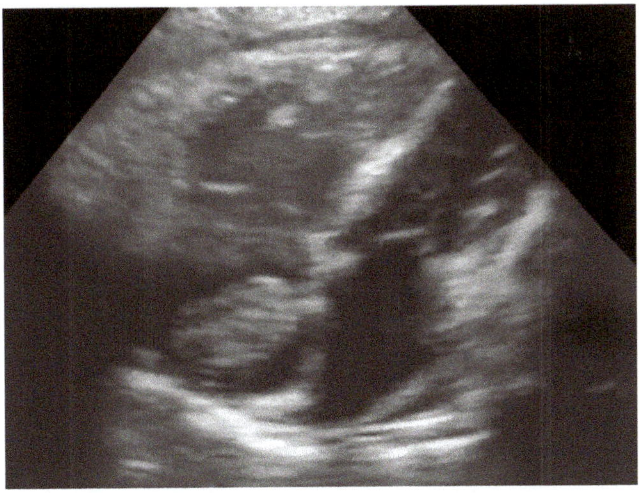

189. 1. What are the dosing regimens for thrombolysis in pulmonary embolism?
2. What is the current evidence for low-dose thrombolysis in ICU?

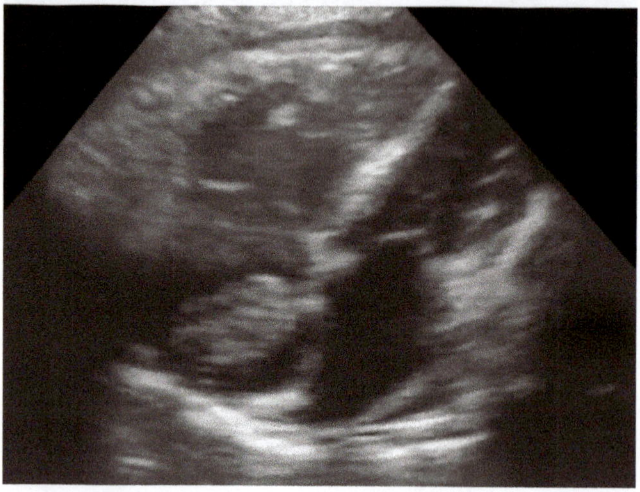

190. 1. Comment on the computed tomography (CT) image shown.
2. What are the treatment options for this patient, if the patient is with stable hemodynamics?

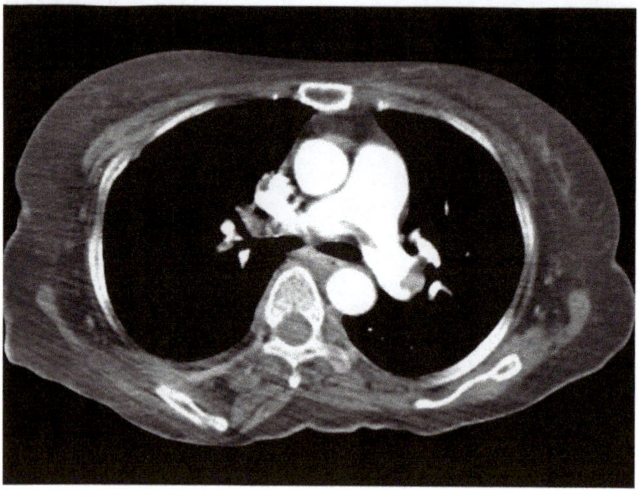

191. What is the investigation of choice in a pregnant female coming with suspicion of pulmonary embolism?

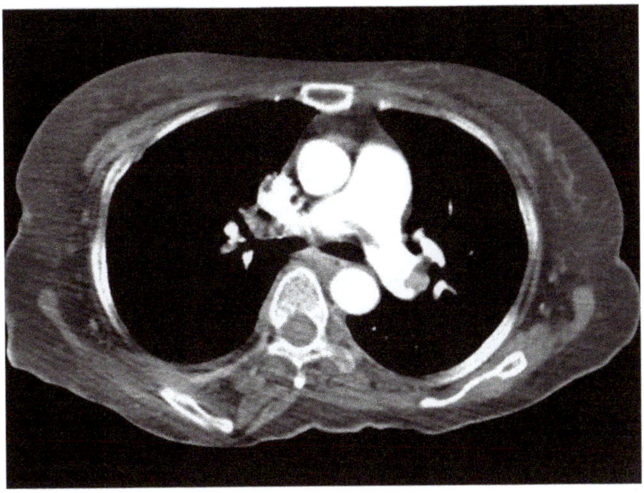

192. 1. Comment on the arterial line tracing.
   2. What test will you use to confirm the finding?
   3. What are the most common causes for this waveform in the ICU?

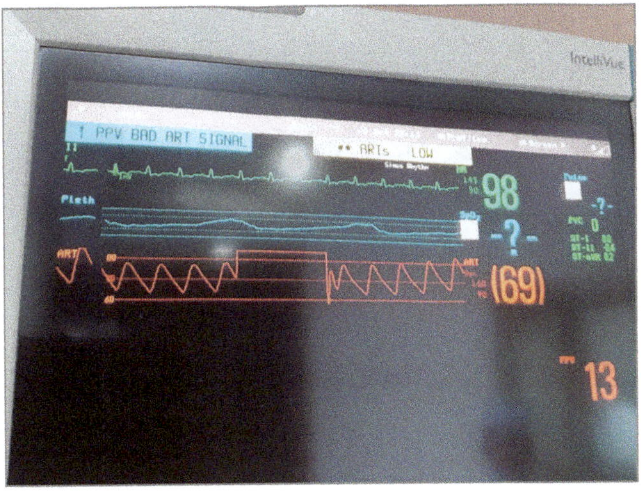

193. 1. What is stroke volume variation (SVV)?
    2. What are the conditions where SVV becomes unreliable?

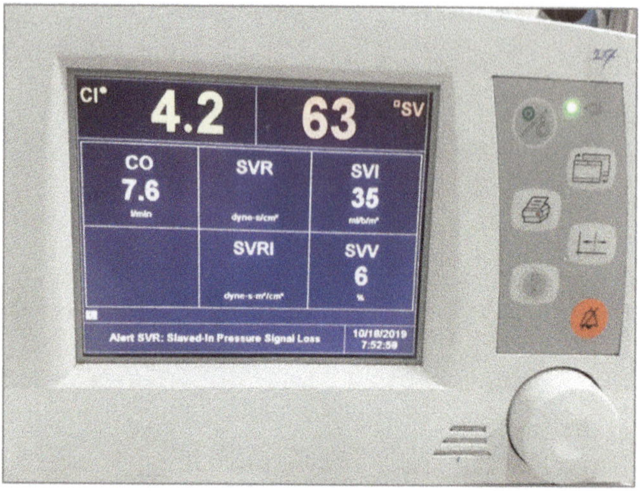

194. Identify the image and its uses in ICU.

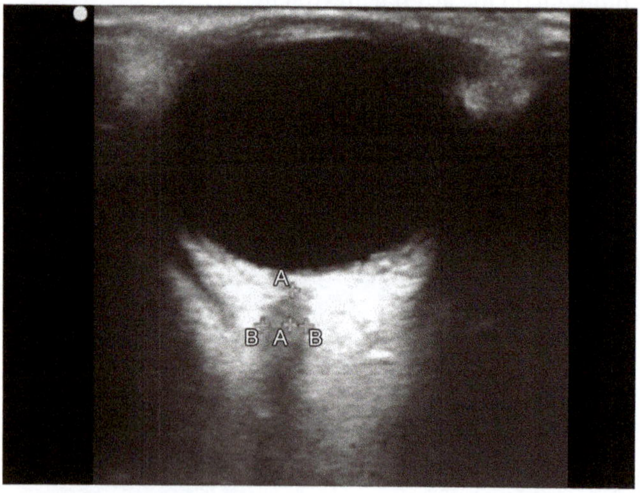

195.

1. Identify the device.
2. What is the current evidence and recommendation for use in ICU?
3. What are the absolute contraindications for use in ICU?

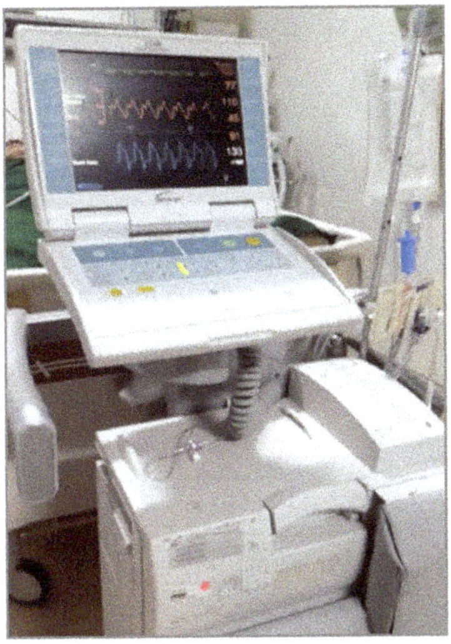

196.

1. What is the ideal location for tip of intra-aortic balloon pump (IABP) balloon?
2. What is the significance of monitoring urine output in a patient on IABP?

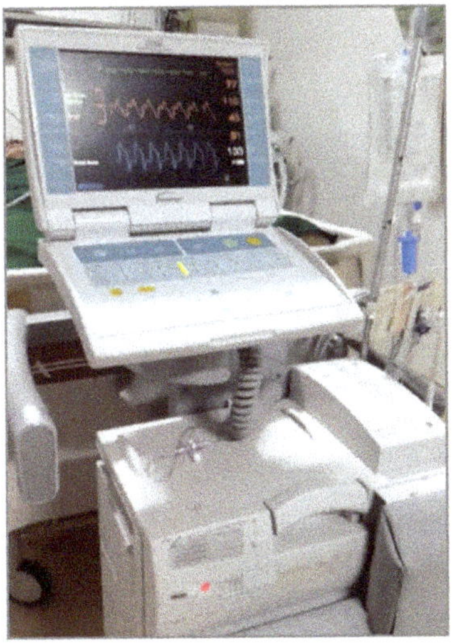

197. Comment on the IABP graph given below.

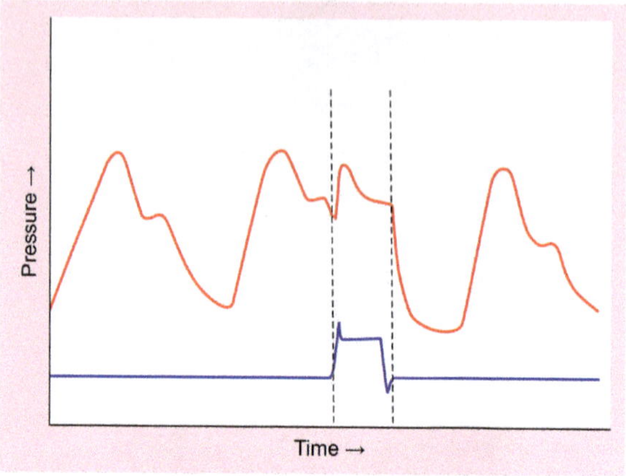

198. Comment on the IABP graph given below.

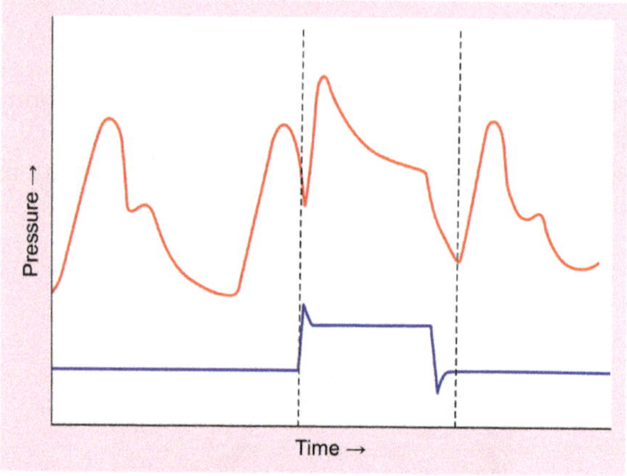

199. Comment on the IABP graph given below.

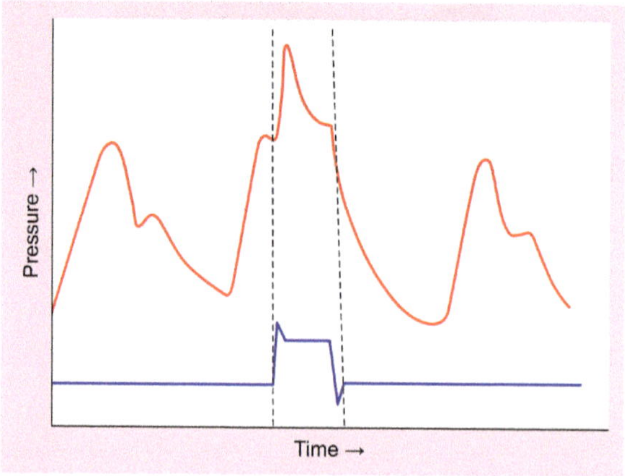

200. Comment on the IABP graph given below.

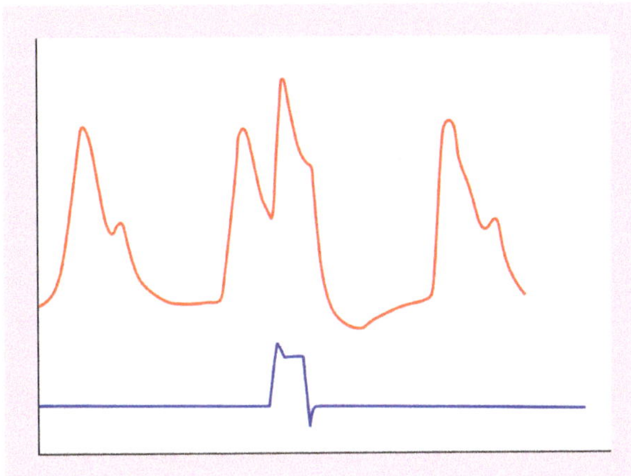

201. 1. Identify the image.
2. What do you understand when the images are described in the following? Expand the terms.
    - PPV%
    - MFI
    - hPPV%

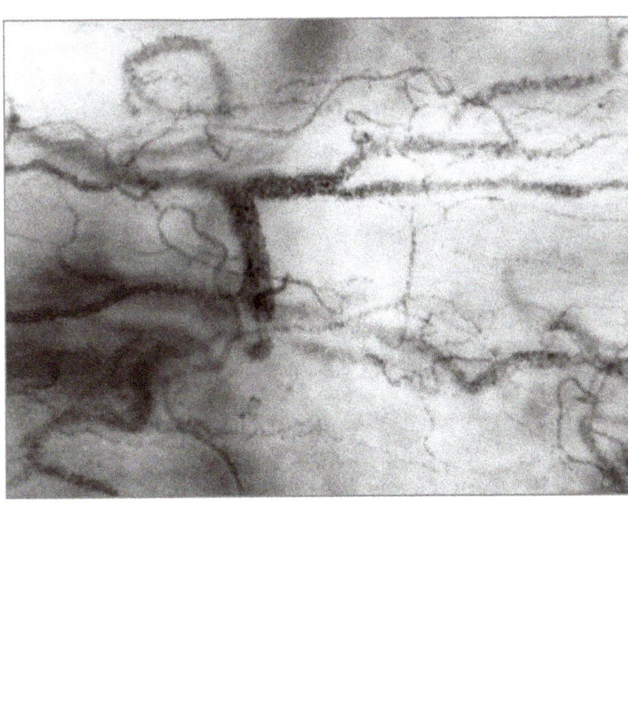

202. 1. Identify the device.
2. What is it used for?

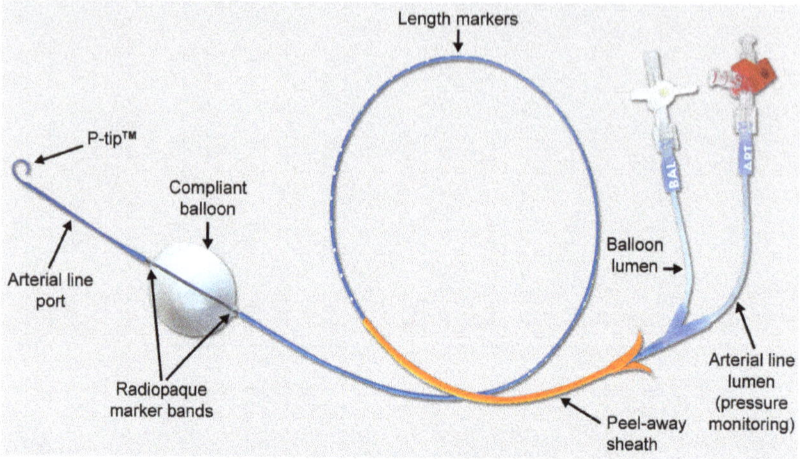

203. 1. Identify the procedure being attempted in this image.
2. Enumerate the indications and contraindications for its use.

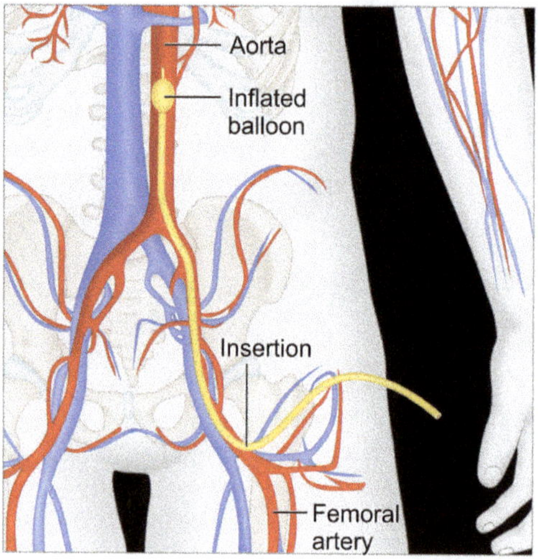

204. A 50-year-old patient is a known case of (k/c/o) diabetes mellitus (DM), hypertension (HTN) with left leg cellulitis and septic shock is intubated and is on mechanical ventilation. Echocardiogram (echo) is done which is shown in the Figure below. What is the current evidence for use of this echo parameter in intensive care unit (ICU).

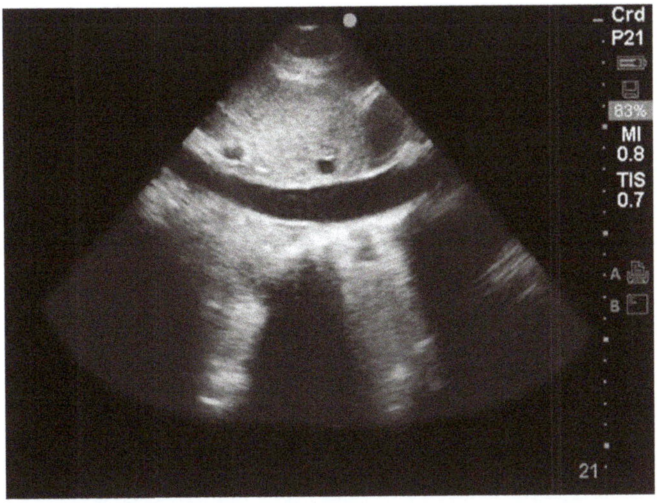

205. A 65-year-old diabetic patient is admitted to the ICU, with diagnosis of left thigh necrotizing fasciitis; she is on infusion of noradrenaline of 0.05 μg/kg/h and her arterial line shows a mean arterial pressure (MAP) of 55 mm Hg. She is on invasive ventilation. A passive leg raising (PLR) test was done along with a recording of transthoracic echo to assess for fluid responsiveness. The Figure is shown below. Identify the Figure and what parameter is being recorded. What is utility of measurement of this parameter in the critically ill along with PLR maneuver?

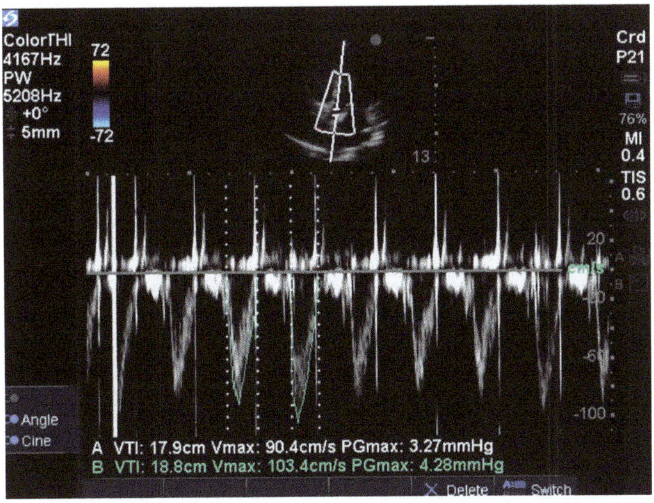

206. A 54-year-old patient, a known case of (k/c/o) DM, HTN, and chronic kidney disease on regular dialysis was admitted to the ICU with complaints of breathlessness for past 2 days. There was no history of (h/o) fever. Her last dialysis was on the day of admission to ICU. On admission to ICU, she was breathless with peripheral capillary oxygen saturation (SpO_2) of 88% on 10 L O_2. BP was 210/90 mm Hg. She was initiated on noninvasive ventilation (NIV) and an echocardiographic recording was done and a finding was measured. Identify the same and enumerate its uses in ICU.

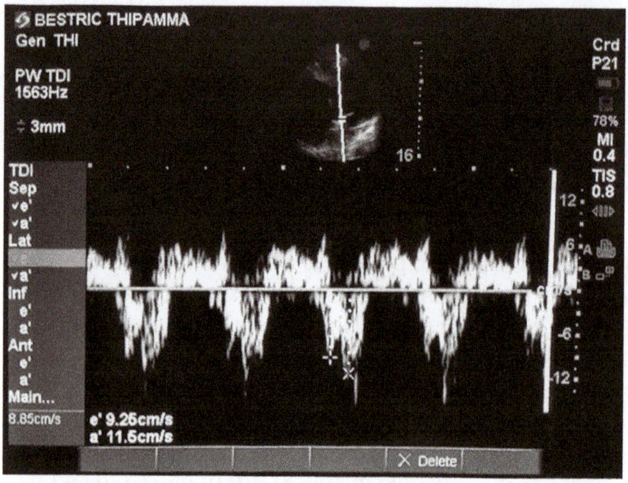

207. What assessment is being done in the echo? What is the utility of this measurement in ICU?

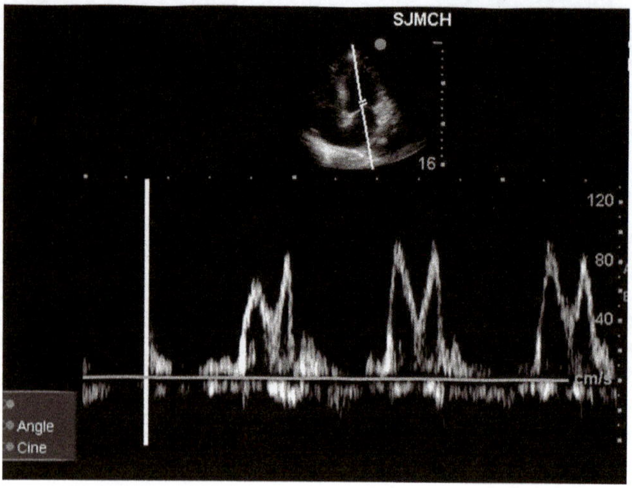

208. A 30-year-old patient presented with history of fever for 2 months and breathlessness for past 5 days and was admitted to ICU. He was breathless and required invasive ventilation. An echo was performed, which is shown in the Figure below. Identify the abnormality and further management of the patient in the ICU.

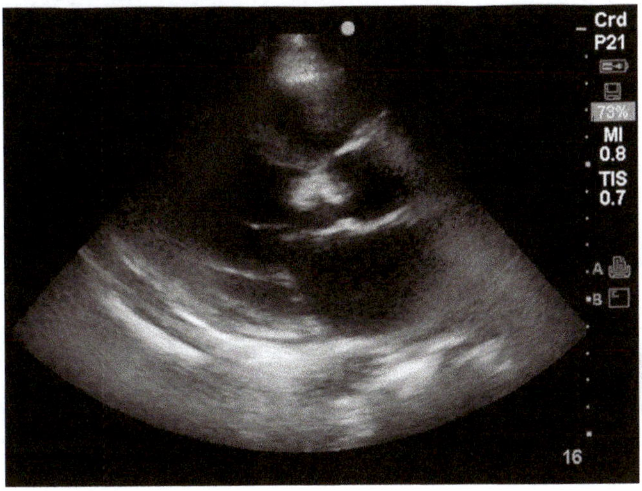

209. A 30-year-old patient had severe traumatic brain injury and was admitted to the ICU 12 days back. He had sudden onset breathlessness and hypotension and an echo assessment was done. What measurement is being done? Enumerate its uses in ICU.

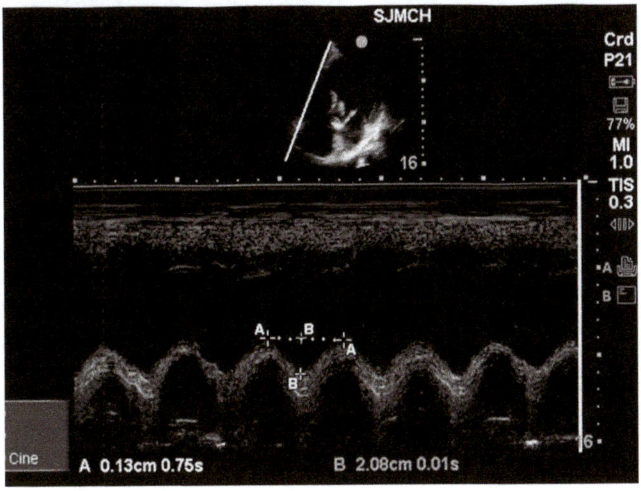

210. A 50-year-old chronic obstructive pulmonary disease (COPD) patient admitted to the ICU with history of breathlessness was intubated and initiated on invasive ventilation. On echo assessment, he had right ventricular dilation. Identify the Figure and its uses in ICU.

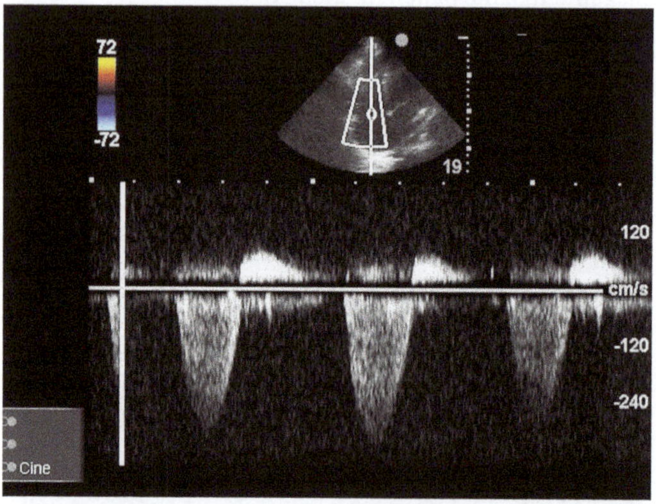

211. A 50-year-old diabetic patient was recently diagnosed as pulmonary tuberculosis. He had progressive breathlessness for 5 days and was admitted to the ICU. Echo was done, which showed the finding. Identify the abnormality and its management.

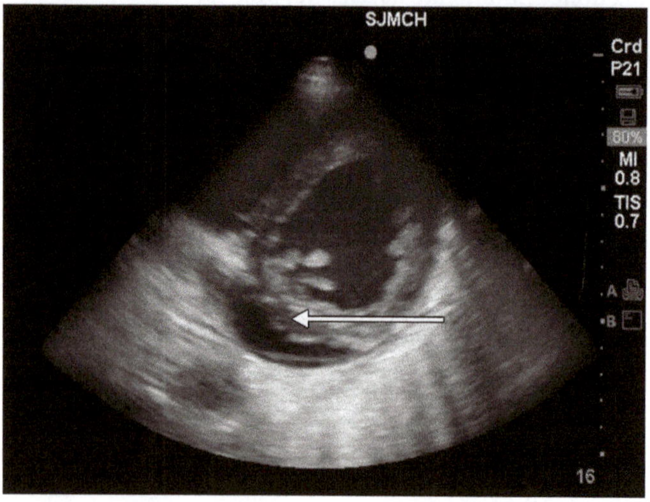

212. A 35-year-old was admitted to the ICU with history of fever, cough with expectoration, and body ache for 5 days. She was intubated and was diagnosed as viral pneumonia; she had sudden onset of desaturation and increase in peak pressures with hypotension. A lung ultrasound was done as shown in Figure below. Describe the finding in the Figure and its use in assessment of the patient.

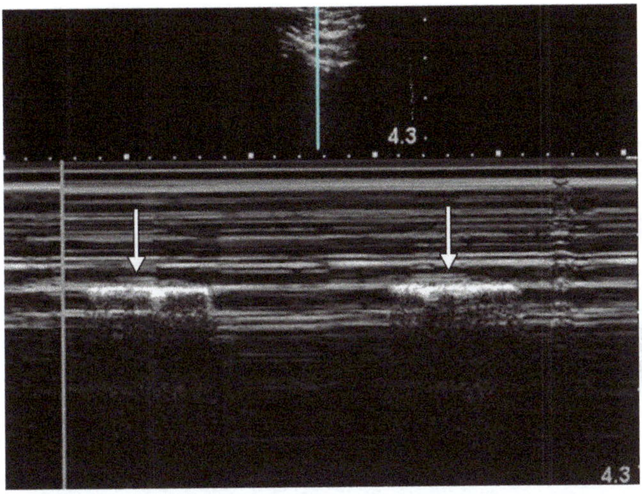

213. A 72-year-old chronic kidney disease patient on regular hemodialysis was admitted to the ICU with history of breathlessness; a lung ultrasound was done. Identify the abnormality. Describe the Figure and indications of treatment for the same.

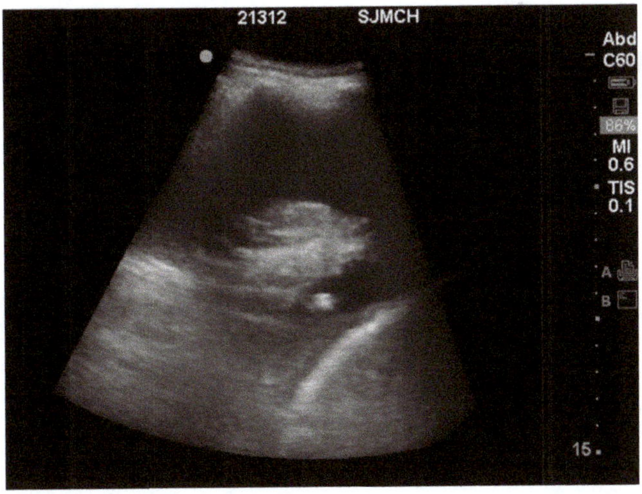

214. A 43-year-old patient was admitted with right-sided middle cerebral artery (MCA) territory stroke and had an ICU stay of 8 days during which he had decompressive craniectomy and underwent tracheotomy. An assessment of diaphragm was done with ultrasound. Identify and comment on the measurement. What are the uses of the diaphragm ultrasound in ICU?

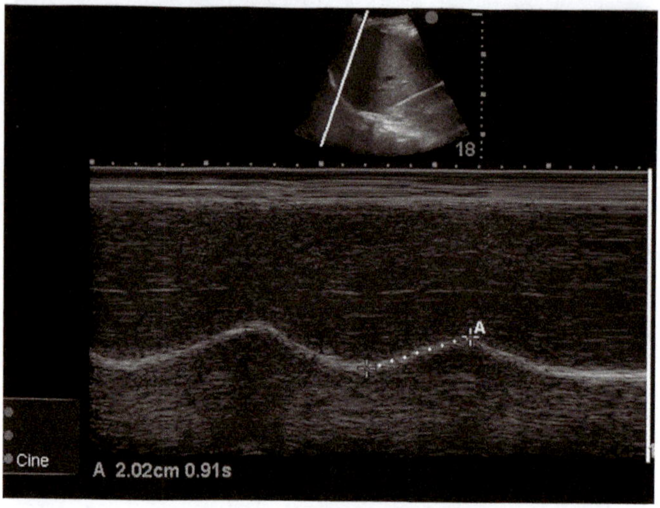

215. The ultrasound lung finding of a patient with pulmonary edema is shown in Figure. Describe the findings. How will you differentiate between ARDS and cardiogenic pulmonary edema using lung ultrasound?

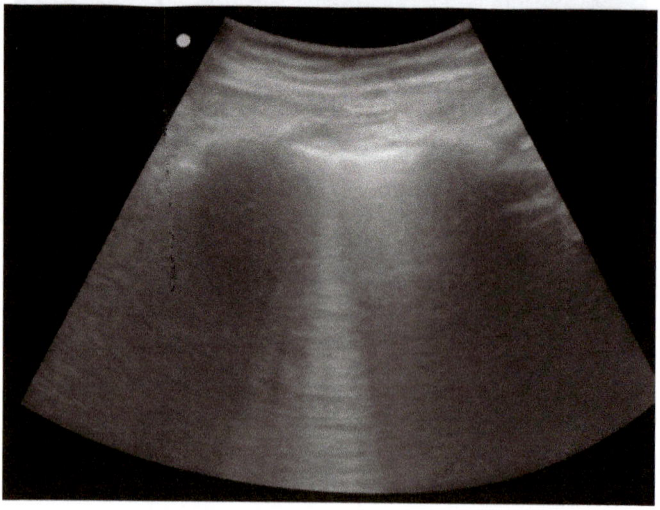

216. A 22-year-old patient with history of chronic ethanol use is admitted to ICU with history of abdominal pain. He was breathless and hypoxic and was intubated. In the ICU, he had worsening of hypoxemia and a recruitment maneuver was used. Describe the use of ultrasound for the same.

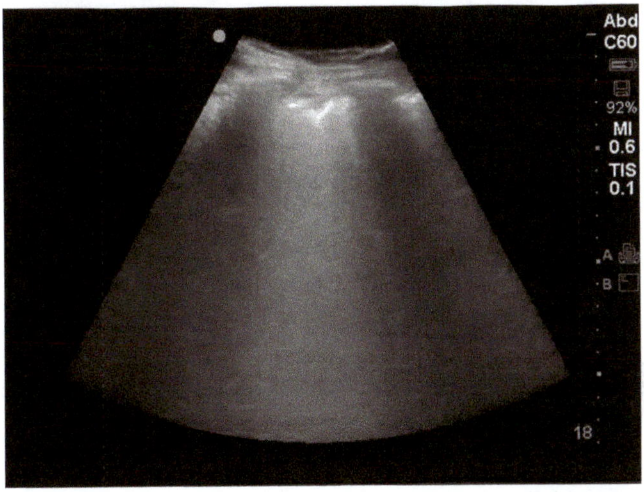

217. Compute a lung ultrasound score (LUS) in the ultrasound Figures given below.

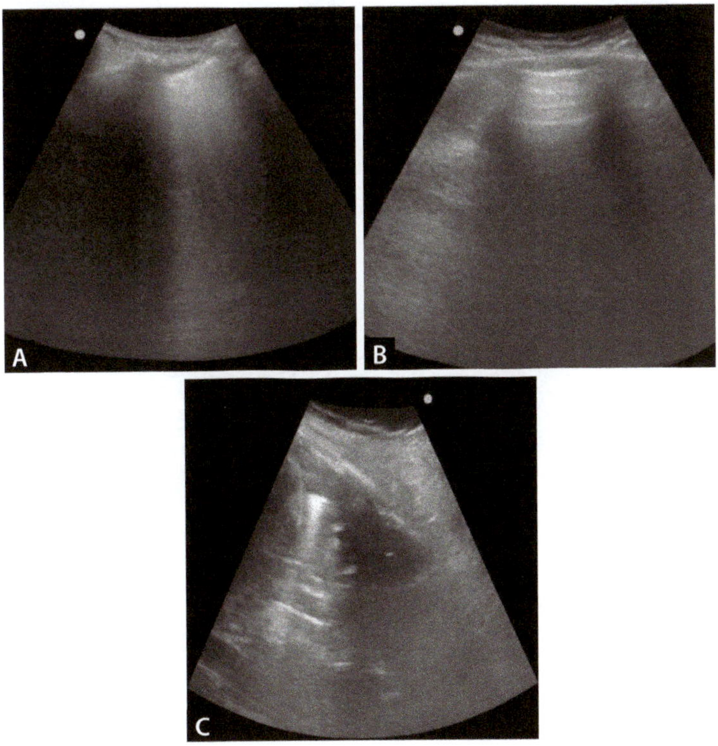

218. Identify the echo image and its view. Enumerate the uses of this view. How will you identify regional wall motional abnormality in this view?

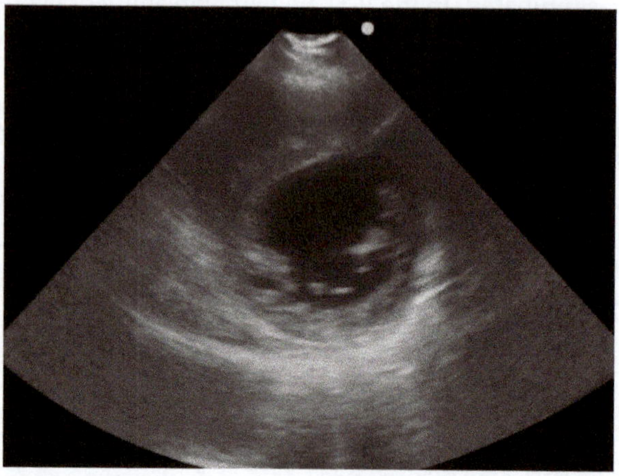

219. Identify the procedure done. Explain the steps of the procedure.

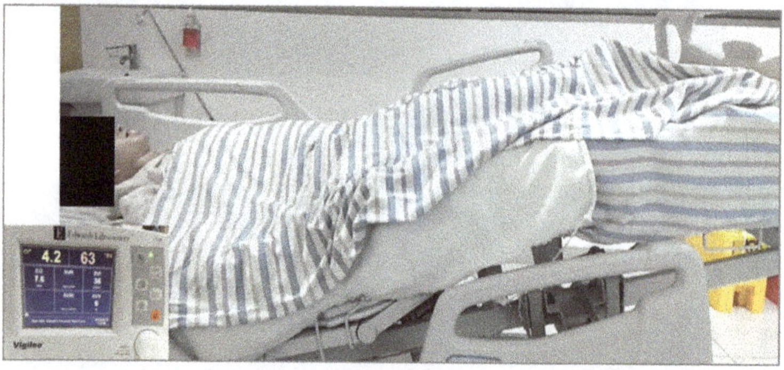

220. What are the hemodynamic utilities of this in intensive care unit (ICU)?

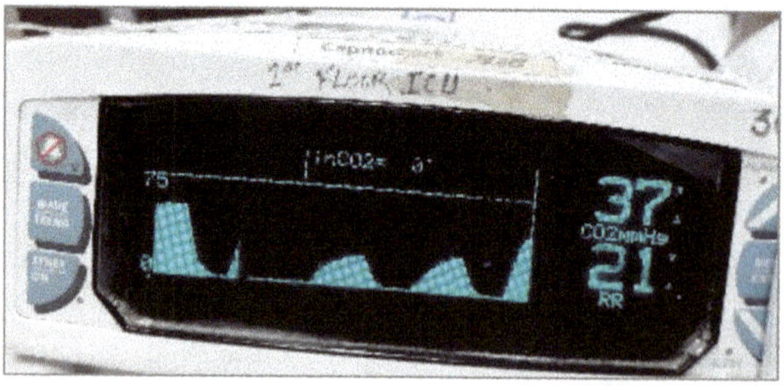

221. Identify the test being done. What are the advantages and disadvantages?

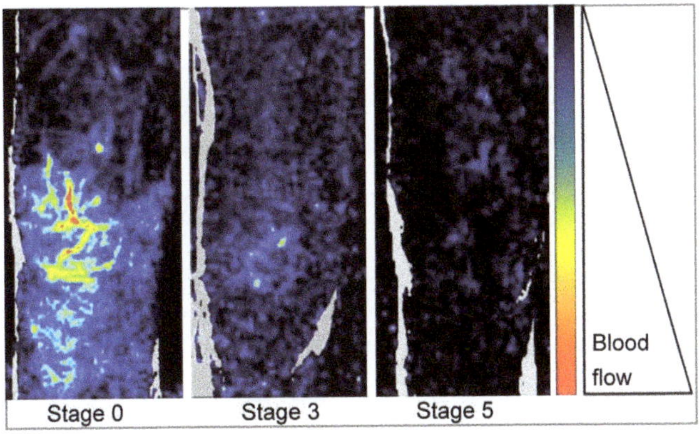

Source: Ait-Oufella H, Bourcier S, Alves M, Galbois A, Baudel JL, Margetis D, et al. Alteration of skin perfusion in mottling area during septic shock. Ann Intensive Care. 2013;3(1):31.

222. What is the use of peripheral perfusion index in hemodynamic monitoring?

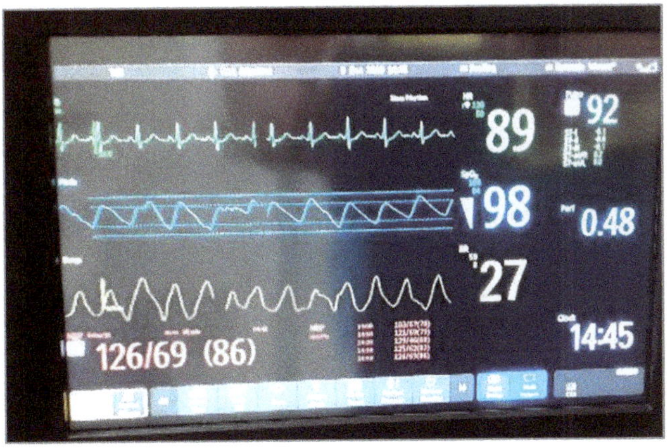

223.

1. What is the current evidence for the role automated chest compression devices in cardiopulmonary resuscitation (CPR)?

2. What is head-up CPR?

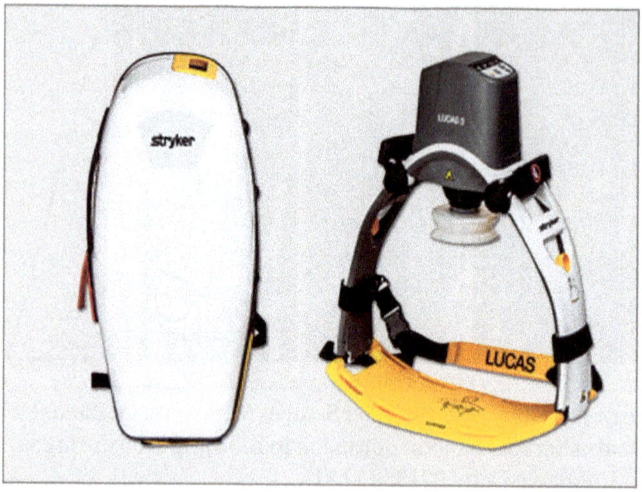

224. Describe head-up position (HUP) CPR.

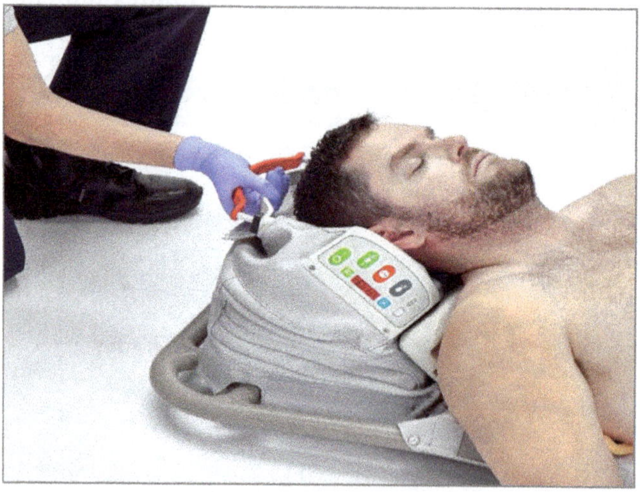

225. A 52-year-old male brought to the casualty with alleged history of assault and stab in the left flank half an hour prior. On arrival, he had a heart rate of 132 beats/min, respiratory rate (RR) of 28 breaths/min, blood pressure (BP) of 90/56 mm Hg and oxygen saturation 96% on 4 L

face mask. He is appearing pale and drowsy. The initial fast examination was negative and the computed tomography (CT) scan taken is given a follows.

- What is the diagnosis?
- What are the causes of a negative test scan?
- How will you classify hemorrhagic shock?

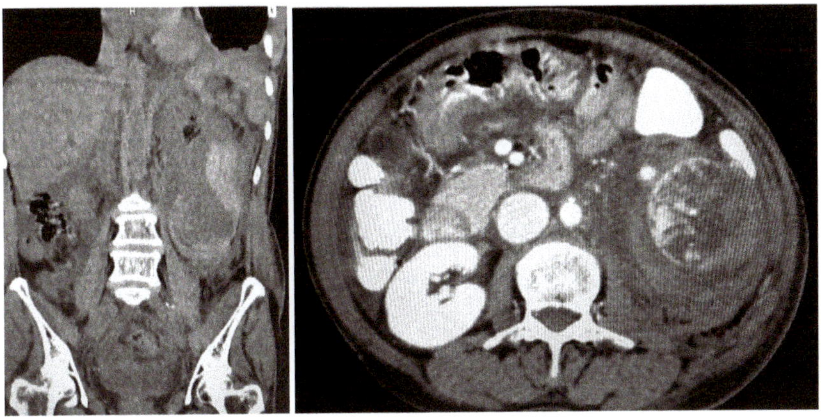

226.

1. Identify the mode of ventilation.
2. How will you improve oxygenation in this mode?
3. How will you improve ventilation and carbon dioxide (CO_2) washout?
4. What will be strategy for paralysis for a patient with acute respiratory distress syndrome (ARDS) and worsening hypoxia on this mode of ventilation?

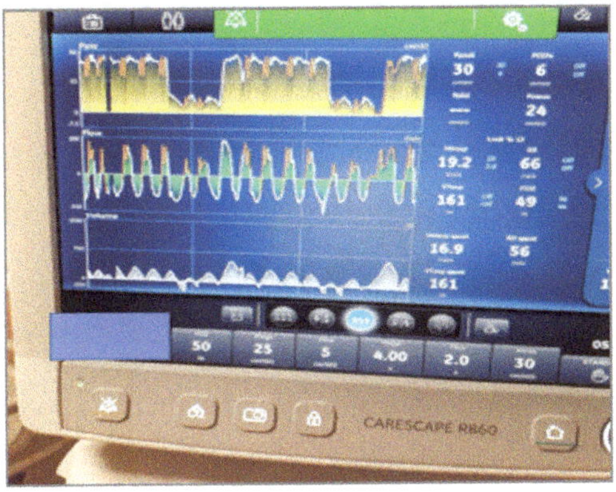

DRUGS

227. What is World Health Organization (WHO) step ladder for pain management in intensive care unit (ICU)?
    - What are the steps in the ladder?

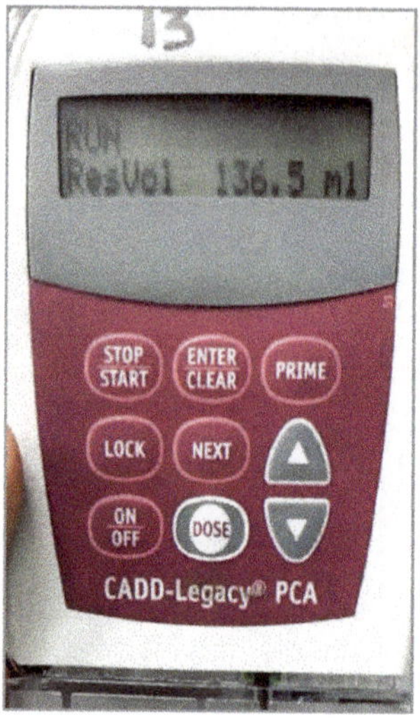

228. What is the evidence for acetaminophen in managing fever in ICU? Describe in brief.

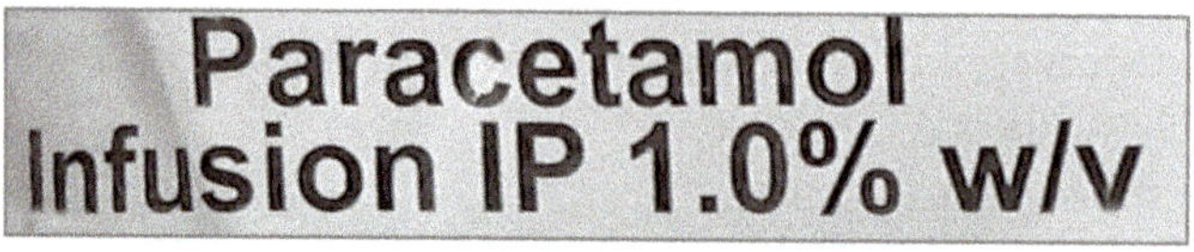

229. What are the uses of sodium bicarbonate in ICU?

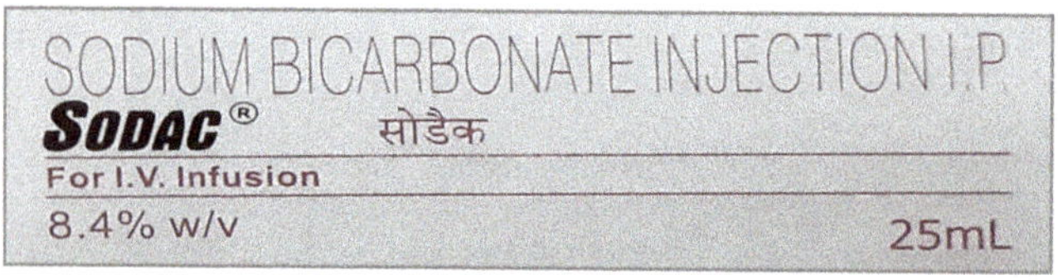

230. What is the recommended strength of soda bicarbonate for managing hyperkalemia?

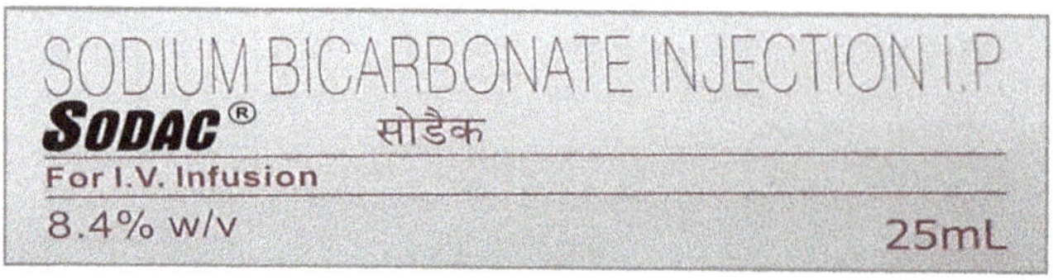

231. What is the KDIGO?
- What is the KDIGO recommendation for use of soda bicarbonate in managing contrast-induced nephropathy?
- What is the evidence for the same?

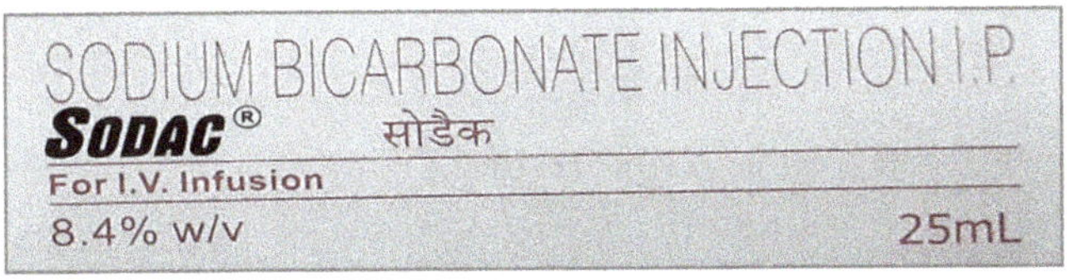

232. What are the major receptors for action and the effects of noradrenaline on immune system?

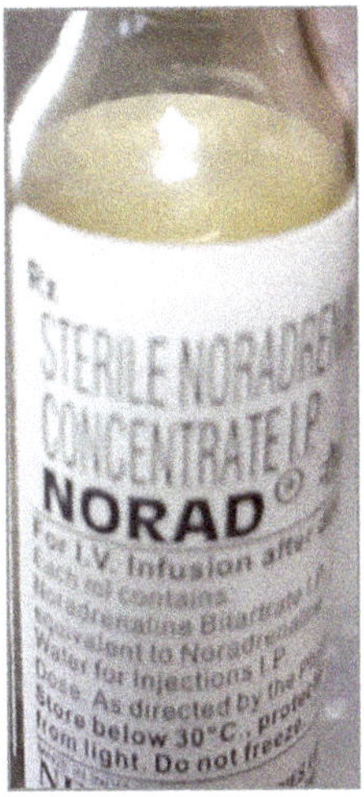

233. What are the common ECG changes in digoxin toxicity?

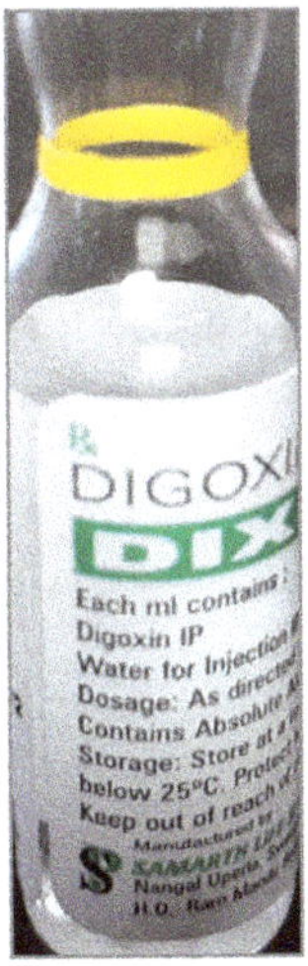

234. Discuss the uses of protamine sulfate in ICU. How is it manufactured? How will you administer it?
   - What are the adverse effects? What precautions are to be taken? Discuss the uses of protamine sulfate in ICU.

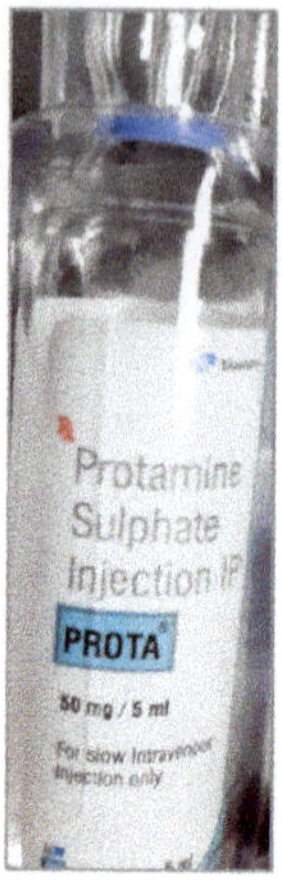

235. What is Andexanet alfa? What is its use and at what dose is it used?

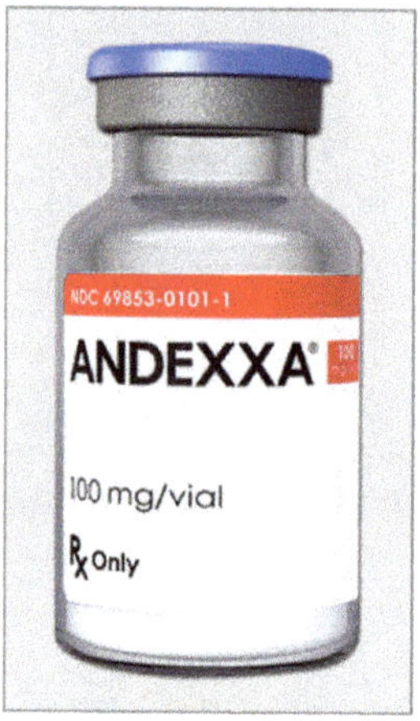

236. By which route will you administer adenosine in ICU?
   - What are the contraindications for adenosine administration?

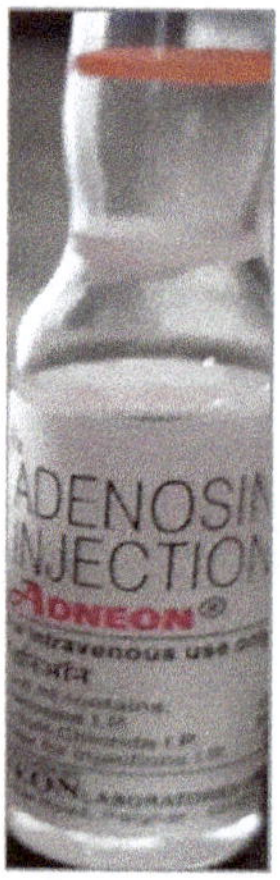

237. What is the mechanism of action of dexmedetomidine?
- What are the uses?
- What is the dosing? What are the common adverse effects?

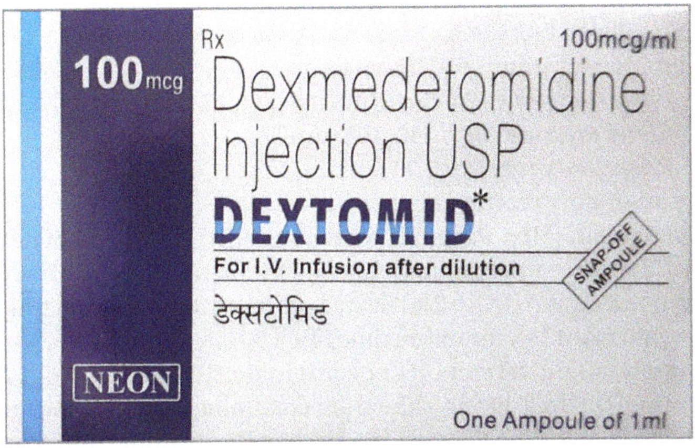

238. How will you administer adrenalin in case of:
- Cardiac arrest
- Status asthmaticus
- Anaphylactic shock

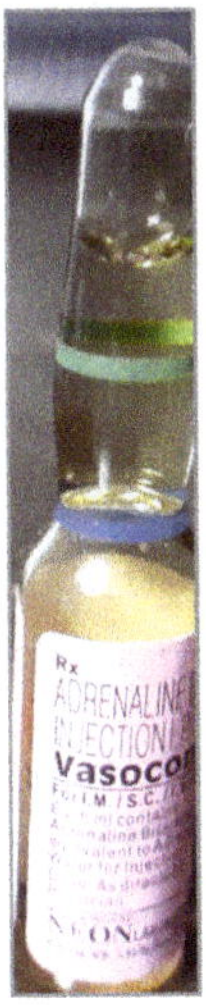

BIOCHEMISTRY

239. A 30-year-old male is shifted to the intensive care unit (ICU) following an episode of generalized tonic-clonic seizure (GTCS) which lasted for 30 seconds after which he regained normal sensorium. He is an otherwise healthy person, with no comorbidities, and no previous history of any medical illness. He had come to the hospital for voluntary platelet donation. During pheresis, he felt a bit uneasy with mild perioral numbness and he developed seizure just prior to the termination of pheresis. How will you investigate the patient and what is the management?

240. A 75-year-old male, a known case of diabetes mellitus, chronic obstructive pulmonary disease, dilated cardiomyopathy with atrial fibrillation on oral anticoagulant treatment presents with accelerated hypertension and epistaxis. His daughter suspects drug automatism, as the medicine box she had refilled 4 days back was empty.
In emergency room (ER) his vitals are:
- *Pulse rate (PR)*: 72 beats/min, irregularly, irregular
- *Blood pressure (BP)*: 140/104 mm Hg
- *Respiratory rate (RR)*: 30 breaths/min

The laboratory reports sent have come as:
Hemoglobin (Hb): 8.2 g/dL; total count (TC): 9600/cc; platelet count (Plt): 2.6 lakhs; prothrombin time (PT): 23 s (normal 15 s); International normalized ratio (INR): 2, activated partial thromboplastin time (aPTT): 55 s (normal 45 s); thrombin time (TT): 90 s; sodium (Na): 138 mmol/L; potassium (K): 4.8 mmol/L; bicarbonate: 19 mmol/L; and chloride: 88 mmol/L. Urea: 60 mg/dL; serum creatinine (S Cr): 2.3 mg/dL; Bb 1.8; aspartate aminotransferase (AST): 32 IU/L; alanine aminotransferase (ALT): 27 IU/L; total protein 6.8 g/dL; albumin: 4 g/dL; lactate: 8 mmol/L; base excess: -6.
How will you manage this patient?

241. A 34-year-old male is brought to the ER with complaints of irritability and altered mentation of 2 days duration. There is no history of fever or any other prodromal symptoms. Toxicology screening in emergency department is negative.
- *On examination (O/E)*: PR: 120 beats/min; BP: 130/84 mm Hg; chest: bilaterally (B/L) clear; abdomen: healed midline incision present, rest within normal limits (WNL).
- *Arterial-blood gas (ABG) on room air*: pH: 7.2; partial pressure of oxygen (pO_2): 74 mm Hg; partial pressure of carbon dioxide (pCO_2): 34 mm Hg; bicarbonate (HCO_3): 14 mmol/L; lactate: 1.2 mmol/L; Na: 130; K: 3.4; chloride (Cl): 100 B; glucose (Glu): 140 mg/dL; blood urea: 50 mg/dL; S Cr: 1.2 mg/dL; albumin: 2 g/dL.
- *Urine ketones*: Absent.
- *Previous history*: Blunt trauma abdomen, laparotomy with extensive small intestine resection and splenectomy done 1 month back.

What is the possible diagnosis and management?

242. A 30-year-old female, software professional while disembarking a 2-hour flight developed acute onset of severe right-sided chest pain and breathlessness and cough. She had one episode of mild blood stain in sputum. In the airport, the documented vitals are: PR: 140 beats/min; BP: 124/70 mm Hg; chest: B/L clear; RR: 26 breaths/min; peripheral oxygen saturation (SpO_2) on room air: 92%, afebrile.
- *Chest radiography (CXR)*: Appeared normal and a 12-lead electrocardiography (ECG) showed sinus tachycardia, right axis deviation with right ventricular (RV) strain pattern. The patient was

started on intravenous heparin before referral to the ICU. In the ICU, screening echo revealed a dilated RV dilated, with normal left ventricular (LV) function.

- Deep venous thrombosis (DVT) screening revealed right-sided DVT in femoral region.

How will you manage the patient?

243. A 50-year-old alcoholic male was brought to the emergency department by relatives who found him unconscious in his room in the afternoon. No prior significant history.
   - *On examination*: PR: 110 beats/min; BP: 130/85; RR: 30 breaths/min; SpO_2: 98 on RA; rectal temperature: 33°C.
   - *Arterial blood gas on room air*: pH: 6.9; pO_2: 80 mm Hg; pCO_2: 34 mm Hg; HCO_3: 6 mmol/L; base excess: -20; lactate: 16 mmol/L; Na: 128 mmol/L; K: 5.4 mol/L; Cl: 96 mmol/L; Glu: 90 mg/dL.
   - Other laboratory investigations include a blood urea of 136 mg/dL; S Cr: 1.8 mg/dL; serum thyroid stimulating hormone (S TSH): 1.4 (WNL); S Ca: 6.4 mg/dL; serum osmolality (S Osm): 350 mOsm/kg H_2O.
   - A serum lactate sent to laboratory has been informed as 2 mmol/L.

   What is the diagnosis and urgent management?

244. A 75-year-old female patient is admitted to the ICU after she was found drowsy and not arousable at home.
   - On arrival in ER, the vitals documented include: PR: 40 beats/min; sinus rhythm; BP: 100/60 mm Hg; RR: 14 breaths/min; pupils: B/L equal and reacting; temperature: 95 °F.
   - Toxicology screen—negative, computed tomography (CT) brain taken revealed only normal age-related atrophy.
   - *Arterial blood gas*: pH: 7.2; pO_2: 85 mm Hg; pCO_2: 42 mm Hg; HCO_3: 20 mmol/L; lactate: 1.5 mmol/L; Na: 130 mmol/L; K: 4.4 mEq/L; calcium (Ca): 9 mg/dL; Glu: 60 mg/dL.
   - Renal function urea 65 mg/dL; S Cr: 1.8 mg/dL; S Ammonia: 15 µmol/dL; normal liver function tests.
   - Her lipid profile showed elevated total cholesterol and triglycerides. Her chest X-ray showed cardiomegaly and minimal pleural effusions bilaterally.
   - *12-lead ECG*: Low-voltage complexes with Osborn waves.
   - *Past history*: Admitted to ICU 6 months back in July for syncope—diagnosed to have atrial fibrillation with fast ventricular rate. Currently on amiodarone and rivaroxaban.

   What is the likely diagnosis? How will you do further workup?

245. A 65-year-old man with known diabetes mellitus, hypertension and dyslipidemia on treatment with losartan-hydrochlorothiazide, metformin, glimepiride arrived in the emergency department with history of generalized weakness and fatigue for 3 days.

- In the ER he had one episode of GTCS. There is no history of fever, any focal neurological deficit.
- Arterial blood gas immediately after seizure revealed: pH: 7.20; pO_2: 67 mm Hg; pCO_2: 34 mm Hg; HCO_3: 15 mmol/L; lactate: 4.2 mmol/L; Na: 111 mEq/L; K: 4.5 mEq/L; Cl: 77 mEq/L; ionized Ca: 1.1 mmol/L; Glu: 350 mg/dL.

What is the possible diagnosis and initial workup?

246. A 65-year-old man on treatment with losartan-hydrochlorothiazide, metformin, glimepiride arrived in the emergency department with history of generalized weakness and fatigue for 3 days.
    - In the ER he had one episode of GTCS which is suspected to be due to drug-induced hyponatremia.
    - A bolus of 150 mL of 3% saline is infused over 20 minutes. However the patient remained comatose and threw a second episode of seizure in ER.

    What will be the approach to management now?

247. A destitute is brought into the ER of your hospital after he was found on roadside in a weak semiconscious debilitated state.
    - *In ER, the vitals recorded are*: PR: 100 beats/min; BP: 110/60 mm Hg; RR: 34 breaths/min; SpO_2: 95%.
    - *Arterial blood gas*: pH: 7.15; pO_2: 78 mm Hg; pCO_2: 32 mm Hg; HCO_3: 15 mEq/L; Na: 134 mEq/L; K: 3.6 mEq/L; Cl: 98 mEq/L; lactate: 2 mmol/L; Glu: 65 mg/dL.
    - *Other investigations*: Urea: 65 mg/dL; S Cr: 1.4 mg/dL; Mg: 1.4 mg/dL; phosphate (PO_4): 3.5 mg/dL; albumin: 1.8 mg/dL. He was shifted to ICU with a diagnosis of pre-renal acute kidney injury (AKI) secondary to hypovolemia. He was started on intravenous dextrose-normal saline, along with RT feed. He showed signs of clinical improvement, with improvement in sensorium and urine output. As he was tolerating enteral feed, the intravenous fluids were stopped and enteral feeds were increased to 1,500 kcal/day. On the third day of ICU admission, he was noted to be drowsy and he had a sudden run of ventricular tachycardia and cardiac arrest from which he could not be revived.
    - Arterial blood gas taken immediately prior to cardiac arrest showed: pH: 7.2; pO_2: 60 mm Hg; pCO_2: 46 mm Hg; HCO_3: 16 mmol/L; Na: 128 mEq/L; K: 2.5 mEq/L; Cl: 103 mEq/L; lactate: 4.5 mmol/L. Biochemistry samples sent revealed: urea: 50 mg/dL; S Cr: 1.5 mg/dL; Mg: 1 mg/dL; PO_4: 1.5 mmol/L; Glu: 200 mg/dL.
    - What is the diagnosis and what adjustments ideally needed in the management of such cases?

248. A 23-year-old male patient was brought to the emergency department with acute onset breathing difficulty and noisy breathing of 2 days duration. A chest X-ray obtained showed mediastinal widening, and a CT scan suggested mediastinal lymphadenopathy causing vascular

obstruction of the superior vena cava and other great veins. The patient was admitted to ICU for observation in view of imminent respiratory distress. As the patient had inspiratory and expiratory wheeze, the ER registrar had also called for intravenous dexamethasone along with nebulization with salbutamol.

After 1 hour of ICU admission, the nurse notes a sudden run of ventricular tachycardia with pulse. ABG taken at that point showed: pH: 7.25; pO_2: 60 mm Hg on 5 L/min of O_2 via facemask; pCO_2: 30 mm HG; HCO_3: 18 mEq/L; lactate: 2.4 mmol/L; Na: 133 mEq/L; K: 6.4 mEq/L; Cl: 97 mEq/dL; Ca: 6.7 mg/dL. What is the possible diagnosis and management?

249. Laboratory reports of a patient admitted with tumor lysis syndrome: Na: 131 mEq/L; K: 6.7 mEq/L; Ca: 6 mg/dL; PO_4: 14 mg/dL; UA: 21 mg/dL.
    - How will you manage the patient?

250. A patient is admitted to ICU with SVC syndrome, mediastinal mass, and tumor lysis syndrome. He is being managed aggressively for tumor lysis syndrome (TLS) with antihyperkalemic measures, hydration, and rasburicase has also been administered. Blood sample was repeated after 4 hours of hydration and rasburicase shows values: Na: 133 mEq/L; K: 4.2 mEq/L; Ca: 6.7 mg/dL; PO_4: 11 mg/dL; UA: 0.2 mg/dL.
    - How will you interpret the results?

251. A 23-year-old female, with an uneventful antenatal history underwent normal delivery 3 days back. The puerperal period also remained uneventful and a discharge was planned on the 4th day. On day 4 of her delivery she developed acute onset of GTCS which resolved spontaneously.
    - Investigations after seizures: Hb: 6 g/dL; total leukocyte count (TLC): 17,000; Plt: 50,000; Na: 142; K: 4; Ca: 9.3; Mg: 3; Glu: 150 mg/dL. Liver function tests were within normal limits.
    - Computed tomography (CT) brain: WNL.

    What investigation would you do? What will be the management?

252. A 40-year-old gymnasium trainer has been brought to ER when he was found inside the bathroom, unconscious with frothing from mouth with garlic odor.
    - *On examination*: PR: 140 beats/min; BP: 60/30 mm Hg; RR: 30 breaths/min; cold extremities.
    - *Bedside ECG*: Normal right-sided chamber function.
    - Global hypokinesia of LV with very poor ejection fraction.
    - *Arterial blood gas*: pH: 6.9; 40 mm Hg on O_2 with Hudson mask; pCO_2: 70 mm Hg; HCO_3: 15 mmol/L; lactate: 8 mmol/L; Na: 140 mEq/L; K: 4 mEq/L; Cl: 100 mEq/L; Glu: 120. mg/dL.
    - Suspecting poisoning gastric lavage done, gastric lavage turns silver nitrate and lead acetate paper black.

    What is the diagnosis and management?

253. A 60-year-old male patient (no comorbidities) with 1 month history of fever, 20 days backache reported to accident and emergency (A&E) department with altered mentation.
- *Biochemistry*: S Na: 130 mEq/L; Cl: 110 mEq/L; K: 4.5 mEq/L; Ca: 15 mg/dL; blood urea: 80 mg/dL; S Cr: 2.1 mg/dL; serum bilirubin (S Bil): 1.2 mg/dL; S protein: 9 g/dL; S albumin: 2.5 g/dL.
- *Arterial blood gas*: pH: 7.28; pCO_2: 35 mm Hg; pO_2: 80 mm Hg on RA; HCO_3: 18 mmol/L; lactate: 2.4 mmol/L.

What is the diagnosis and management?

MISCELLANEOUS

254. Give an example of drugs acting on each phase of the cardiac action potential.

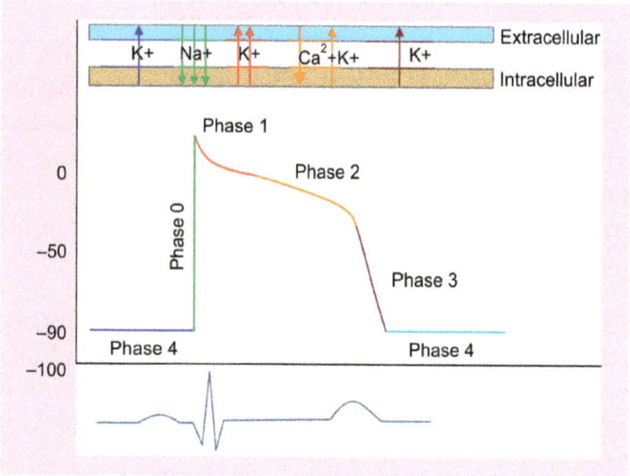

255. Drug kinetics

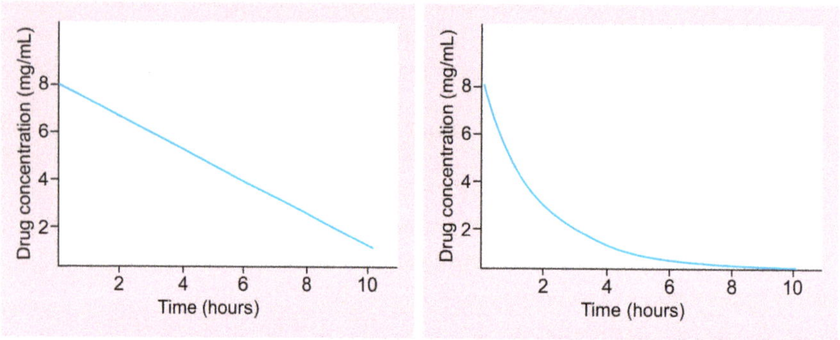

- A patient is admitted to the intensive care unit (ICU) following overdose of phenytoin tablets. Based on the pharmacokinetic principles, which image is representative of drug elimination?
- Name a few other drugs which follow the same order of pharmacokinetics.

256. A 63-year-old diabetic and hypertensive patient is shifted back from the OT after undergoing on pump coronary artery bypass grafting (CABG).

- Intraoperative and immediate postoperative period was uneventful and on postoperative day 2, deep venous thrombosis (DVT) prophylaxis with low-molecular weight heparins (LMWH) was suggested.
- However the clinical pharmacist pointed out that the platelet count which was 3.45×10^9/L has dropped to 1.45×10^9/L and is concerned regarding addition of LMWH.
- A platelet factor 4 (PF4) enzyme-linked immunosorbent assay (ELISA) test was ordered and came as 1.45 (cut off <0.60).

What will be the drug of choice for DVT prophylaxis in this patient?

257. A 45-year-old male, known case of esophageal carcinoma underwent neoadjuvant chemotherapy and Ivor Lewis esophagectomy.
    - Postoperative, he was started on parenteral nutrition, targeting 1,000 kcal and 40 g protein, via peripheral line.
    - 3 days later, he was found to be drowsy and shifted to ICU.
    - Laboratory reports are shown.

    Hemoglobin (Hb): 8.9; total count (TC): 12,000; platelet (Plt): 1,15,000; International normalized ratio (INR): 1.8; urea: 18; serum creatinine (S Cr): 0.8; Na: 128 mmol/dL; K: 1.4 mmol/dL; Ca: 6.4 g/dL; Mg: 1.1 mg/dL; Cl: 96 mmol/dL; phosphate (PO_4): 1.15 mg/dL; Bb: 2.1; aspartate transaminase (AST): 26; alanine transaminase (ALT): 41; alkaline phosphatase (ALP): 114; protein: 4.6; albumin: 1.8
    - Possible diagnosis?
    - What are the causes of hypophosphatemia? How will you correct it?

258. A 26-year-old female, known case of papillary carcinoma thyroid—status post-thyroidectomy was noted to have noisy breathing on routine postoperative rounds by day 3 with a clinical suspicion of laryngospasm, an arterial blood gas (ABG) taken which is given in the image.
    - How will you manage the patient?

Tata Hospital, 2nd Floor ICU

Pat ID

First name

Blood Type Arterial

Blood Gas values (measured at 37. 0C)		
pH	7.46	(7.350 - 7.450)
PCO_2	34.6 mmHg	(35.0 - 45.0)
PO_2	86.4 mmHg	(80.0 - 100.0)
$cHCO_3$	24.45 mmol/L	
BE	0.5 mmol/L	
BE(ecf)	0.9 mmol/L	
tHb	11.3 g/dl	(11.5 - 17.40)
SO_2	98.8 %	(75.0 - 100)
SO_2 (c)	99.4 %	
Electrolytes		
Na^+	135.8 mmol/L	(135.0 - 148.0)
K^+	3.38 mmol/L	(3.50 - 4.50)
Cl^-	96.3 mmol/L	(98.0 - 107.0)
Ca^{++}	0.85 mmol/L	(1.15 - 1.29)
Metabolites		
Glu	110.9 mg/dl	(70 - 110)
Lac	0.6 mmol/L	(0.44 - 2.2)

259. A graphical representation of the pharmacokinetics/pharmacodynamics (PK/PD) properties of common antibiotics used in the ICU is given below. Identify examples for the same and mention how the drug delivery can be improved in each case.

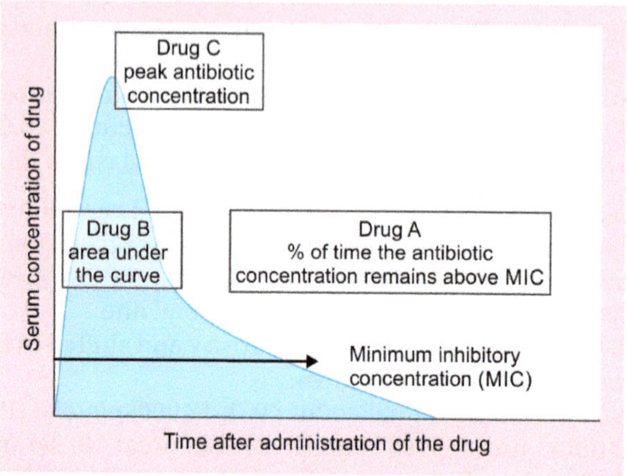

260. What are the devices used for inhalational sedation in ICU?
- How is the anesthesia gas conserved in these devices?

261. Identify the class of drugs it belongs to?
Name other drugs of the same class.
What are the indications?

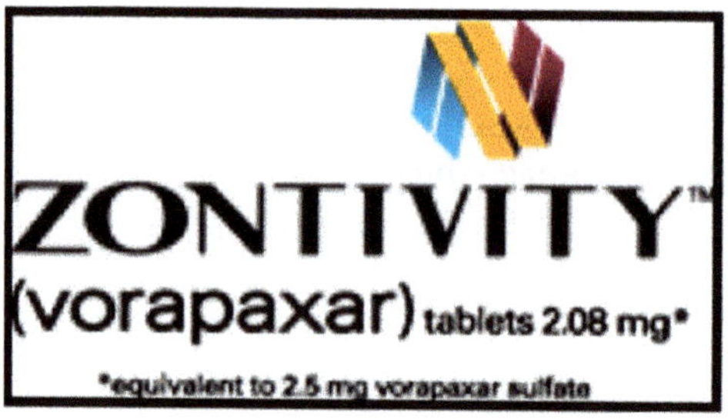

262. Identify the devices.
- What are they used for?

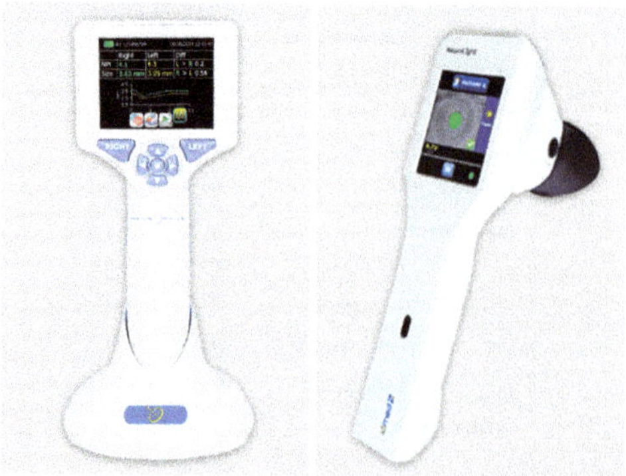

263. A 64-year-old male, diabetic, on treatment in ICU for community-acquired pneumonia (CAP) and septic shock, was on broad-spectrum antibiotics for 10 days, now recovering, currently off vasopressors and on pressure support mode of ventilation. Full enteral feeds started targeting a calories requirement of 1,800 kcal/day and 60 g protein. The next day, during ICU rounds, it was noticed that the patient had four episodes of loose stools. He is afebrile, white blood cell (WBC) count 12,200/cc with neutrophil/lymphocyte ratio (NLR) of 11. How do you classify diarrhea in ICU? What is motor diarrhea?

264. Comment on the contrast-enhanced computed tomography (CECT) abdomen of a patient who presented with severe abdominal pain and vomiting.

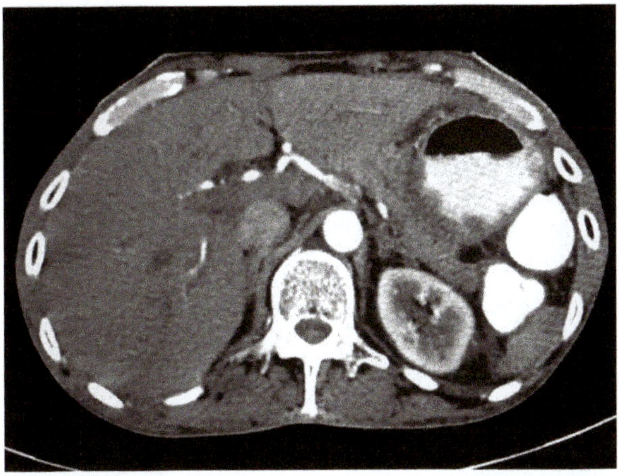

265. A 43-year-old male, otherwise American Society of Anesthesiologists (ASA) 1, is admitted to the ICU after being operated for carcinoma head of pancreas. He is having persistent ileus and is on watchful expectancy for postoperative leak. His calculated APACHE II (Acute Physiology and Chronic Health Evaluation II) score is 3 and calculated SOFA (Sequential Organ Failure Assessment) score is 4. He has been in ICU for the past 3 days and is not expected to tolerate enteral nutrition in the next 1 week.
- How will you assess for the need of nutritional support in him?
- What is his modified NUTRIC (Nutrition Risk in Critically Ill) score?
- What is the role for immunonutrition in postoperative patients?

266. During ICU audit, you have found that your ICU has a Standardized Mortality Ratio (SMR) of 1.5.
- How do you calculate SMR?
- What is the ideal SMR an ICU can get?
- What are the causes for a high SMR?

267. In your ICU for the month of February, 12 cases were reported as ventilator-associated pneumonia (VAP).
If there were 36 patients in total who received mechanical ventilation, during February, and assuming that each patient was ventilated for an approximate of 5 days, what is the ICU's VAP rate?

268. • A 16-year-old male admitted to ICU as a case of perforation peritonitis and septic shock following appendicitis. Currently on ventilator for the past 3 days requiring vasopressors (Noradrenaline @ 0.2 µg/kg/min). Has fever of 38.6°C, intermittent that responds to paracetamol.
- What is the definition of fever in ICU?
- Enumerate a few causes for noninfectious cause of fever in ICU.

269. A 36-year-old primigravida, at 32 weeks of gestation presented to emergency room with one episode of seizure. on examination, she had a pulse rate (PR) of 102/min, blood pressure (BP) of 160/110 mm Hg, respiratory rate (RR) of 22/min, and saturation of 96% on room air. The laboratory findings are a Hb of 7.4 g/dL; WBC of 12,000/cc; Platelet count of 98,000/cc; Bilirubin of 2.4 mg/dL; ALT: 246 IU/L; AST: 446 IU/L; LDH: 800. A peripheral smear was sent and the image is shown below. What is the possible diagnosis and management?

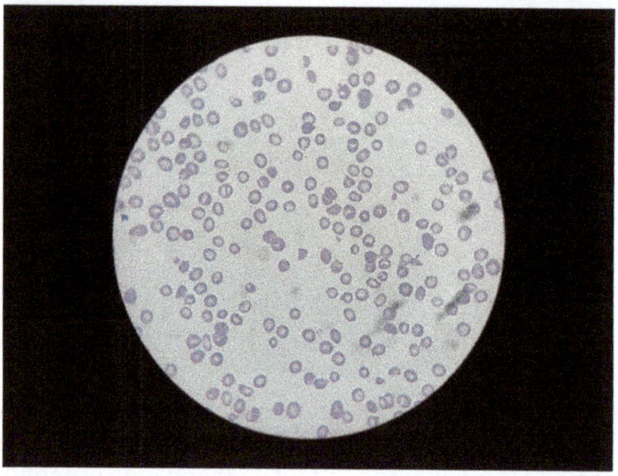

270. The peripheral smear of a patient admitted with severe community acquired pneumonia is as given in the image. The laboratory values of the patient are as follows—Hb: 8.2 g/dL; TC 8,800/cc; Plt: 2,48,000/microliter; Bilirubin of: 3.2 mg/dL; LDH: 1,100 IU/L; AST: 32 IU/L; ALT 26 IU/L; Urea: 48 mg/dL; S Cr: 0.9 mg/dL; K: 5.1 mmol/L. From the laboratory picture, what is the possible organism implicated in the disease?

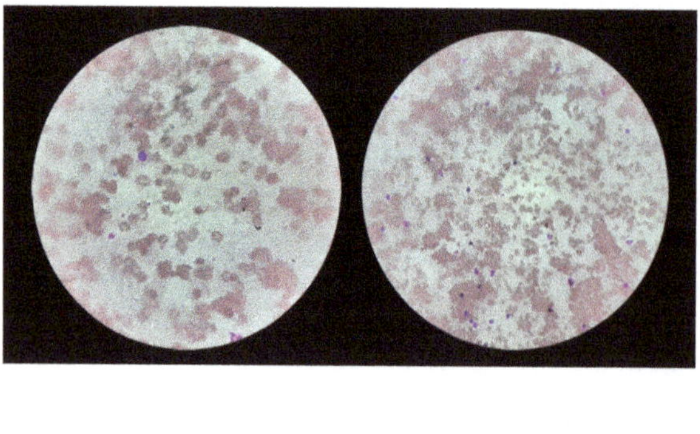

271. The consort diagram of a trial evaluating the Transfusion Requirements in Critical Care (TRICC trial) is given in the image. After going through the diagram, comment on how you will accept the results of this trail in your practice?

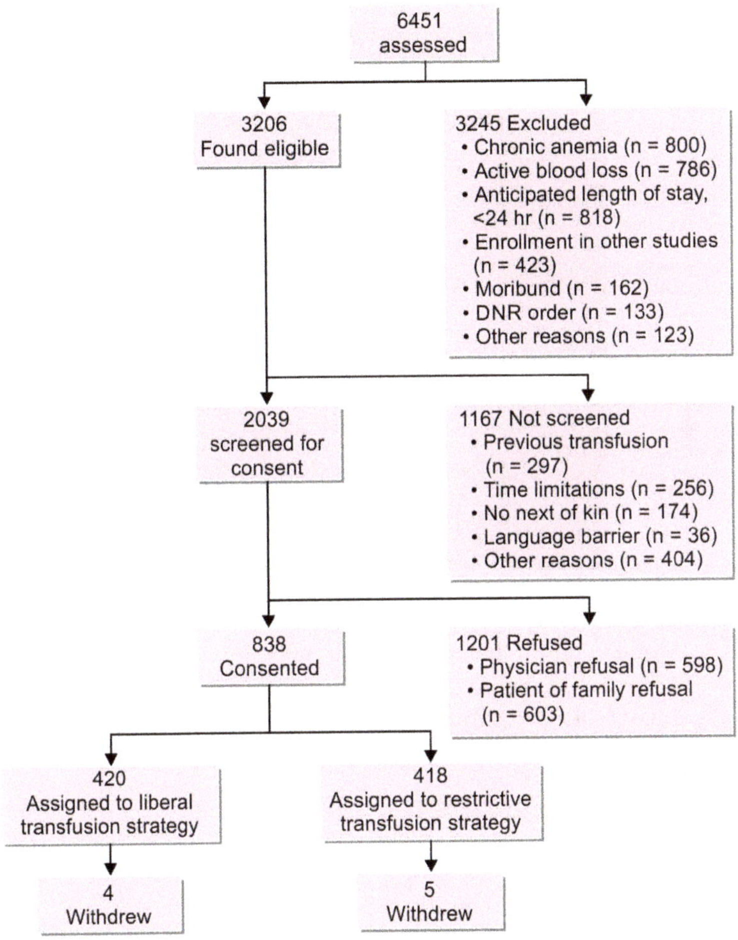

272. • What is discriminative ability of a test?
• What is Youden index (J)?

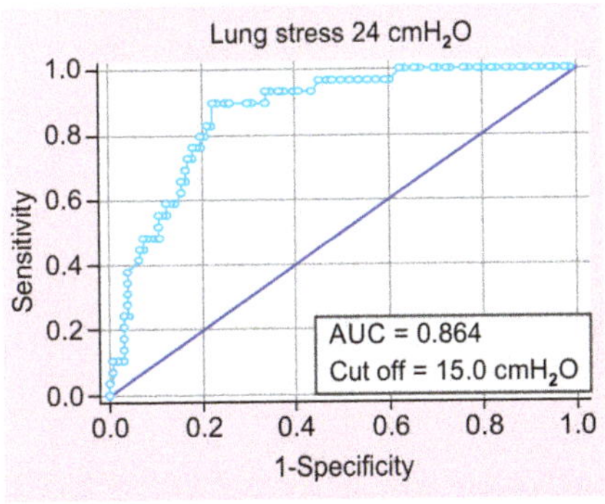

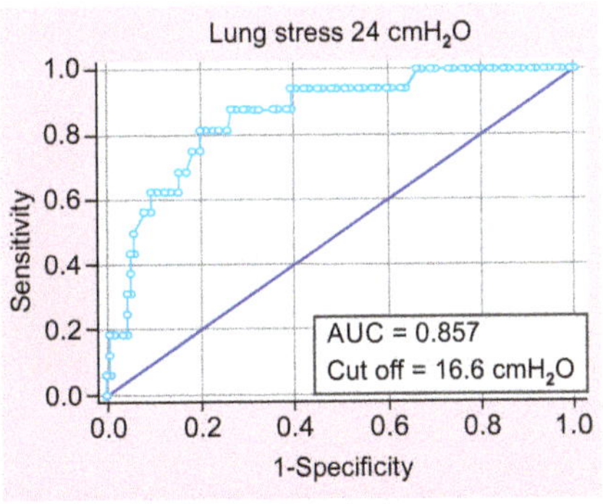

273. An 8-year-old child with past history of obstructive hydrocephalus due to meningitis which required operative management now presented to emergency room (ER) with decreased sensorium, 3 days after discharge from hospital. The magnetic resonance imaging (MRI) taken is given in the image.
- What is diagnosis and management?

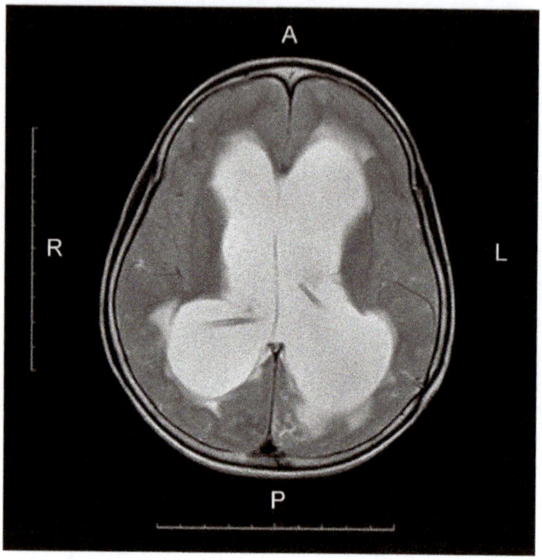

274. • Patient admitted with breathing difficulty
- Given is the angiogram before and after a drug is administered.
- Identify the procedure done.
- Mention dose for the same.

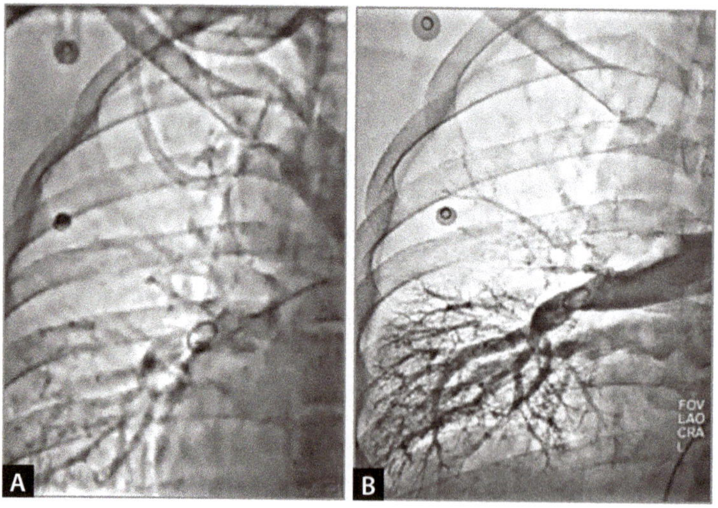

275. What is the use of Pitt score in intensive care unit (ICU)?

*The Pitt Bacteremia Score**

Criterion	*Points*
• Fever (oral temperature)	
– ≤35 °C or ≥40 °C	2
– 35.1–36.0 °C or 39.0–39.9 °C	1
– 36.1–38.9 °C	0
• Hypotension	2
– Acute hypotensive event with drop in systolic blood pressure >30 mm Hg and diastolic blood pressure >20 mm Hg	
or	
– Requirement for intravenous vasopressor agents	
or	
– Systolic blood pressure <90 mm Hg	
• Mechanical ventilation	2
• Cardiac arrest	4
• Mental status	
– Alert	0
– Disoriented	1
– Stuporous	2
– Comatose	4

*All criteria are graded within 48 hours before or on the day of first positive blood culture. The highest point score during that time is recorded

276. • Case of sepsis, septic shock, being managed with fluids resuscitation and noradrenalin at 0.3 μg/kg/min. In-between he is requiring fluid boluses for hypotension.
- Ventilator graphics trend over 8 hours is shown.
- What is possible diagnosis and management?

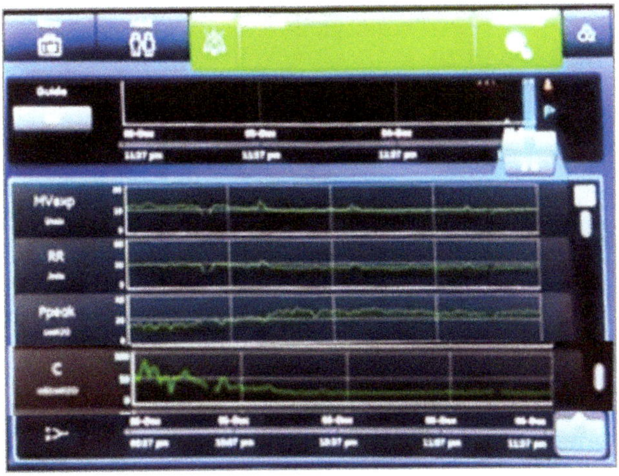

277. • A 78-year-old male, diabetic, admitted with complaints of fever, chills, and breathing difficulty of 2 days duration.
- Admitted to ICU as he was confused.
- In ICU, sinus tachycardia of 128 beats/min, blood pressure (BP) was 88/60 mm Hg, and respiratory rate (RR) was 25 breaths/min. He maintained a saturation of 90% on 4 L oxygen.
- Laboratory investigation is significant for hypoalbuminemia of 2.2 g/dL.
- Arterial blood gas (ABG) on room air shows a partial pressure of oxygen (PaO_2) of 90 mm Hg with pH of 7.42 and partial pressure of carbon dioxide (pCO_2) of 30 mm Hg.

How will you predict the need for intensive respiratory care and vasopressor support in this patient?

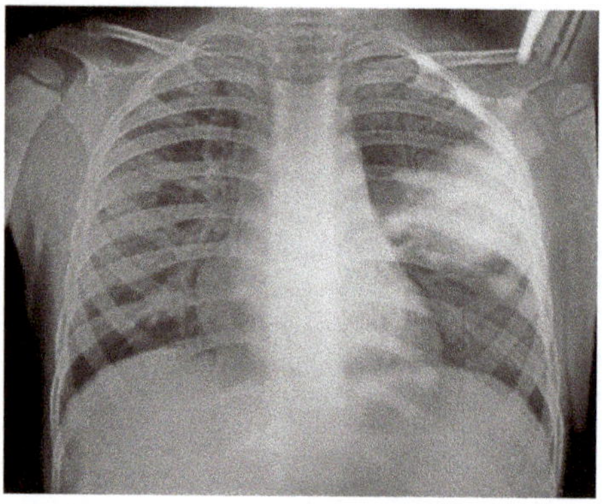

278. How will you calculate the dilution of N-acetyl cysteine (NAC) for paracetamol poisoning in a 14-year child weighing 50 kg, given that it is available as 20% w/v 5 mL vial?

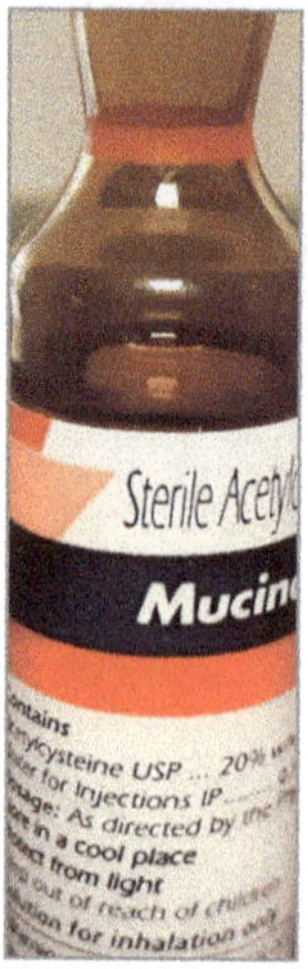

279. A 75-year-old male patient admitted with acute urinary retention after administration of ipratropium bromide nebulization. Post-catheterization, the urine output dropped and the patient developed abdominal pain, and anuria. A computed tomography (CT) scan was taken which is shown in the image.
   - What is diagnosis and management?

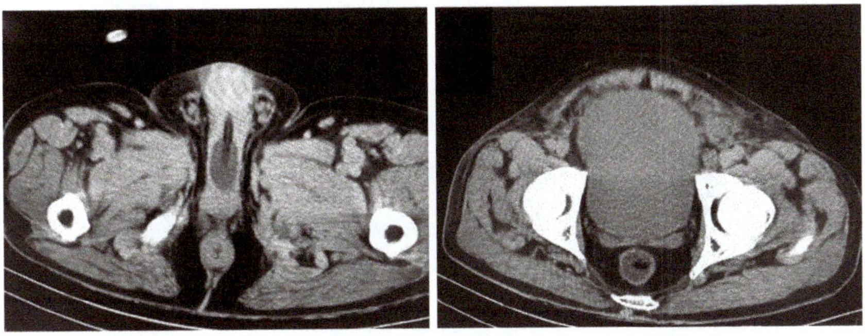

280. A patient presents to ER with polytrauma and continues to remain hemodynamically unstable, despite resuscitation.
   - His X-ray pelvis is given here.
   - What is the diagnosis? Enumerate important point in the management.

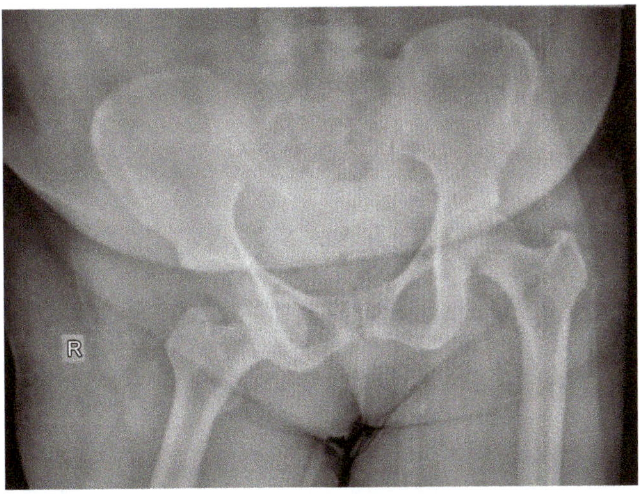

281. This 28-year-old victim of road traffic accident (RTA) presented in class 2 hemorrhagic shock. His X-ray is as given here. Assuming hypovolemia due to a calf muscle collection, how much blood volume can accumulate in calf?
   - Four hours after admission, the nurse reports severe pain of the injured limb, requiring escalating doses of analgesics. His urine

output has been trailing since admission, and for the last 1 hour he is anuric.

- What is the diagnosis? How will you investigate and confirm the diagnosis? Enumerate the steps in management.

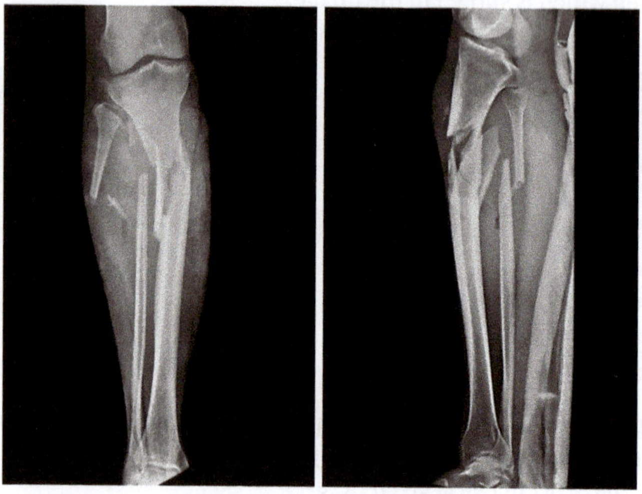

282. *Case continued:* Bedside fasciotomy was done on an urgent basis and the patient was taken up for surgery 3 days after initial stabilization. In the postoperative period, he developed sudden hypoxia, confusion, and became tachycardic.
    - What are the differential diagnoses? How will you confirm the diagnosis?
    - Discuss management.

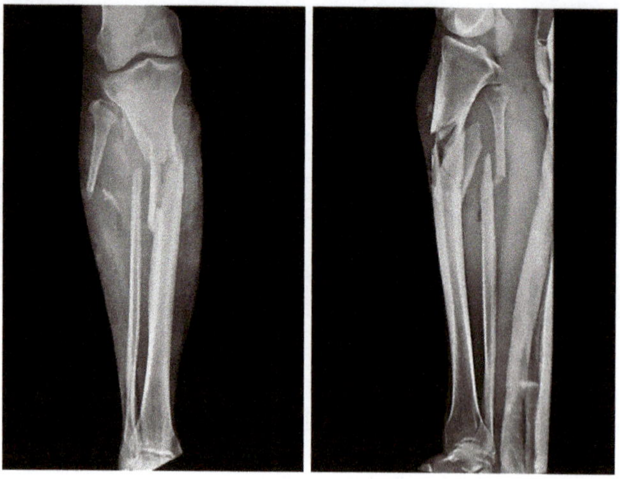

283. Computed tomography of abdomen of a patient with persistent fever and tachycardia, 4 days after being diagnosed with pancreatitis.
    - What is the diagnosis?
    - What is the radiological classification for this?

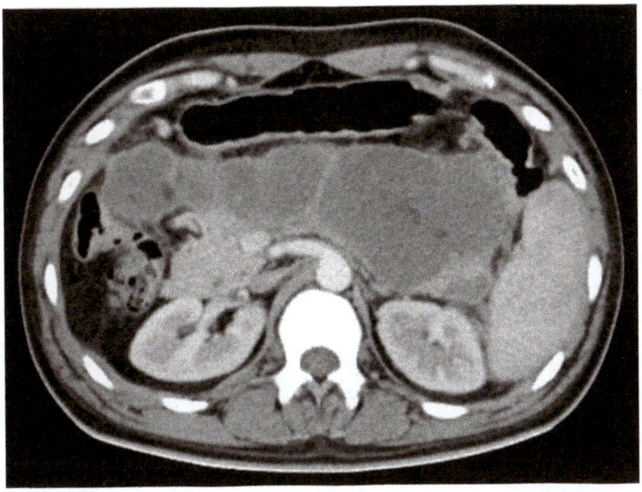

284. A 64-year-old male diabetic patient on treatment for urinary tract infection (UTI), presented with septic shock.

- Computed tomography is shown.
- What is the diagnosis? What is the management?

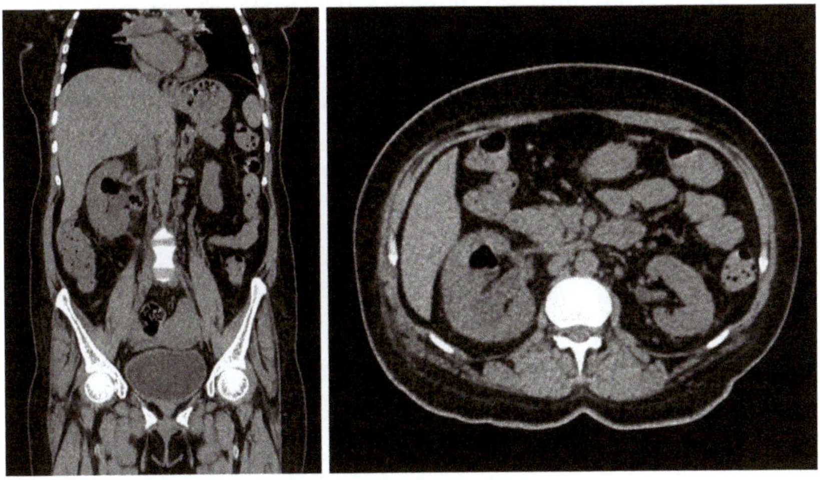

285. Thromboelastography (TEG) of a patient with RTA shifted to ICU from ER.

- What is the diagnosis? Discuss management.

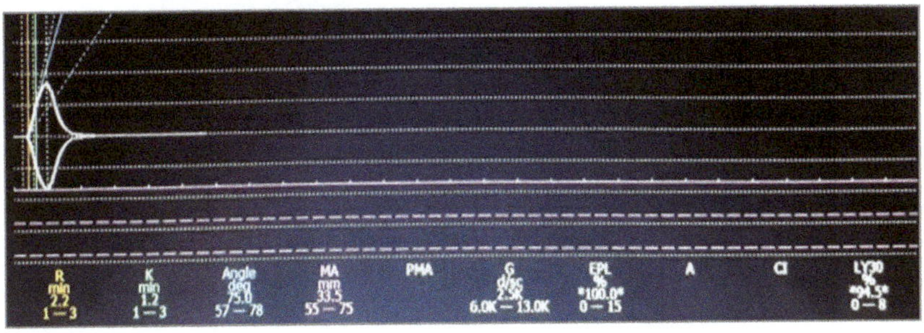

286. How will we differentiate between primary and secondary fibrinolysis?

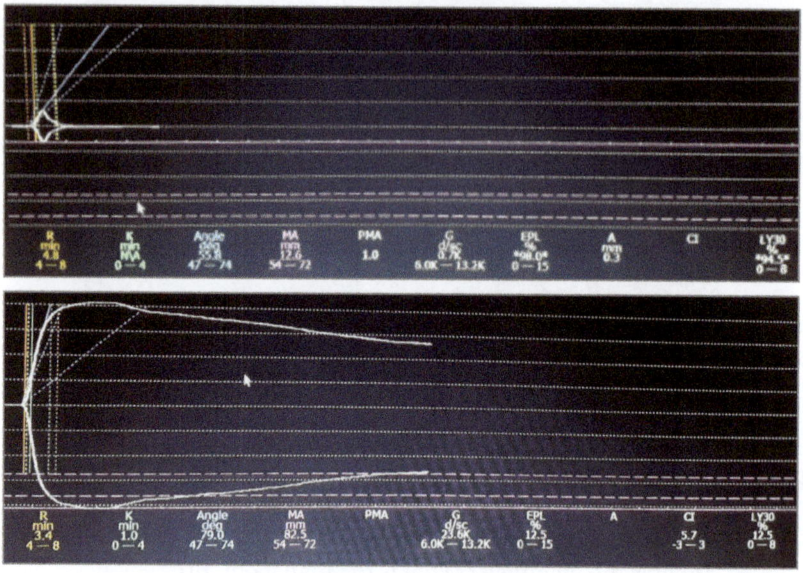

287. When will you consider proning in acute respiratory distress syndrome (ARDS)?
- What are the contraindications for proning?
- What are the possible complications of proning?

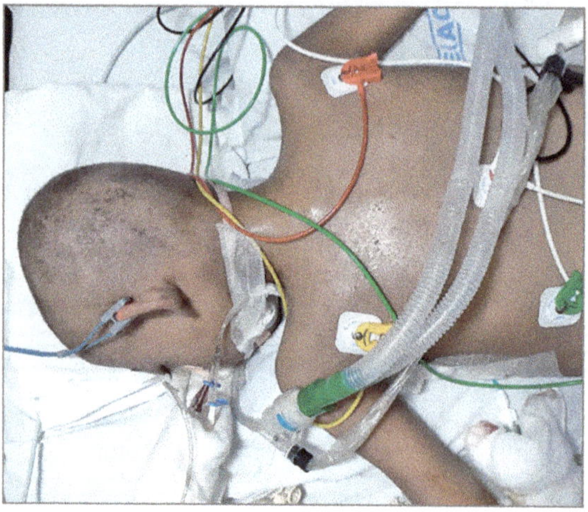

288. Enumerate the possible mechanisms by which proning improves oxygenation?

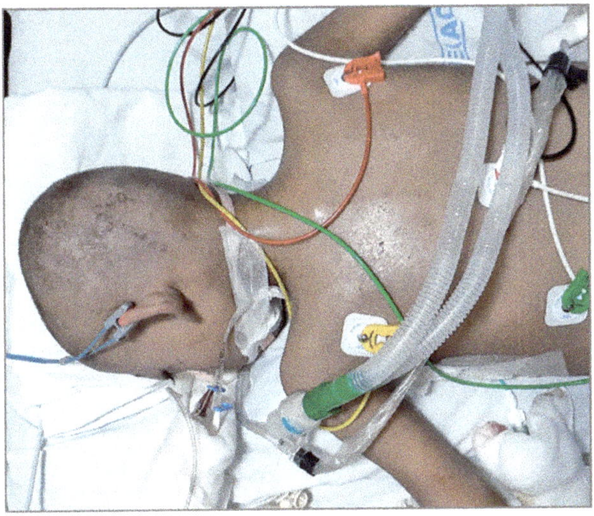

289. When will you consider to stop prone positioning in ARDS?

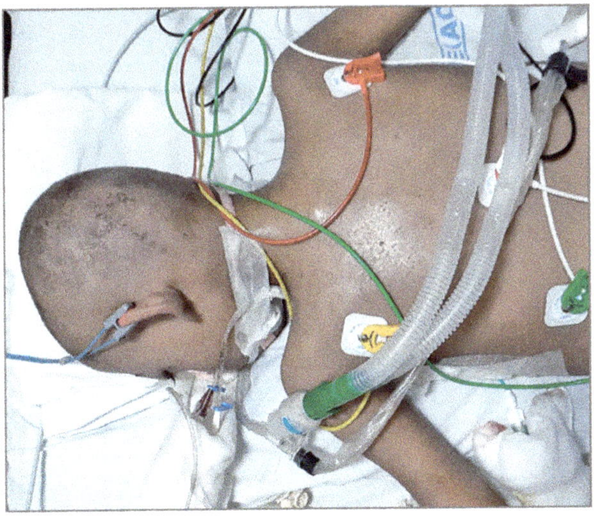

290. Identify the phase variables and the mode of ventilation given in the image.

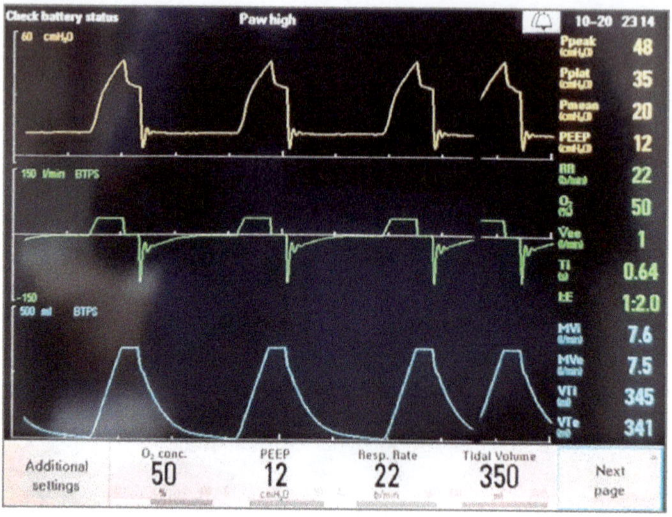

291. What is the significance of this value?

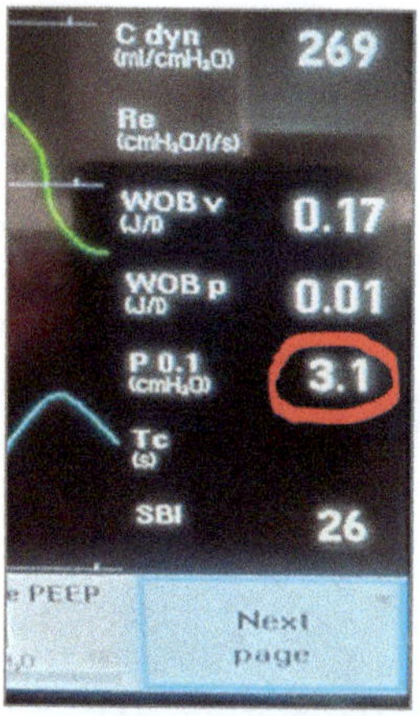

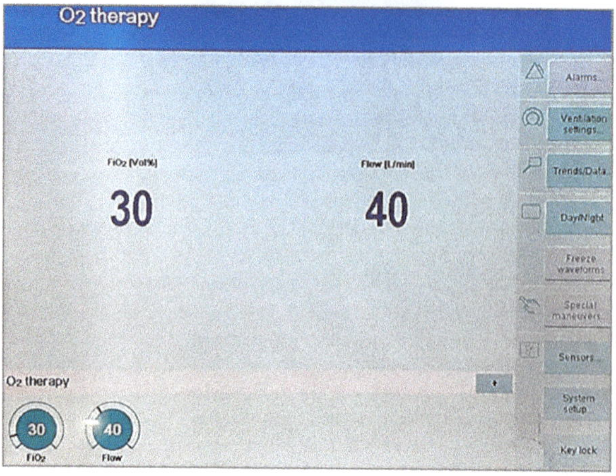

292. Enumerate the physiological benefits of high-flow nasal cannula (HFNC).

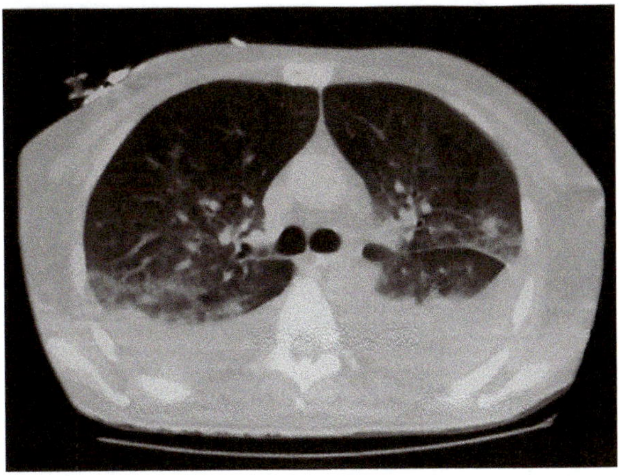

293. What is time constant?
   - What are slow or fast alveoli?

294. Calculate the static compliance, dynamic compliance, and power of mechanical ventilation for this patient.

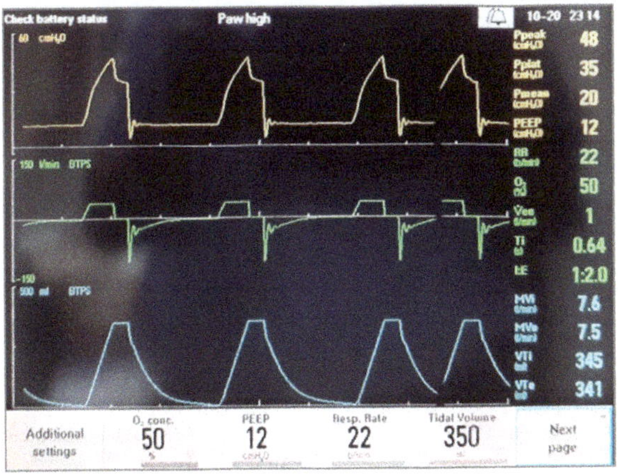

295. Identify the abnormality in this flow volume loop.

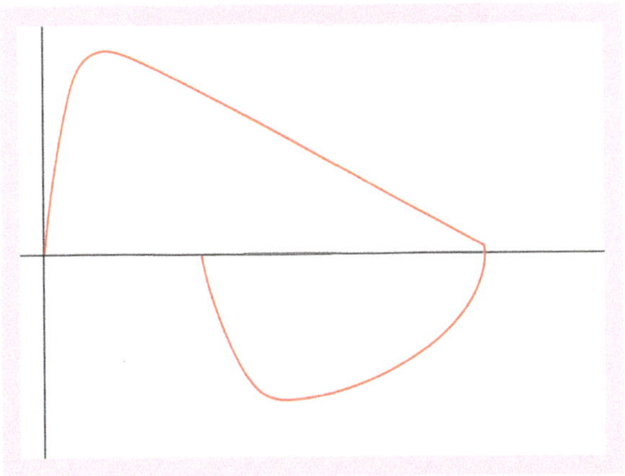

296. Identify the abnormality in the flow-time scalar.

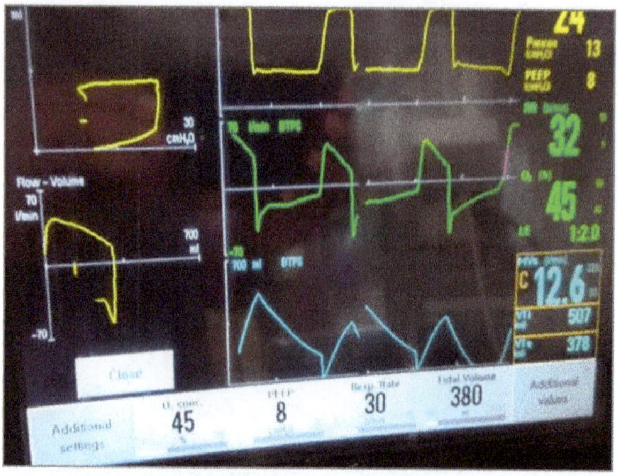

297. Identify the abnormality in the pressure-time scalar.

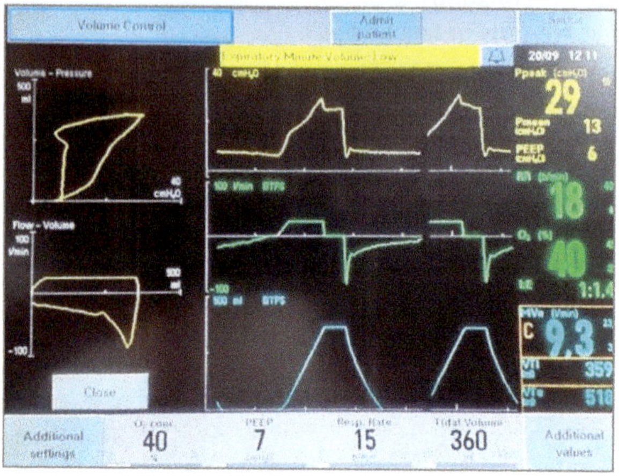

298. • What is the driving pressure in this case?
• What are the implications of driving pressure at the bed side?

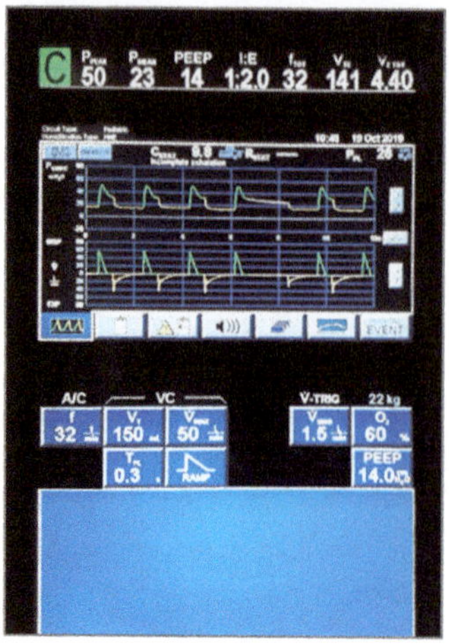

299. Write the equation of motion for a patient on mechanical ventilation.

300. What are the uses of capnography in ICU?

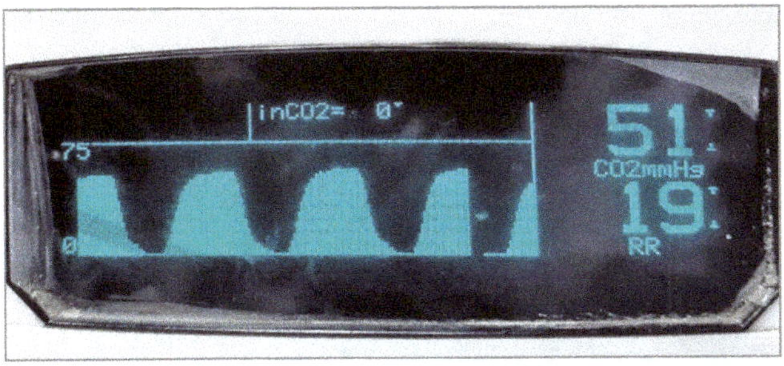

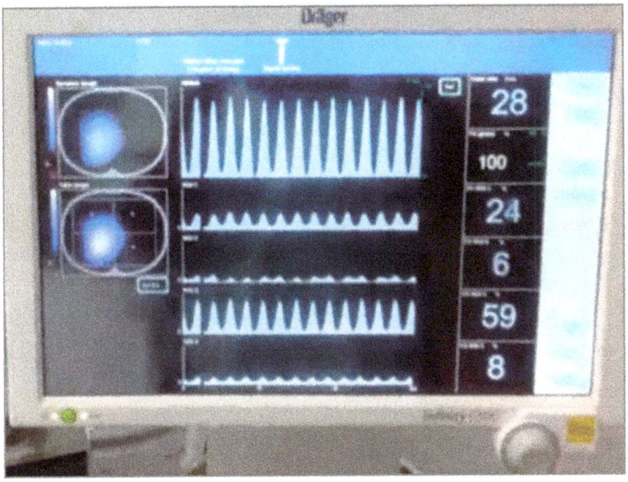

301. Identify the image and comment upon the current ventilation strategy.

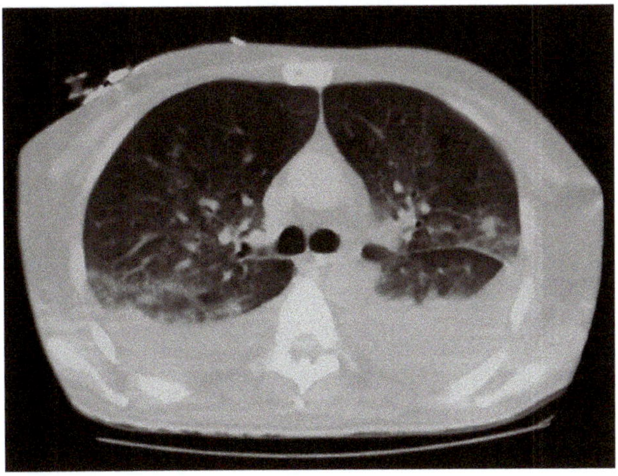

302. • What is recruitment maneuver?
- What are the ways it is done at bedside?
- How will you monitor a patient during recruitment?

303. Identify the type of asynchrony.

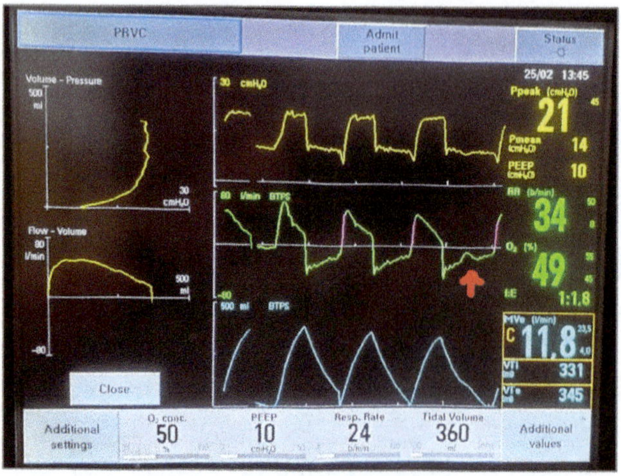

304. Identify the asynchrony in this Figure.

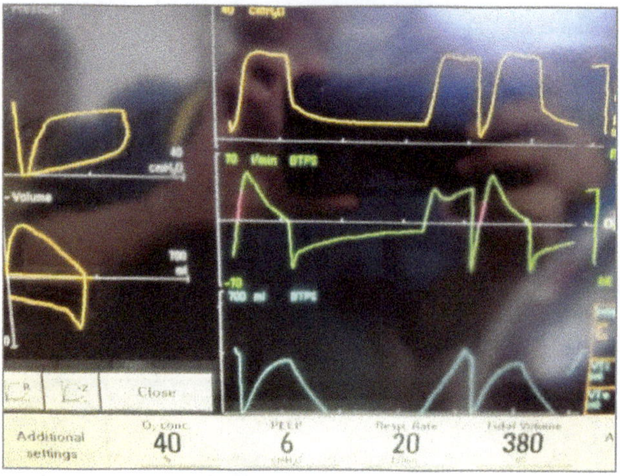

305. Your patient is on pressure-support ventilation as a part of weaning. Your respiratory therapist is worried about the set flow trigger. Do you agree? What are the problems with low- or high-sensitivity trigger?

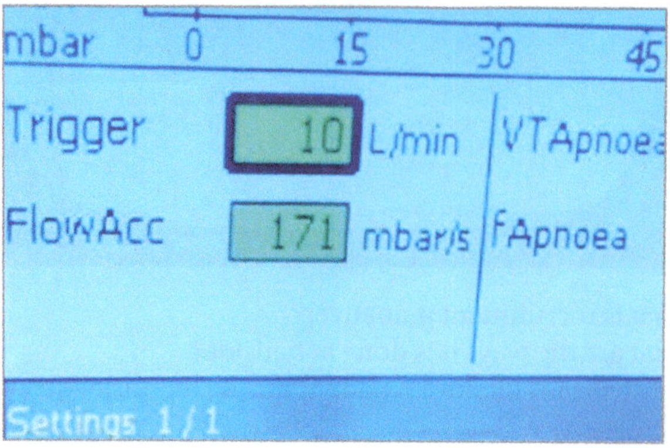

CASE SCENARIOS

306.

- A 24-year old male, is being referred to your intensive care unit (ICU) as a case of worsening hypoxia due to bilateral pneumonia. He was intubated 5 days back for type 1 respiratory failure and has been worsening, despite lung protective ventilation strategy over 3 days.
- There is a history of influenza A (H1N1) pneumonia 2 weeks back, and he was recovering when he developed fever and worsening of dyspnea.
- On arrival pulse rate (PR) 130/min, warm to touch, respiratory rate (RR) 32/min, blood pressure (BP) 90/70 mm Hg, oxygen saturation (SpO_2) 70%.
- Patient is being sedated and paralyzed and ventilated with 6 mL/kg predicted body weight (PBW) tidal volume, positive end-expiratory pressure (PEEP): 14, fraction of inspired oxygen (FiO_2): 1, and RR 32/min with plateau pressure (Pplat) 32 cmH_2O.
- Chest X-ray, arterial blood gas (ABG), bronchoalveolar lavage (BAL) specimen C/S reports are shown in images 1 to 3.
- Currently, he is on piperacillin tazobactam 4.5 g intravenous (IV) q6h.

Tata Hospital, 2 Floor ICU

Pat ID

First name

Blood Type Arterial

Blood Gas values (measured at 37. 0C)		
pH	7.05	(7.350 - 7.450)
PCO_2	90.6 mmHg	(35.0 - 45.0)
PO_2	37.4 mmHg	(80.0 - 100.0)
$cHCO_3$	24.15 mmol/L	
BE	-5 mmol/L	
BE(ecf)	-5.54 mmol/L	
tHb	9.3 g/dl	(11.5 - 17.40)
SO_2	70.8 %	(75.0 - 100)
SO_2 (c)	72.4 %	
Electrolytes		
Na^+	140.8 mmol/L	(135.0 - 148.0)
K^+	3.38 mmol/L	(3.50 - 4.50)
Cl^-	110.3 mmol/L	(98.0 - 107.0)
Ca^{++}	1.14 mmol/L	(1.15 - 1.29)
Metabolites		
Glu	114.9 mg/dl	(70 - 110)
Lac	2.6 mmol/L	(0.44 - 2.2)

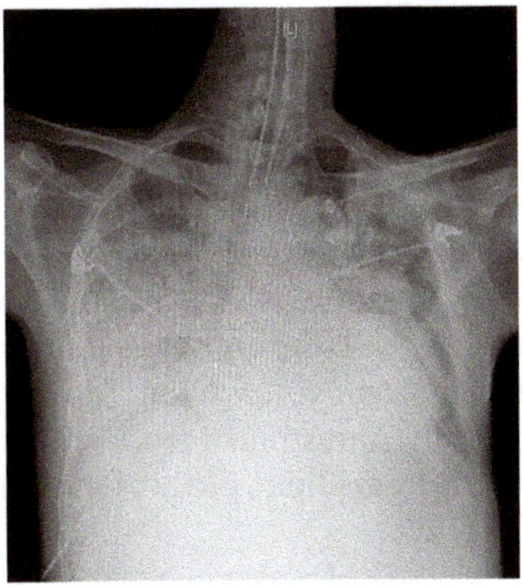

Methicillin	S
Erythromycin	S
Clindamycin	S
Amoxicillin clavulanate	S
Piperacillin tazobactam	S
Cefazolin	S
Ceftriaxone	S
Tetracycline	S
Ofloxacin	R
Imipenem	S
Inducible clindamycin resistance	Negative

- How will you optimize ventilation?
- What is the current evidence for recruitment maneuver, high-frequency oscillatory ventilation (HFOV), and proning?
- What is the role of bicarbonate in this case?
- What is your opinion on ECMO—in light of the recent evidence?

307.
- It was decided to initiate ECMO for this patient.
- Which configuration of ECMO do you prefer? Venoarterial (VA) or venovenous (VV)?
- What will be the preferred route of cannulation?
- What will be the initial ECMO set up?

308.
- Identify the ECMO circuit—VV/VA?
- What is the arrow pointing toward?

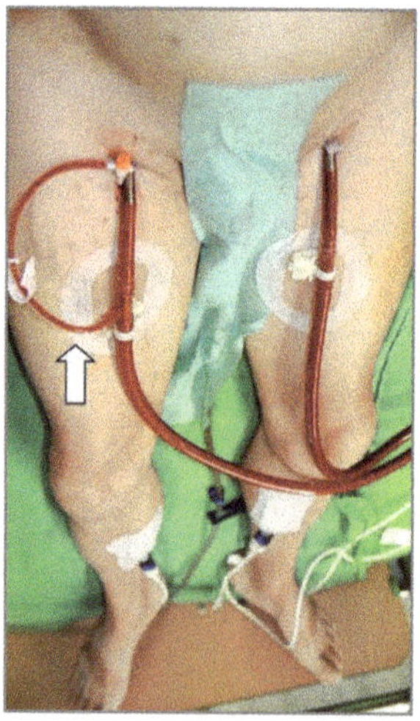

Source: Rupprecht L, Lunz D, Philipp A, Lubnow M, Schmid C. Pitfalls in percutaneous ECMO cannulation. Heart Lung Vessel. 2015;7(4):320-6.

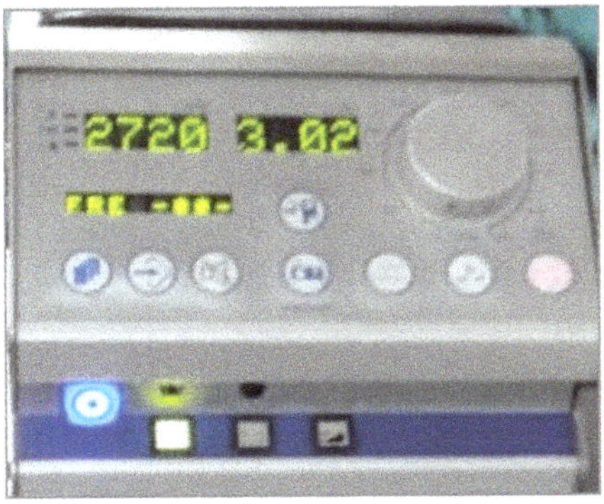

309. What is the difference in the initial blood flows in VA-ECMO vs. VV-ECMO?

310. Extracorporeal membrane oxygenation has been initiated and despite initiation of ECMO at 4.5 L/min, he has persistent hypoxemia—SpO_2 80%.
How will you troubleshoot the problem?

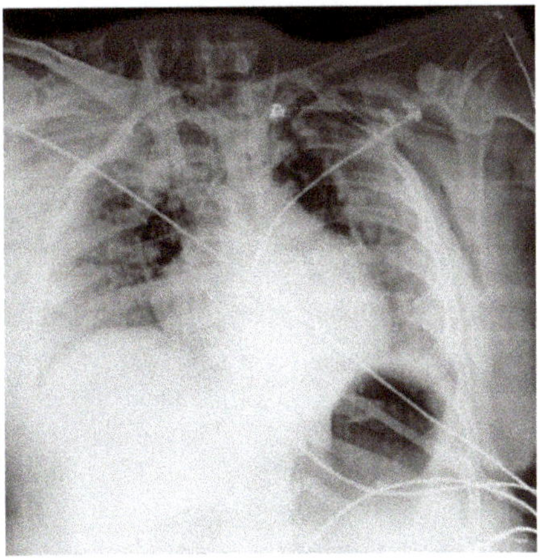

311. Recirculation was suspected and the cannulas were widely separated without compromising the ECMO flow. Saturation improved and the patient was continued with minimal ventilation along with ECMO.
    - How will you improve the CO_2 levels in this patient on ECMO?
    - What complications can occur in cases of wrong sweep gas flows?

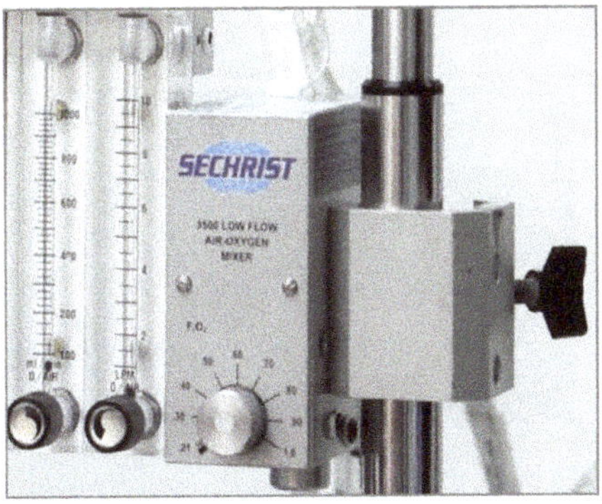

312. How will you monitor anticoagulation for a patient on ECMO?

313.
- After stable ventilation parameters, on the 4th day, the patient had a spike of fever—102°.
- His oxygen saturation also started to fall and is currently at 90% despite same ECMO flows and 100% FiO_2 on ECMO.

How will you optimize the situation? What is the current cause of the hypoxia?

314. Based on the available culture reports, how should the antibiotics be dosed on ECMO?

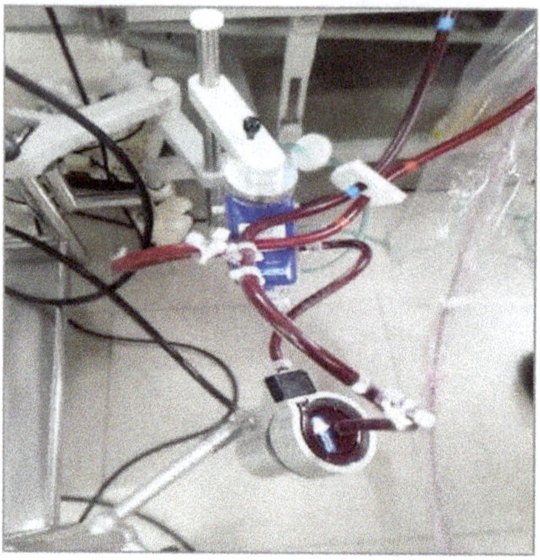

315.
- Both blood and BAL culture grew methicillin-sensitive *Staphylococcus aureus* (MSSA).
- Computed tomography (CT) thorax taken is shown in the image. Antibiotics were continued. However, he continued to have continuous high-grade fever.

What measures need to be taken urgently?

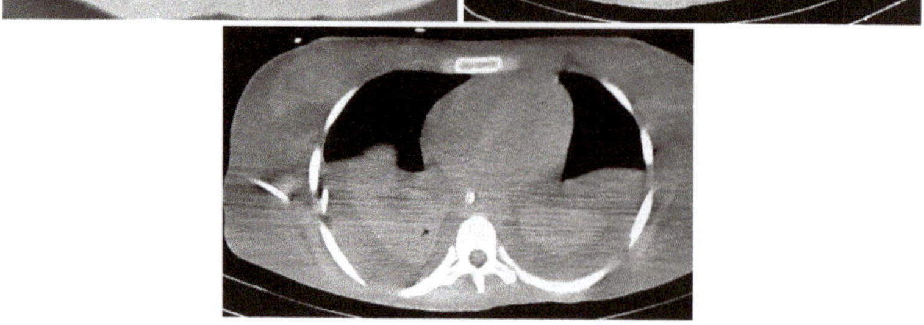

316. • What are Light's criteria for pleural effusion?
 • What are the indications for thoracocentesis in bilateral pleural effusion?
 • What all investigations need to be done on the pleural fluid?

317. • Bedside transesophageal echocardiography did not reveal any vegetation.
 • Bilateral implantable cardioverter defibrillators (ICDs) were inserted and empyema drained.
 • The fever settled and gradually patient improved.
 • How will you wean the patient?
 • What is the difference between weaning from ECMO in VA versus VV-ECMO?

318. What is Harlequin syndrome?

319. A patient is shifted back to the intensive care unit (ICU) after right-extended hepatectomy for elective ventilation, due to massive intraoperative blood loss. In the ICU, the registrar notices that all drains are oozy and patient is appearing pale with cold peripheries, and has trailing urine output.
 • On controlled ventilation, on noradrenalin of 0.3 μg/kg/min, he is having a regular heart rate (HR) of 140 beats/min, and a blood pressure of 100/76 mm Hg. Arterial blood gas (ABG) taken shows a combined metabolic and respiratory acidosis with a base excess of - 8 mmol/L and lactates of 5 mmol/L.
 • A thromboelastography (TEG) taken in the ICU is as shown. What is the possible cause of bleeding?
 • How will you manage the case?

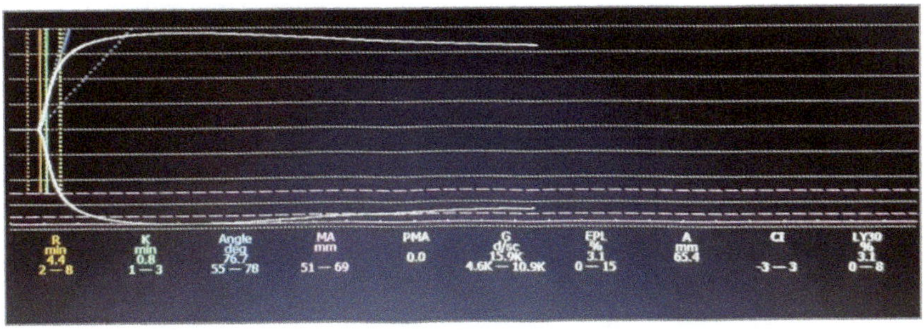

320. In the case of the patient discussed in Question 315, it was concluded that the patient was bleeding from a surgical cause and needs urgent exploration. Urgent blood is called for and massive transfusion protocol is initiated. What are the pretransfusion checklists undertaken by ICU team before transfusing blood products?

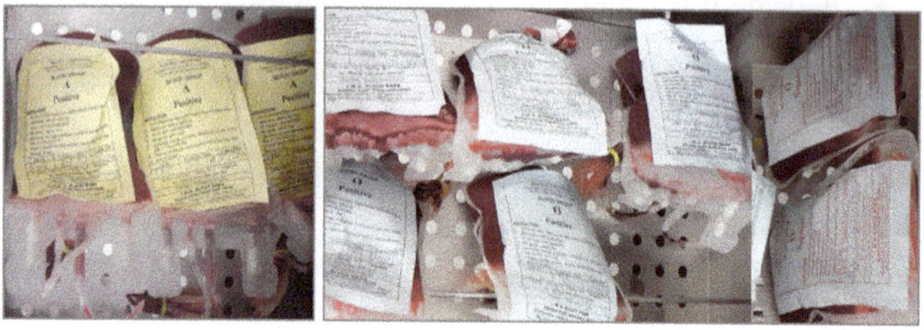

321. When and how will you initiate massive transfusion protocol? What will be the blood group of choice for packed red blood cell (PRBC) and plasma?

322. In the operating room (OR), an arterial bleeder was found and ligated. Blood and blood products were transfused as required in the OT. What are the complications of massive blood transfusion? How will you prevent them?

323. Postoperative period was significant as the patient required fraction of inspired oxygen (FiO_2) 0.8 and a PEEP of 12 cmH_2O to maintain peripheral capillary oxygen saturation (SpO_2) of 94%. How will you classify TRALI?

324. The peak pressure alarms on the mechanical ventilator started to go off frequently and the urine output also started to trail. He started to become hypotensive, not responding to fluid boluses of 250 mL given twice. ABG shows worsening of metabolic acidosis, hypoxia, and hypercarbia. The attending nurse notices that abdomen has become more tense. What is the diagnosis? How will you classify the condition? How will you explain oliguria despite maintained mean arterial pressure (MAP) and fluid boluses?

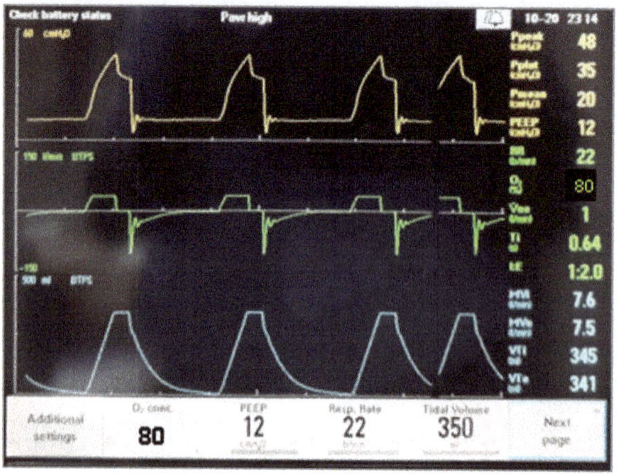

325. How will you measure IAP?

326. A 26-year-old male, teetotaler, with no addictions and no significant past history, presented to the out-patient department (OPD) with complaints of weakness of both legs and difficulty in walking of 24-hour duration. 6 weeks back, he had history of upper respiratory infection for 5 days, for which no medicines were taken. Clinical examination is significant for weakness in both lower limb—(power 3/5 bilateral) and a tonic pupil. Bilateral reflexes were mute. How will you interpret the electromyogram (EMG)?

Department of Neurosciences
Electrophysiology Lab
Nerve Conduction Study Report

Name:

Age:

Gender:

Reported by:

Diagnosis:

This Electrophysiological study includes

	Sampled nerve/muscles
Motor conduction Study	Right median, right ulnar, left Median, left ulnar, right peroneal, left peroneal, right tibial, left tibial, right femoral, left femoral
F waves study	Right median, right ulnar, left median, left ulnar, right peroneal, left peroneal, right tibial, left tibial
Sensory conduction study	Right median, right ulnar, left median, left ulnar, right sural, left sural, right superficial peroneal, left superficial peroneal

Interpretations

Motor conduction study showed reduced CMAP amplitude from bilateral median, ulnar, peroneal, and tibial nerves. Distal latencies were prolonged from bilateral median, ulnar and bilateral tibial nerves. Conduction velocities were normal from bilateral median, ulnar peroneal and tibial nerves.

F waves were absent from right peroneal and prolonged from bilateral median, ulnar, tibial and left peroneal nerves.

Sensory conduction study showed normal peak latency, normal amplitude and normal conduction velocity from bilateral sural, superficial peroneal, median and ulnar nerves.

327. It was decided to start plasmapheresis for the patient. How will you calculate the dosage of plasmapheresis in this patient? What are the other indications for plasmapheresis in ICU?

328. What is the KDIGO classification of AKI in iCU?

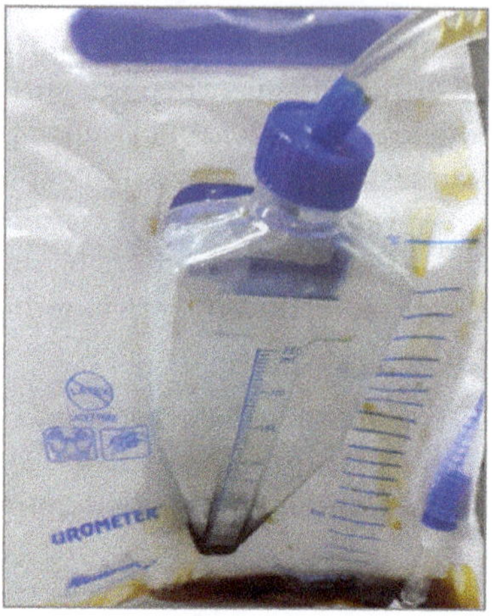

329. PF ratio reduced by 180, PEEP 5, FiO_2 40
- Leukocytosis: WBC 13,000/cm^3
- BAL sent grew *Enterococcus*
- The quality control asked your opinion whether this can be considered as a VAP or not. how will you opine?

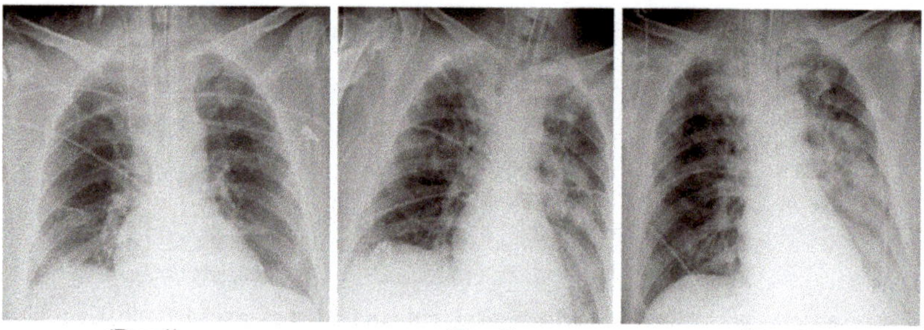

(Day 1)	(Day 2)	(Day 3)
PF ratio 380	PF ratio 260	PF Ratio 200
WBC count 9,800/cm^3	WBC count 8,600/cm^3	WBC count 13,000/cm^3

330. Identify the device kit.
- What is it used for?

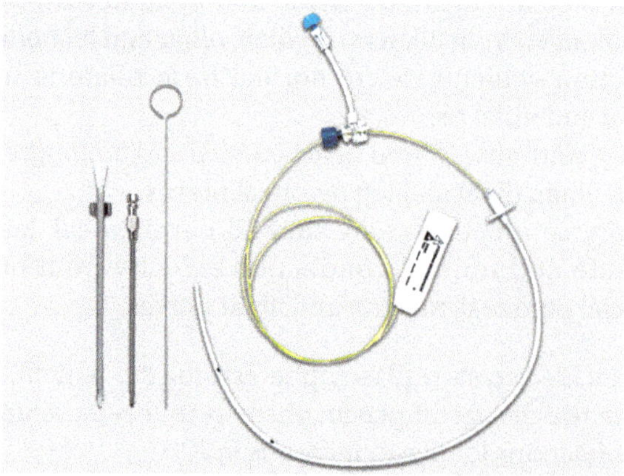

ANSWERS

RESPIRATORY MEDICINE

Ans. 1

- Chest X-ray shows bilateral pneumothorax with subcutaneous emphysema, pneumopericardium, and pneumoperitoneum. The patient needs to be evaluated for the risk of perforated hollow viscus and raised intra-abdominal pressure.
- Pneumoperitoneum can occur with bilateral pneumothoraxes in the absence of visceral injury and may need just observation.
- In this case, as the patient is having issues with ventilation, bilateral ICD may be placed and pneumothoraxes needs to be drained out. If no visceral injury is suspected, the patient may just be observed as pneumoperitoneum will resolve once pneumothorax is resolved and the intrathoracic pressure is decompressed.

Further Reading

Hakim SY, Abdelrahman H, Mudali IN, El-Menyar A, Peralta R, Al-Thani H. Pneumoperitoneum in a patient with pneumothorax and blunt neck trauma. Int J Surg Case Rep. 2014;5(12):1106-9.

Nishina M, Fujii C, Ogino R, Kobayashi R, Kohama A. Pneumoperitoneum and pneumoretroperitoneum in blunt trauma patients. J Trauma. 2000;49:565-6.

Ans. 2

- Chest X-ray shows tracheostomy tube *in situ* and ECG leads crossing the film.
- There is haziness of the left side suggestive of left-sided consolidation.
- The 4th rib appears fractured in the posterior aspect.
- There is left pneumothorax with an ICD *in situ* although the lung remains collapsed.

Ans. 3

- Deep sulcus sign.
- In the supine position, pneumothorax collects within the nondependent portions of the pleural space while in the upright position, the pneumothorax collects in the apicolateral location.
- In the ICU, collection of pneumothorax laterally deepens the lateral costophrenic angle and produces the deep sulcus sign.

Further Reading

Kong A. The deep sulcus sign. Radiology. 2003;228(2):415-6.

Ans. 4

- Image shows dissection of the ascending aorta with intimal flap. Dissections of the ascending aorta is to be treated as a surgical emergency with a mortality of 50% within the first 48 hours if surgery is not performed, while dissection of the descending thoracic and/or the abdominal aorta can often be managed medically.

- Management includes preparing for emergency by insertion of two large bore intravenous (IV) cannula, arterial line placement, and controlling the heart rate and blood pressure (target heart rate of <60 beats/min and systolic blood pressure between 100 and 120 mm Hg). This can be achieved by IV esmolol or labetalol or verapamil or diltiazem (if beta blockers are not tolerated).
- Once heart rate is controlled, sodium nitroprusside infusion or nicardipine infusion may be started for vasodilation and further blood pressure control.
- Pain needs to be managed with adequate analgesia.
- End organ perfusion needs to be monitored continuously.

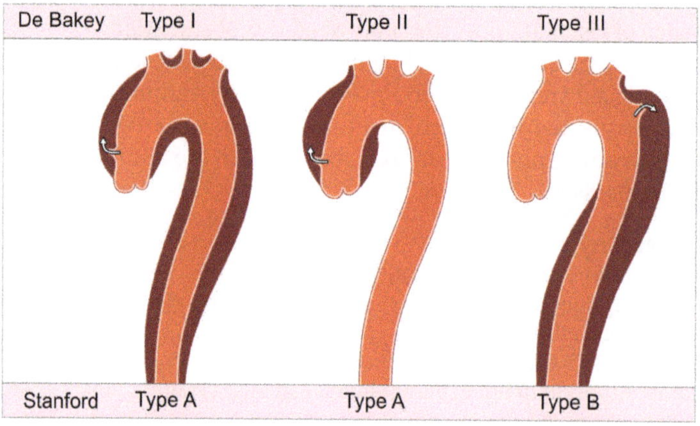

Further Reading

Fukui T. Management of acute aortic dissection and thoracic aortic rupture. J Intensive Care. 2018;6:15.

Ans. 5

CT shows a fistulous track between trachea and esophagus suggestive of trachea esophageal fistula. Initial general measures include oxygenation with supplemental oxygenation, restricted oral intake, elevating the head of the bed to 45°, prokinetic therapy, repeated oral suctioning, treating aspiration pneumonia, and removal of nasogastric tubes. The definitive treatment should be a consensus between experts of thoracic surgery, oncology, gastroenterology, and interventional pulmonary.

Further Reading

Chauhan SS, Long JD. Management of tracheoesophageal fistulas in adults. Curr Treat Options Gastro. 2004;7:31-40.

Ans. 6

- Although the PF ratio is <200, the CT scan shows mainly nodules which are probably metastatic in the background of choriocarcinoma.
- As per the Berlin definition, the presence of bilateral nodules does not classify under the definition of ARDS.

Further Reading

The ARDS Definition Task Force. Acute Respiratory Distress Syndrome: The Berlin Definition. JAMA. 2012;307(23):2526-33.

Ans. 7

- Lobar pneumonia—community acquired.
- CURB-65, PSI, ATS criteria for severe CAP
- *FLORALI study:* There is no significant reduction in intubation rate overall. More than 80% of these patients had pneumonia and type 1 failure.
- Subgroup analysis of patients with PaO_2:FiO_2 ≤200 mm Hg had a significant reduction in intubation rates with high-flow oxygen therapy. ICU and 90-day mortality rates were significantly lower in the HFNC group compared to NIV and oxygen alone groups.

Further Reading

Frat JP, Thille AW, Mercat A, Girault C, Ragot S, Perbet S, et al. High-flow oxygen through nasal cannula in acute hypoxemic respiratory failure. New Engl J Med. 2015;372(23):2185-96.

Ans. 8

- Cardiogenic pulmonary edema.
- In patients with cardiogenic pulmonary edema, the positive pressure aids in the inspiratory and expiratory flow, and supports the failing inspiratory muscles. By improving the functional residual capacity, CPAP decreases dead space ventilation, improves minute ventilation, and re-expands flooded alveoli thereby placing the respiratory pressure volume characteristics in a more favorable position.
- During systole, the intrathoracic positive pressure reduces the venous return, reduces transmural pressure facilitating left ventricular contractility, and thus decreases the intrathoracic volume. CPAP also causes a significant decrease in the heart rate, by increased parasympathetic tone in response to lung inflation.

Further Reading

Agarwal R, Aggarwal AN, Gupta D, Jindal S. Non-invasive ventilation in acute cardiogenic pulmonary oedema. Postgrad Med J. 2005;81(960):637-43.

Ans. 9

- The patient is having worsening of respiratory status within a week of known insult, having a PF ratio of 86 on PEEP of 16.
- As per the Berlin definition, he is having severe ARDS as the chest X-ray shows bilateral opacities that are unlikely to be collapse, effusion or nodules. In the absence of any known risk factors, a cardiac origin of edema is to be excluded by echocardiography.
- ARDS is classified as mild, moderate, and severe if the PaO_2/FiO_2 ratio is between 300–200 mm Hg, 200–100 mm Hg, and <100 mm Hg, respectively with a PEEP of at least 5 cm H_2O.

Further Reading

Fanelli V, Vlachou A, Ghannadian S, Simonetti U, Slutsky AS, Zhang H. Acute respiratory distress syndrome: new definition, current and future therapeutic options. J Thorac Dis. 2013;5(3):326-34.

Ans. 10

- The chest X-ray shows central line in situ in the correct position. The endotracheal tube has migrated inside the right main stem bronchus with resultant right main stem intubation which explains the high peak and plateau pressures due to a single lung ventilation.
- The worsening hypoxia may be due to impending left lung collapse.
- The endotracheal tube needs to be pulled out urgently.

Further Reading

Ganti L, Shivdat J, Bawany S. Back to Basics: Endotracheal Tube Too Deep, Too Shallow, Then Just Right. Cureus. 2018;10(5):e2706.

Ans. 11. Dual chamber pacing.

Class 1 indications	• Documented symptomatic sinus bradycardia or • Symptomatic chronotropic incompetence
	• Third-degree AV block • Symptomatic second-degree AV block • Mobitz II with widened QRS complex • Recurrent syncope caused by spontaneously occurring carotid sinus stimulation

Further Reading

Dalia T, Amr BS. Pacemaker Indications. Treasure Island (FL): StatPearls Publishing; 2020.

Ans. 12

- Poor quality of chest X-ray that shows ECG leads, bilateral perihilar consolidation right more than left, appropriately positioned endotracheal tube, and deep sulcus sign left side.
- The right side also shows the guidewire coiled inside the thorax suggestive of guidewire embolization.
- Ultrasound to rule out left-sided pneumothorax, interventional radiology consult for retrieving the guidewire.
- Incident reporting and formulation of guidelines for central line insertion including training and use of ultrasound guidance for central line insertion, and management protocols for treating complications are required.

Further Reading

Kusminsky RE. Complications of central venous catheterization. J Am Coll Surg. 2007;204(4):681-96.

Ans. 13

- Ultrasound of the thorax showing homogeneous pleural effusion (PLEFF) with no internal echoes or septations and collapse of the lung which is also seen floating in the effusion. No air bronchogram is seen.
- An interpleural distance of >45 mm at the right thoracic base or >50 mm at the left thoracic base predicted PLEFF of >800 mL.
- Differential diagnosis transudative effusion versus malignant effusion.

Further Reading

Brogi E, Gargani L, Bignami E, Barbariol F, Marra A, Forfori F, et al. Thoracic ultrasound for pleural effusion in the intensive care unit: a narrative review from diagnosis to treatment. Crit Care. 2017;21(1):325.

Ans. 14

- HeartMate (left ventricular assist device) with pacemaker
- The new generation cardiac assist devices use the continuous-flow pumps and generate a pulseless flow and pulseless state. Identifying a cardiac arrest may be difficult in these patients and the examination findings like skin color and capillary refill are reasonable predictors of the presence of adequate flow and perfusion. In cases of inadequate perfusion, unresponsiveness, or other altered mental state, the ventricular assist device (VAD) function should be assessed by looking and listening for alarms, VAD hum on the left chest and left hypochondrium, and checking the device connections and adequate power for the VAD.
- Waveform capnography can also be used to track perfusion in patients in whom the physical findings that are commonly used to assess perfusion are not reliable.

Further Reading

Peberdy MA, Gluck JA, Ornato JP, Bermudez CA, Griffin RE, Kasirajan V, et al. Cardiopulmonary Resuscitation in Adults and Children With Mechanical Circulatory Support: A Scientific Statement From the American Heart Association. Circulation. 2017;135:e1115-34.

Sen A, Larson JS, Kashani KB, Libricz SL, Patel BM, Guru PK, et al. Mechanical circulatory assist devices: a primer for critical care and emergency physicians. Crit Care. 2016;20(1):153.

Ans. 15

- The chest X-ray shows extensive subcutaneous emphysema, presence of ECG leads, and bilateral intercostal tube drainage with unexpanded right lung.
- The Ryles tube is also mispositioned with the tip still inside the thorax. The placement of Ryles tube, whether intrapulmonary or intraesophageal, needs to be confirmed prior to administering anything through it.

Ans. 16

- Chest X-ray of the patient shows bilateral cavities with surrounding consolidation and air fluid level.
- Differential diagnosis incudes infection by anaerobic organisms causing lung abscess due to aspiration, tuberculosis, septic emboli, and metastatic lesions.
- Initial management includes sending sputum for Gram stain, AFB stain and culture, and blood for culture, measuring lactate levels, and initiation of broad-spectrum antibiotics along with chest physiotherapy and drainage. Patient needs isolation for airborne infection until tuberculosis is ruled out.
- Preferably avoid fluoroquinolones as empiric therapy in these patients till TB is ruled out.

Further Reading

Gadkowski LB, Stout JE. Cavitary pulmonary disease. Clin Microbiol Rev. 2008;21(2):305-33.

Ans. 17

Chest X-ray shows massive right-sided pleural effusion with Ellis curve. Light's criteria for exudative effusion is any one of the following:

Presence of:

- Pleural fluid protein/serum protein >0.5
- Pleural fluid LDH/serum LDH >0.6
- Pleural fluid LDH more than two-thirds of upper limit of serum LDH value. Recently two-thirds has been changed to .45.

In all cases of effusion, diagnostic workup includes a thoracocentesis and fluid should be sent for pleural fluid protein, LDH, sugar, Gram stain and culture, AFB smear, and fungal smear. Presence of pus, low pH, and low sugar should raise the suspicion of empyema and intercostal drainage may be required.

For suspected cases of TB, pleural fluid should be sent for biochemistry, cytology, ADA, interferon gamma levels, and pleural fluid culture.

Further Reading

Saguil A, Wyrick K, Hallgren J. Diagnostic approach to pleural effusion. Am Fam Physician. 2014;90(2):99-104.

Ans. 18

Chest X-ray showing right-sided hydropneumothorax—possibly iatrogenic during coughing thereby causing respiratory distress. The patient needs to be observed closely with monitoring of respiration and saturation. In case of clinical worsening, intercostal drainage via chest tubes or pigtail can be inserted.

Further Reading

Gordon CE, Feller-Kopman D, Balk EM, Smetana GW. Pneumothorax following thoracentesis: a systematic review and meta-analysis. Arch Intern Med. 2010;170(4):332-9.

Ans. 19

CT chest shows diffuse interstitial opacification and ground glassing/mosaic appearance of both lungs.

Differentials for such pattern include:

- *Pneumocystis carinii* pneumonia
- *Mycobacterium tuberculosis,* atypical mycobacteria
- Viral pneumonia
- Mixed infections
- Fungal infections like *Cryptococcus*
- Noninfectious causes such as nonspecific interstitial pneumonia, lymphocytic interstitial pneumonitis, and Kaposi sarcoma.

Management will include investigations preferably a bronchoalveolar lavage with samples sent for Gram stain and special stains, cultures, PCR and broad-spectrum antibiotics, therapeutic dose of cotrimoxazole and oseltamivir. Corticosteroids need to be added early in the disease course for widened A-a dO_2 gap.

Further Reading

Allen CM, Al-Jahdali HH, Irion KL, Al Ghanem S, Gouda A, Khan AN. Imaging lung manifestations of HIV/AIDS. Ann Thorac Med. 2010;5(4):201-16.

Ans. 20

CT image shows diffuse small nodules distributed randomly.

Differentials include:

- Miliary tuberculosis
- *Cytomegalovirus* infection
- Histoplasmosis
- Healed varicella infection
- Pneumoconiosis like silicosis, coal workers pneumoconiosis
- Hypersensitivity pneumonitis
- Sarcoidosis, etc.

Further Reading

Sharma BB. Miliary nodules on chest radiographs: A diagnostic dilemma. Lung India. 2015;32(5):518-20.

Ans. 21

- CT angiogram showing filling defect in the bifurcation of the main pulmonary artery and left pulmonary artery suggestive of saddle thrombus and left-sided pulmonary thromboembolism.
- The indication for thrombolysis is hemodynamic instability defined as cardiac arrest needing resuscitation or persistent hypotension not caused by other pathologies.
- Hypotension in pulmonary embolism is managed by cautious volume loading with saline or Ringer's lactate in patients with normal or low central venous pressure.
- Norepinephrine in doses of 0.2–1.0 mg/kg/min increases RV inotropy and systemic blood pressure and promotes positive ventricular interactions, and restores coronary perfusion gradient while dobutamine in doses of 2–20 mg/kg/min may increase RV inotropy, lowers filling pressures although there is risk of systemic vasodilation and hypotension.

Ans. 22

- Left-sided pneumothorax with subclavian cannula *in situ.*
- Pneumothorax is the most common complications of central line insertions with an incidence 1-6.6%.
- The incidence of pneumothorax goes up with the number of needle passes from 4.3% in single pass insertion to 24% after second insertion.
- The treatment strategy for pneumothorax in this case will depend upon the size of the pneumothorax, patient's symptoms, whether breathing spontaneously or on mechanical ventilation, and a clinical diagnosis of tension pneumothorax. Pneumothoraces in asymptomatic patients who are not on positive pressure ventilation may be observed closely and with repeat X-rays. In patients who are symptomatic, or at risk of developing tension pneumothorax, a Heimlich valve or intercoastal tube drainage may be considered.

Further Reading

Kusminsky RE. Complications of central venous catheterization. J Am Coll Surg. 2007;204(4):681-96.

Tsotsolis N, Tsirgogianni K, Kioumis I, Pitsiou G, Baka S, Papaiwannou A, et al. Pneumothorax as a complication of central venous catheter insertion. Ann Transl Med. 2015;3(3):40.

Ans. 23

- Ultrasound image showing multiple B lines across all lung fields suggestive of interstitial thickening or edema. Although up to 3 B lines can be normal, presence of confluent bilateral B lines suggests development of pulmonary edema.
- In ARDS, apart from bilateral B lines of pulmonary edema, the presence of heterogeneously spared areas of lung posterior lung consolidations with air bronchograms, and coarse appearance of pleural line may suggest ARDS.

Further Reading

Copetti R, Soldati G, Copetti P. Chest sonography: a useful tool to differentiate acute cardiogenic pulmonary edema from acute respiratory distress syndrome. Cardiovasc Ultrasound. 2008;6:16.

Ans. 24

- *First image:* LUS aeration 2; Second image: LUS 2; Third image: LUS 1.
- Score of 0 is assigned to a lung region if all of the intercostal spaces show normal aeration pattern—lung sliding, horizontal A lines, and less than 3 B lines.
- Score of 1 is assigned if the intercostal spaces show multiple B lines that originate from pleural line or from juxta-pleural consolidations.
- Score of 2 is assigned to the examined region if there are coalescent B lines.
- Score of 3 is assigned if there is lung consolidation, with static or dynamic air bronchograms.
- The scores of the 12 examined regions are summed to calculate the LUS score, which ranges between 0 and 36.

Further Reading

Bouhemad B, Brisson H, Le-Guen M, Arbelot C, Lu Q, Rouby JJ. Bedside ultrasound assessment of positive end-expiratory pressure-induced lung recruitment. Am J Respir Crit Care Med. 2011;183:341-7.

Ans. 25

- RR = 30/min
- IE ratio 1:1
- Ti = 1 second
- Te = 1 second
- For constant flow-volume ventilation, with triangular airway pressure waveform Paw can be calculated as:
  Paw = 0.5 × (PIP – PEEP) × (TI /Ttot) + PEEP (assuming similar resistance during inspiration and expiration)
  $0.5 \times (36 - 16) \times ½ + 16 = 21\ cmH_2O$
- Oxygenation index (OI) = Mean Airway Pressure × FiO_2 × 100/PaO_2
  = 21 × 1 × 100/80
  = 26.25

Further Reading

Hess DR. Respiratory mechanics in mechanically ventilated patients. Respir Care. 2014;59(11):1773-94.

Ans. 26

- RR = 30/min
- IE ratio 1:1
- Ti = 1 second
- Te = 1 second
- In pressure control ventilation, Paw can be estimated as:
  Paw = (PIP – PEEP) × (TI/Ttot) + PEEP
  = (28 – 16) × ½+ 16 = 22 mm Hg
- Oxygenation index = Mean airway pressure × FiO_2 × 100/PaO_2
  .= 22 × 1 × 100/80 = 27.5
  Traditionally, OI has been used to guide escalation of respiratory support to high-frequency ventilation (OI >20) and extracorporeal membrane oxygenation (OI >40) in pediatric ARDS.

Further Reading

Hess DR. Respiratory mechanics in mechanically ventilated patients. Respir Care. 2014;59(11):1773-94.

Ans. 27

- CT scan is showing dense consolidation on the right side with halo sign.
- The halo sign was initially described in immunocompromised patients with angioinvasive *Aspergillus* infection of the lung and is thought to be due to the perilesional hemorrhage around a lung nodule.
- It has also been described in other fungal infections of the lung such as mucormycosis, candidiasis, cryptococcosis, and coccidioidomycosis.
- It has also been described in viral infections such as herpes simplex virus, varicella-zoster virus, and cytomegalovirus and in systemic diseases such as Wegener granulomatosis.
- As this patient has not improved on broad-spectrum empiric therapy, antifungal therapy may be considered as an empiric therapy. Simultaneously a serum or paired serum and BAL galactomannan also may be sent and, if elevated, are suggestive of invasive mold infections.
- Voriconazole is the drug of choice for empiric treatment of aspergillosis and should be administered IV to avoid the variability in bioavailability issues. Liposomal amphotericin B is the preferred drug in case of suspected mucormycosis.

Ans. 28

Acceptability criteria for spirograms are that they should be free from artifacts such as coughing, early glottis closure or early termination submaximal effort, and leak or mouth piece occlusion, have good starts, and should show satisfactory exhalation, i.e. a duration of at least 6 seconds or a plateau in the volume–time curve.

- In this spirogram, looking at the V-T graph, the acceptability criteria of blowing at least 6 seconds or a plateau has not been met.
- The performer has also coughed in the first second with an abrupt end of the expiratory effort and subsequent poor inspiratory effort.
- Hence, this spirogram is not acceptable and should not be used for clinical decision making.

Further Reading

Acceptability criteria in Spirometry (ATS/ERS guidelines Standardisation of Lung function testing. ERJ; 2005.

Miller MR, Hankinson J, Brusasco V, Burgos F, Casaburi R, Coates A, et al. Standardisation of spirometry. Eur Respir J. 2005;26(2):319-38.

Ans. 29

1. Confirm patient data and history
2. Look at the flow-volume loop and the volume time (V-T) graph for acceptability.
   - *Identity:* Concealed
   - *History:* Not provided
   - *Acceptability:* Met
   - *FEV_1/FVC:* >80
   - *FEV_1:* 101%
   - *Impression:* Normal PFT
   - *Comment:* Although the spirometry is reported as normal, during inspiration the flow-volume loop is getting flattened suggesting a variable extrathoracic obstruction of the upper airways, e.g. multinodular goiter. This needs to be correlated with the clinical history.

Ans. 30

The flow-volume loop suggests a flattening of both the inspiratory and expiratory portion of the flow-volume loop which is typically seen in a fixed airway obstruction of the upper airways probably due to fibrotic subglottic stenosis after tracheostomy.

The spirometry values however seem normal.

Ans. 31

- *Identity:* Concealed
- *History:* CCOPD with mMRC grade 3 dyspnea
- *Acceptability:* Met
- *FEV_1/FVC:* 33% suggestive of obstructive pathology
- *FEV_1:* 21% of predicted suggestive of severe obstruction
- *Spirometry classification:* Very severe obstruction
- *Suggestion:* To perform bronchodilator reversibility test
- The grading of COPD now follows the revised ABCD classification as per GOLD 2017 guidelines
- Once COPD is diagnosed, the airflow limitation is assessed—here it is 21.4% which is GOLD grade 4 and then a exacerbation history and current symptom assessment is made. His symptom assessment shows he has a dyspnea grade >2 mMRC. The above patient has >1 hospital admissions which puts him into a exacerbation prone phenotype. He, therefore, is now GOLD grade 4, group D.
- As such he can be given a long-acting muscarinic agent as first choice. Additional long-acting beta-2 agonist (LABA) can be given since he is very symptomatic. Inhaled steroid along with the LABA can be given if the absolute eosinophil count is >300/mm^3, the patient should be advised regarding adequate vaccination (pneumococcal and influenza vaccines). ROFLUMILAST is also another option to reduce frequency of exacerbations.

Further Reading

Gold guidelines 2019.

Ans. 32

- *Identity:* Concealed
- *History:* Not provided
- *Acceptability:* Met
- *FEV_1/FVC:* 93% suggestive of normal or restrictive pathology
- *FEV_1:* 76% suggesting normal spirometry

Though the spirometry lung volumes have only mild reduction in volumes, the flow-volume loop suggests a flattening of the inspiratory portion of the flow-volume loop. This is seen in a variable obstruction of the upper airways at the extrathoracic portion, e.g. multinodular goiter.

Ans. 33

- Clinically, this patient is tachycardic, tachypneic with hypotension, and having a low diastolic blood pressure suggestive of a vasodilatory shock.
- For assessing validity of an ABG, we need a simultaneous serum bicarbonate. Using the same bicarbonate in the ABG does not make sense as the machine also has derived it with the same formula you are going to use. The use of validity comes only in cases where there is a possibility of transcription of ABG values and not a point of care result.
- The P/F ratio is more than 400.
- There is an acidosis which is mainly a high anion gap metabolic acidosis (HAGMA) with hyperglycemia, probably spurious hyponatremia and hyperkalemia—anion gap of 31.3 (inclusive of potassium) with appropriate respiratory compensation. Correction for albumin is not provided in the question.
- The delta gap = $(31.3 - 12)/(24 - 3) = 0.9$ which is in normal range ruling out a nonanion metabolic acidosis.
- The likely differentials are diabetic ketoacidosis in the background of a septic shock (due to the severely vasodilated state) with lactic acidosis.
- Hypocalcemia would also point to a differential diagnosis of ethylene glycol toxicity and we need to calculate the osmolar gap and check for urine oxalate crystals.

Further Reading

Adrogué HJ, Madias NE. Management of life-threatening acid-base disorders. First of two parts. N Engl J Med. 1998;338(1):26-34.

Adrogué HJ, Madias NE. Management of life-threatening acid-base disorders. Second of two parts. N Engl J Med. 1998;338(2):107-11.

Ans. 34

- Spurious hyponatremia due to hypertonicity from hyperglycemia—hypertonic hyponatremia.
- The corrected sodium will be $114 + 2.4 \times (886 - 100)/100 = 114 + 19 = 133$ mmol/L.
- This hyponatremia does not need correction and correction of hyperglycemia per se will bring the sodium levels to normal.

Ans. 35

- Dengue disease course

Day	*1–3*	*4–6*	*7–10*
Temperature	Febrile	Afebrile	Afebrile
Course	Stable	Critically ill	Recovery
Laboratory	Viremia HCT, PLC normal	NS1 HCT increase PLC decrease	IgM/IgG Recovery
Issues	Dehydration	Shock and organ damage	Resolution of third spacing

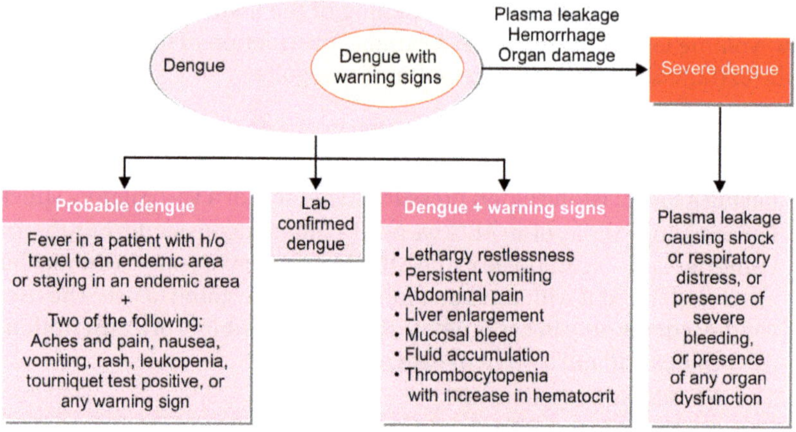

WHO classification of dengue 2009

- PF ratio = 130; moderate ARDS due to plasma leakage—laboratory confirmed severe dengue
- Patient needs guarded fluid resuscitation and respiratory support
- Oxygen, high flow nasal oxygen, and noninvasive ventilation (NIV) may be applied
- The goals of fluid resuscitation include improving central and peripheral circulation which can be detected by a reduction in tachycardia, improvement in pulse pressure, improvement in temperature of the extremities, improvement in blood pressure, improvement in pulse volume, and a markedly improved capillary refill time, without causing fluid overload.
- Obtain a reference hematocrit before fluid therapy.
- Watch out for clinical signs of shock including heart rate, blood pressure, pulse pressure, tissue hypoperfusion such as capillary refill time, lactate, organ dysfunction, etc.
- In case of hypotension or tissue hypoperfusion, start resuscitation with isotonic solutions such as 0.9% saline, Ringer's lactate at a rate of 5–7 mL/kg/h for 1–2 hours, then 3–5 mL/kg/h for 2–4 hours, and then 2–3 mL/kg/h or even less according to the clinical response and oxygen saturation.

During fluid resuscitation:

- Patient's clinical conditions same—hematocrit remains the same or rises minimally—continue with the same rate of fluid administration and reassess

- Patient's clinical condition worsens and develops shock—hematocrit is rising rapidly—increase the rate of fluid administration or colloid administration
- Patient's clinical condition worsens and develops shock with a drop in hematocrit—consider blood transfusion.
- Maintain the minimum intravenous fluid rate so that a good perfusion is maintained and urine output is more than 0.5 mL/kg/h.
- Maintain a detailed intake-output chart.
- Monitor vital signs, perfusion parameters, and organ function.
- During the recovery phase, as the fluids in the third space re-enter the circulation, there will be resolution of pleural effusion and ascites and an improved diuresis. Intravenous fluids need to be reduced or stopped at that point to prevent further fluid overload.
- The clinical signs will be a stable vital sign including normalizing pulse rate, pulse pressure, blood pressure, pulse, and adequate peripheral perfusion.
- The hematocrit decreases in the presence stable vital signs.
- Patient remains afebrile for more than 24–48 days.
- There is resolution of bowel/abdominal symptoms with an improving urine output.
- If the patient is hemodynamically stable and is afebrile for more than 24–48 hours, intravenous fluids may be stopped although he needs to be monitored closely.
- Diuretics may be given for active de-resuscitation.
- However, during the phase of plasma leakage, diuretics are better avoided as it may lead to intravascular volume depletion.

Further Reading

World Health Organization. (2009). Dengue: Guidelines for Diagnosis, Treatment, Prevention and Control. WHO/HTM/NTD/DEN/2009.1. [online] Available from https://apps.who.int/iris/handle/10665/44188 [Last accessed February, 2020].

Ans. 36

- In the ABG, assessment of oxygenation indicates a P/F ratio of 133. There is a normal anion gap metabolic acidosis due to hyperchloremia, anion gap of 9, with an additional respiratory acidosis. Although there is a high lactates it is not reflected in the calculation, probably as albumin is not included in the calculation.
- A-a gradient = 621.4 - 107 = 514.4
- The expected A-a gradient is approximately 14. A very wide A-a gradient is seen. The response of the A-a gradient to increasing levels of FiO_2 needs to be assessed to differentiate between a shunt or a VQ mismatch.

Further Reading

Masotti L, Ceccarelli E, Cappelli R, Barabesi L, Forconi S. Arterial blood gas analysis and alveolar-arterial oxygen gradient in diagnosis and prognosis of elderly patients with suspected pulmonary embolism. J Gerontology. 2000;55(12):M761-4.

Ans. 37

- *pH:* Reduced
- *PCO_2:* Reduced

- *HCO_3:* Reduced
- Suggesting a metabolic acidosis with respiratory compensation
- Expected compensation = 9.4 × 1.5 + 8 = 22.1 ± 2
  Hence, there is added respiratory acidosis also.
- ABG shows normal PaO_2 levels, PF ratio, and A-a DO_2 cannot be calculated as FiO_2 is not given
- High anion gap metabolic acidosis with an anion gap of 26.6 (probably due to lactic acidosis) along with a respiratory acidosis—assuming normal albumin levels
- Delta AG = 14.6/14.6 = 1
- There is no hidden metabolic alkalosis
- From the history, the patient is in a state of altered mentation, and is tachypneic; satisfying 2/3 of the q-SOFA score for a possible diagnosis of sepsis
- *Management includes:*
  - Measurement of lactates; remeasure lactates as here it is already more than 2 mmol/L
  - Obtain cultures—from local site and blood
  - Administer broad-spectrum antibiotics
  - Initiate administration of 30 mL/kg fluids as there is lactate >4 mmol/L
  - Measure blood pressure and initiate vasopressors if MAP <65 mm Hg, during or after fluid resuscitation
  - Surgical consult for urgent source control.

Further Reading

Levy MM, Evans LE, Rhodes A. The Surviving Sepsis Campaign Bundle: 2018 update. Intensive Care Med. 2018;44(6):925-8.

Ans. 38

- Severe acidemia can lead to reduced left ventricular contractility, arterial vasodilation, arrhythmias, and a blunted response to catecholamines. The current practice is to initiate bicarbonate therapy in metabolic acidosis, when acidosis is severe (pH <7.1) or pH is 7.1–7.2. A similar strategy has been used in ARDSNET trial also for acidosis with pH less than 7.15 during lung protective ventilation.
- Sodium bicarbonate is usually available as 8.4% (50 mEq/50 mL) or 7.2% (44.6 mEq/50 mL).
- In a randomized trial (BICAR-ICU), in a select group of patients (metabolic acidosis with pH < 7.20, HCO_3 < 20 and $PaCO_2$ < 45, with lactate > 2 mmol/L and SOFA score > 4), targeting a pH of 7.30 with administration of 4.2% soda bicarbonate (a maximum of 1 L in 24 hours)—although the mortality was not reduced, in patients with AKIN score II–III, bicarbonate therapy seemed to reduce mortality (46% vs. 63%) at 28 days with a significant reduction in need of dialysis from 52 to 35% and reduced incidence of hyperkalemia.

Further Reading

Jaber S, Paugam C, Futier E, Lefrant JY, Lescot T, Pottecher J, et al. Sodium bicarbonate therapy for patients with severe metabolic acidaemia in the intensive care unit (BICAR-ICU): a multicentre, open-label, randomised controlled, phase 3 trial. Lancet. 2018;392(10141):31-40.

Ans. 39

- *ABG:* Acidosis
- *PCO_2:* Respiratory acidosis
- *Bicarbonate:* Reduced—added metabolic acidosis
- Change in PCO_2 = 86 mm Hg
- Expected change in pH in the acute respiratory acidosis is 8.64 × 0.08 = 0.69, expected pH = 7.4 - 0.69 = 6.7
- In case of chronic respiratory failure, expected change in pH = 8.64 × 0.03 = 0.26, and expected pH = 7.4 - 0.26 = 7.14.
- Anion gap = 32.07—HAGMA
- Change in anion gap AG = 20
- Change in HCO_3 = 6.6
- Delta ratio > 2 suggesting a chronic respiratory acidosis or a superadded metabolic alkalosis
- Oxygenation - PF ratio >316
- PAO_2 = 285.2 - 157.5 = 127.7
- A-a DO_2 = 127.7 - 88 = 39.8
- Expected A-a DO_2 for 72 years = 22
- Mild increase in A-a DO_2
- The patient is having acute on chronic respiratory acidosis with a HAGMA with normal sugars and lactates, the remaining differentials are:
  - Ketoacidosis
  - Uremia
  - Salicylate poisoning
  - Toxins
- Respiratory acidosis is usually rare and terminal in salicylate poisoning. In the absence of laboratory parameters to support the diagnosis of uremia or ketoacidosis, toxicology needs to be considered.
- Here the pH is suggestive of acute on chronic respiratory acidosis with added metabolic acidosis and hypocalcemia. As the lactates in ABG are high, in the appropriate scenarios, it needs to be confirmed by measuring serum lactate by a different method. If present, a lactate gap will be highly suggestive of ethylene glycol toxicity.

Further Reading

Adrogué HJ, Madias NE. Management of life-threatening acid-base disorders. First of two parts. N Engl J Med. 1998;338(1):26-34.

Adrogué HJ, Madias NE. Management of life-threatening acid-base disorders. Second of two parts. N Engl J Med. 1998;338(2):107-11.

Ans. 40

- *ABG:* Acidosis
- Respiratory acidosis with metabolic acidosis
- *Anion gap:* 9.64 (normal)
- A laboratory error, underestimation of sodium (in cases of hypernatremia or hypertriglyceridemia), overestimation of serum chloride and bicarbonate, hypoalbuminemia, bromide intoxication, iodide intoxication, multiple myeloma, lithium intoxication, hypercalcemia, hypermagnesemia, and use of polymyxin B are the causes of low anion gap.

- A negative anion gap is seen in cases of laboratory errors, bromide or iodide intoxication, multiple myeloma, etc.
- Urine anion gap (UAG) is the difference between urine cations and urine anions (normal value +20). The main cations measured are Na^+ and K^+ and main anion is Cl^-. In contrast to serum anions, bicarbonate is not excreted in urine.
- UC include NH_4^+, Ca^{2+}, and Mg^{2+} and the UA in urine are sulfate, phosphate, and organic anions.
- In hyperchloremic metabolic acidosis, body loses sodium and potassium from gastrointestinal (GI) tract along with bicarbonate. Thus, in urine, the compensation will be with excreting ammonia, which is not calculated, and the UAG will be negative.
- In chronic respiratory alkalosis, the UAG is increased or positive, reflecting low ammonium excretion, which is an appropriate compensatory response to the prevailing alkalemia.

Further Reading

Kraut JA, Madias NE. Serum anion gap: Its uses and limitations in clinical medicine. CJASN. 2007;2(1):162-74.

Ans. 41

- Standard refers to standard conditions. It is the concentration of HCO_3^- in plasma when the blood is equilibrated at 37°C at a pCO_2 of 40 mm Hg and hemoglobin fully saturated with oxygen. It gives an approximate idea of the patient's bicarbonate and acid-base milieu, if they were being ventilated properly.
- Actual bicarbonate is estimated by the ABG analyzer from the Henderson–Hasselbalch equation using values of pH and pCO_2. It is rarely used at the bedside as it is not a good marker of the respiratory or metabolic acid-base disturbance. However, *it is the value to be taken for calculating the rules of compensation* and calculating the bicarbonate replacement.
- Actual base excess is the amount of base required to titrate the blood to a normal pH of 7.40, at ambient conditions (pCO_2 40 mm Hg, temperature 37°C, and actual oxygen saturation). The adjustment of base excess to normal conditions ensures that the actual base excess indicates the metabolic component of the ABG.
- The actual base excess adjusted to a hemoglobin of 5 g/dL is called base excess (ecf). This value is used for the compensation rules of Copenhagen school of thought.

Further Reading

Kofstad J. All about base excess - to BE or not to BE. [online] Available from https://acutecaretesting.org/en/articles/all-about-base-excess--to-be-or-not-to-be [Last accessed February, 2020].

Ans. 42

- As per the Stewarts approach, the independent variables for pH determination are SID, pCO_2, and the total protein concentration or a ATOT total weak non-volatile acids. SID = Na + K – Cl = (147.8 + 4.24) – 109.3 = 42.74

- SIG = (Base Deficit) + (SID – 38) + 2.5 [4.2 – Albumin (g/dL)] – Lactate
  –9.6 + 4 + 2.5 × 1.2 – 10.48 = 13
  SIG >2, *this is a SIG metabolic acidosis* causes of a positive strong ion gap include uremia, diabetic ketoacidosis, toxins like methanol, ethylene glycol, propylene glycol, iron, INH, and paraldehyde and conditions such as lactic acidosis.
- Conditions producing a negative SIG include hypercalcemia, hypermagnesemia, hyperkalemia, immunoglobulins, bromide, nitrates, lithium overdose.

Further Reading

Acid base sheet. [online] Available from http://emcrit.org/wp-content/uploads/acid_base_sheet_2-2011.pdf [Last accessed February, 2020].

Ans. 43

- A low mixed venous sample obtained from a pulmonary artery catheter showing very low venous oxygen saturations suggests increased peripheral utilization of oxygen. Changes in central venous oxygen saturation track the changes in mixed venous oxygen saturation in case of sepsis and thus can be used interchangeably. In a patient with shock/sepsis, a low $ScvO_2$ warrants augmentation of oxygen delivery either by fluid resuscitation, inotropic agents or by blood transfusion. However, in cases of meningitis, a low $ScvO_2$ may suggest increased oxygen utilization in brain secondary to meningitis alone.
- Steps to be undertaken immediately include clinical assessment of the patient for signs of shock such as cold peripheries, prolonged capillary refill time, and elevated lactate. If shock is present, patient needs urgent resuscitation for shock.
- *Plan:* CT to rule out a raised ICP, followed by a lumbar puncture, CSF studies including culture and biochemical analysis, meningitis dose of antibiotics, augmentation of cardiac output by fluid resuscitation, inotropic support if patient is not fluid responsive, and blood transfusion if HCT falls after fluid resuscitation.

Ans. 44

- *ABG:* Acidosis
- Metabolic acidosis
- *Expected PCO_2:* 33.6 ± 2 (not compensated)
- *Anion gap:* (147.8 + 4.24) – (109.3 + 17.1) = 25.64 [HAGMA, assuming normal albumin level]
- Delta gap = 13.64/6.9 = 1.97 (approximately 2)
- *Suggesting additional underlying problem:* Metabolic alkalosis or chronic respiratory acidosis
- *Issues:* Hyperlactatemia—suggestive of anaerobic metabolism
- Low $ScvO_2$—suggestive of increased oxygen extraction in peripheries
- In this patient with hyperlactatemia and reduced $ScvO_2$, as the PCO_2 gap is less than 6 mm Hg, further optimization of cardiac output may not be fruitful. In this case, improving oxygen delivery by increasing FiO_2 and hemoglobin needs to be considered.

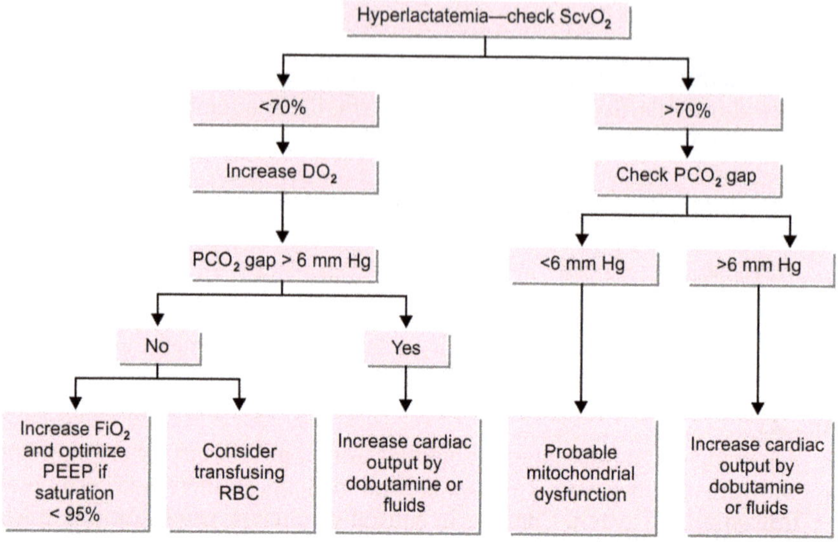

Further Reading

Mallat J, Lemyze M, Tronchon L, Vallet B, Thevenin D. Use of venous-to-arterial carbon dioxide tension difference to guide resuscitation therapy in septic shock. World J Crit Care Med. 2016;5(1):47-56.

Ans. 45

	High anion gap metabolic acidosis "CATMUDPILES"
C	Cyanide poisoning/Carbon monoxide poisoning
	Congestive heart failure
A	Aminoglycosides
T	Toluene
M	Methanol poisoning
U	Uremia
D	Diabetic ketoacidosis
P	Pyroglutamic aciduria/Paraldehyde
I	Iron/INH
L	Lactic acidosis/D lactic acidosis
E	Ethylene glycol
S	Salicylates/Starvation ketoacidosis

Lactic acidosis			
Type A—reduced oxygenation	Type B—normal perfusion and oxygenation		
Regional/systemic hypoperfusion	B1	B2	B3
Severe respiratory failure	Renal failure	Biguanides	Inborn error of metabolism
Anemia	Hepatic failure	Alcohols	

Contd...

Contd...

Carbon monoxide poisoning	Diabetes	Iron
Underutilization of lactate such as liver disease, thiamine deficiency, and uncoupled oxidative phosphorylation	Malignancy	Isoniazid, zidovudine, salicylates

Ans. 46

Metabolic alkalosis can be secondary to infusion of bicarbonate or high citrate from blood transfusion or any process that causes H + loss such as vomiting, NG aspirate or diuretic use.

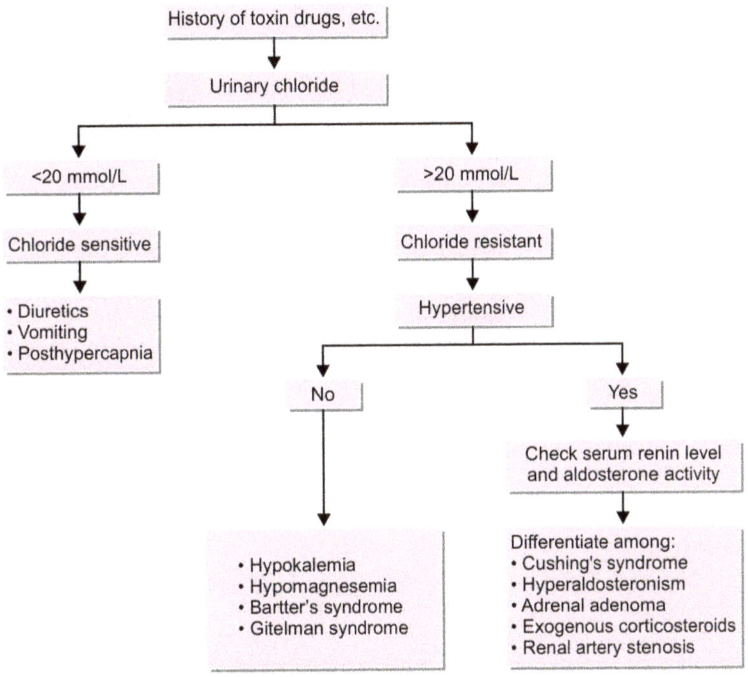

Ans. 47

- Lactate can be measured by either lactate dehydrogenase method or lactate oxidase method.

The lactate oxidase method is commonly used by point-of-care ABG analyzers making them prone for an artefactual very high value of lactate in case of ethylene glycol poisoning.

This is because of a misidentification of glyoxylate as lactate, as both have a similar structure and cannot be differentiated by lactate oxidase method.

In cases of high suspicion, this can be identified by measuring the serum lactate in biochemistry machines which use the lactate dehydrogenase method to detect blood lactate levels, thereby differentiating between lactate and glyoxylate. A gap between the lactates obtained from the ABG analyzer and the biochemistry machines points toward ethylene glycol poisoning.

- Saturation gap is the gap or difference in oxygen saturation between the finger pulse oximeter and the saturation SaO_2 on the ABG report. If it is

>5%, it indicates the presence of abnormal hemoglobin in circulation—methemoglobinemia, carboxyhemoglobinemia or sulfhemoglobinemia. In methemoglobinemia, finger pulse oximetry will detect a low saturation and the ABG analyzer will show normal oxygen saturation.

Further Reading:

Chouksey A, Khurana AK, Goyal A. The girl with the "saturation gap". Lung India. 2018;35(5):448-9.

Hauvik LE, Varghese M, Nielsen EW. Lactate gap: A diagnostic support in severe metabolic acidosis of unknown origin. Case Rep Med. 2018;2018:5238240.

Ans. 48

- The ABG is showing severe combined acidosis, severe hyperkalemia, hyperglycemia, hyperlactatemia, and hypocalcemia. These are the changes that usually occur in stored blood due to the addition of SAGM as preservative. Storage lesion refers to changes in RBC that occur during storage. As time passes, the glucose in stored blood is used up. The 2,3-DPG levels come down and are entirely depleted by the end of 2 weeks causing a left shift of the oxygen carrying capacity of RBC. With time, the RBCs swell due to failure of ion pumps, becoming spherical or hemispherical. This is important clinically as these damaged RBCs are easily deformable as they flow through the splanchnic circulation and the RBC membrane becomes vacuolated. With storage, the potassium levels increase, the RBC membrane gets damaged with changes in the rheological properties. Some amount of hemolysis will be present and release hemoglobin and free iron will be present in the stored blood.
- However, in clinical practice, there has been no proven benefit of fresh blood over stored blood and trials have demonstrated equipoise.

Further Reading:

George J, Myatra S. Blood transfusion in the critically ill patient. Bangladesh Crit Care J. 2018;6(1):40-6.

Shah A, Brunskill SJ, Desborough MJR, Doree C, Trivella M, Stanworth SJ. Transfusion of red blood cells stored for shorter versus longer duration for all conditions. Cochrane Database Syst Rev. 2018;12:CD010801.

Ans. 49

There is a high anion gap metabolic acidosis (30.24) with compensation.

- P/F ratio of 600
- A-a DO_2 of 88.35
- Delta gap = 18/18.3 = approximately 1—HAGMA only

Apneic oxygenation is a step of preoxygenation by which very high oxygen is given without ventilation, during rapid sequence intubation (RSI) along with the attempts of intubation. During apnea, there is a constant removal of oxygen from alveoli into the blood, which creates a pressure gradient for oxygen to move into the alveoli. This oxygen flow is independent of the respiratory effort by the patient, and maintains the oxygen saturation for a considerable time provided airway is maintained patent.

Other measures to reduce hypoxia during intubation include delayed sequence intubation, ketamine only intubation, gentle breaths during RSI etc.

Further Reading

Rudolf B, Hohenhorst W. Use of apneic oxygenation for the performance of panendoscopy. Otolaryngol Head Neck Surg. 2013;149(2):235-9.

Weingart SD, Levitan RM. Preoxygenation and prevention of desaturation during emergency airway management. Ann Emerg Med. 2012;59(3):165-75.

Ans. 50

In hyperoxia, the tissue damage is caused by the development of reactive oxygen species, which develop in excess of antioxidant capabilities leading to cell death and inflammation.

The data on effects of hyperoxia are conflicting.

Earlier data suggest that in cardiac arrest, traumatic brain injury (TBI), stroke, and in myocardial infarction, hyperoxia results in an increased mortality and morbidity.

Wang et al. found that hyperoxia increases the mortality of critically ill patients after cardiac arrest and extracorporeal life support and in the patients with TBI, stroke, and hemorrhage, postcardiac surgery and receiving mechanical ventilation due to mixed primary disease, hyperoxia did not increase mortality.

Further Reading

Ni Y, Wang Y, Liang B, Liang Z. The effect of hyperoxia on mortality in critically ill patients: a systematic review and meta-analysis. BMC Pulm Med. 2019;19:53.

Vincent JL, Taccone FS, He X. Harmful effects of hyperoxia in post cardiac arrest sepsis, traumatic brain injury or stroke: the importance of individualised oxygen therapy in critically ill patients. Can Respir J. 2017;2017:2834956.

Ans. 51

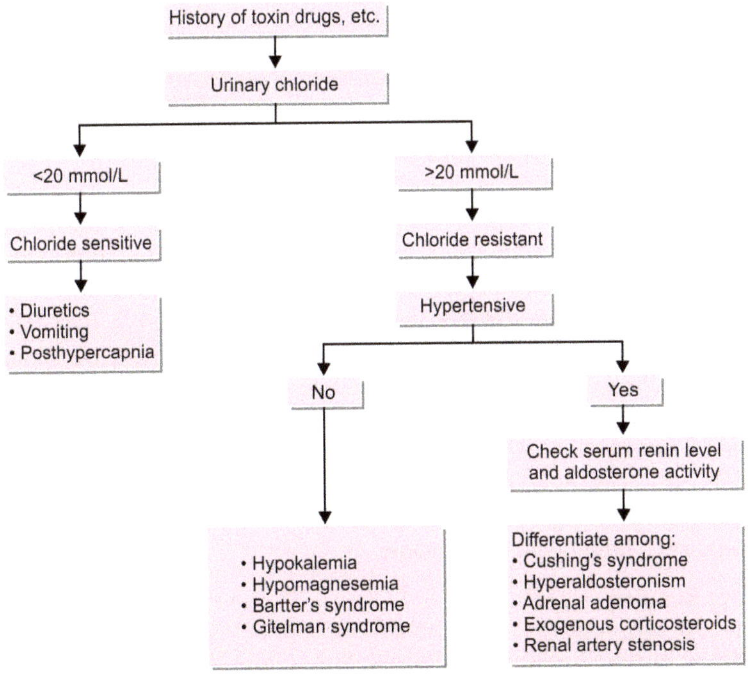

ABG shows a metabolic alkalosis with respiratory acidosis.

Expected respiratory compensation = 0.7 × 85.7 + 21 = 80.99

Presence of electrolyte abnormalities such as hyponatremia, hypokalemia, and hypochloremia, in a case of primary metabolic alkalosis, with no history of drug abuse, vomiting or hypertension suggests Bartter syndrome versus Gitelman syndrome. Bartter syndrome usually manifests in early childhood while Gitelman manifests later. Tetany may be common in Gitelman syndrome. 24-hour urinary calcium is elevated in Bartter while normal or reduced in Gitelman syndrome.

Further Reading

Al Shibli A, Narchi H. Bartter and Gitelman syndromes: Spectrum of clinical manifestations caused by different mutations. World J Methodol. 2015;5(2):55-61.

Ans. 52

According to the alpha-stat principle, we have to interpret the blood gases corrected to the normal body temperature while the pH-stat principle maintains that we have to correct the temperature to the patient body temperature. However, as there is no data available to quantify the balance between oxygen delivery and oxygen demand at temperatures other than 37°C, temperature correction of blood gas samples is not recommended by the American Association for Respiratory Care.

Further Reading

Davis MD, Walsh BK, Sittig SE, D Restrepo R. AARC Clinical Practice Guideline: Blood Gas Analysis and Hemoximetry: 2013. [online] Available from http://rc.rcjournal.com/content/58/10/1694.full.pdf [Last accessed February, 2020].

Ans. 53

Confusion arises due to the units in which calcium is measured and reported. The calcium concentration is reported either as mg/dL or mmol/L or mEq/L. They are interrelated as follows (for calcium):

mmol/L = mg/dL × 1/4

mEq/L = mg/dL × 1/2

Thus, the normal range of total serum calcium concentration is 9 to 11 mg/dL or 2.0 to 2.6 mmol/L or 4.0 to 5.2 mEq/L, of which approximately 45–50% percent is ionized.

For acute symptomatic hypocalcemia, the treatment is 10% calcium gluconate 10 mL (90 mg calcium) in 50 mL of 5% Dextrose or DNS given as a slow IV infusion over 20 minutes followed by an infusion of elemental calcium at a rate of 0.5 mg/kg/h.

This is prepared by adding 110 mL of 10% calcium gluconate to 890 mL of normal saline or 5% dextrose water thus making 1,000 mL of 1 mg/mL solution. Calcium chloride is highly concentrated and 10 mL contains 270 mg of calcium, and requires a larger vein for infusion.

Further Reading

Zaloga GP. Hypocalcemia in critically ill patients. Critical Care Medicine. 1992;20(2):251-62.

Ans. 54

- Arterial phase of CT contrast showing post-traumatic aortic pseudo-aneurysm with mediastinal hematoma.
- Commonly seen in trauma involving sudden deceleration, such as a motor vehicle collision (MVC) at speeds greater than 50 km/h.
- Blunt aortic injuries result in immediate death from aortic transection in majority of the patients with only a small minority surviving till hospital admission. The patients in whom aortic injuries are diagnosed require urgent surgical intervention without which they sustain an aortic rupture within 24 hours.
- CT, angiography, and transesophageal echocardiography are the investigations of choice in whom aortic injury is suspected.

Further Reading

Cullen EL, Lantz EJ, Johnson CM, Young PM. Traumatic aortic injury: CT findings, mimics, and therapeutic options. Cardiovasc Diagn Ther. 2014;4(3):238-44.

Ans. 55

- Percutaneous tracheostomy involves Seldinger technique and dilatation of trachea between rings.
- The described techniques include:
  - Ciaglia technique (multiple sequential dilators)
  - Modified Ciaglia technique (Blue Rhino single dilator)
  - Griggs (forceps) technique
  - Frova and Quintel (PercuTwist) technique
  - Cianchi balloon dilation technique
  - Fantoni translaryngeal (retrograde) technique

Ans. 56

Camel flu is also called as Middle East Respiratory Syndrome Coronavirus (MERS-COV). MERS-CoV outbreak in human population is sustained by zoonotic transmission from dromedary camels. Treatment is mainly supportive and no specific treatment is available.

Further Reading

Kantor S, Chandwani J. Middle East Respiratory Syndrome Coronavirus (MERS-COV). In: Freebairn RC, Kulkarni AP (Eds). Evidence Based Core Topics in Critical Care 2019. New Delhi: Jaypee Brothers Medical Publishers (P) Ltd; 2019.

Ans. 57

Chest X-ray shows nasogastric placed in right lower bronchus which needs to be repositioned urgently.

- Recommended methods for confirmation of appropriate placement of NG tube include:
  - X-ray—gold standard
  - Direct visualization
  - Ultrasound visualization
  - Biochemical markers
  - pH testing
  - Electromagnetic tracing
  - Manometer technique

Methods not recommended any more for confirmation of NG tube:
Auscultatory
Observation for bubbles
Litmus paper

Further Reading

Fan EMP, Tan SB, Ang SY. Nasogastric tube placement confirmation: where we are and where we should be heading. Proceedings of Singapore Healthcare. 2017;26(3):189-95.

Ans. 58

Assessed parameter	*Result*	*Score*
Temperature (°Celsius)	36.5–38.4 °C	0
	38.5–38.9 °C	1
	≤ 36 or ≥ 39 °C	2
Leukocytes in blood (cells/mm^3)	4,000–11,000/mm^3	0
	<4,000 or >11,000/mm^3	1
	≥ 500 Band cells	2
Tracheal secretions (subjective visual scale)	None	0
	Mild/non-purulent	1
	Purulent	2
Radiographic findings (on chest radiography, excluding CHF and ARDS)	No infiltrate	0
	Diffuse/patchy infiltrate	1
	Localized infiltrate	2
Culture results (endotracheal aspirate)	No or mild growth	0
	Moderate or florid growth	1
	Moderate or florid growth AND pathogen consistent with Gram stain	2
Oxygenation status (defined by PaO_2 FiO_2	>24D or ARDS	0
	≤240 and absence of ARDS	2

Temperature: 0
Leukocytes: 1
Tracheal secretions: 1
CXR: 2
Culture: NA
PF ratio: 2
CPIS score: 6
A CPIS score more than 6 suggests higher likelihood of VAP although the utility of the score remain is not clear.

Further Reading

Kalanuria AA, Zai W, Mirski M. Ventilator-associated pneumonia in the ICU. Crit Care. 2014;18:208.

Ans. 59

Recommended tests:

- BAL for CB-NAAT and PJP PCR
- BAL for MGIT culture
- Urine lipoarabinomannan assay (LF-LAM)

In seriously ill HIV positive patients, regardless of CD4 count or with unknown CD4 count, and in patients with CD4 count <100 cells/μL, lateral flow urine lipoarabinomannan assay (LF-LAM) may be used to aid in diagnosing tuberculosis.

Lipoarabinomannan antigen is a lipopolysaccharide present in the cell walls of mycobacteria. It gets into the circulation in the presence of both metabolically active bacteria or degenerating bacterial cells and can be detected in urine, thereby avoiding the need of noninvasive procedures like BAL. As it appears only in cases of active TB disease, it may be used for screening seriously ill patients. However owing to a low sensitivity and specificity, it cannot be recommended as a screening test for all.

Further Reading

Kulkarni AP, Sengar M, Chinnaswamy G, Hegde A, Rodrigues C, Soman R, et al. Indian Antimicrobial Prescription Guidelines in Critically Ill Immunocompromised Patients. Indian J Crit Care Med. 2019;23(Suppl 1):S64-96.

World Health Organization. The use of lateral flow urine lipoarabinomannan assay (LF-LAM) for the diagnosis and screening of active tuberculosis in people living with HIV. [online] Available from https://apps.who.int/iris/bitstream/handle/10665/193633/9789241509633_eng.pdf;jsessionid=7DF95A8AD413B0B085AFAAE65B157E1C?sequence=1 [Last accessed February, 2020].

Ans. 60

Both ATT and ART need to be initiated keeping in mind side effect profile and drug interactions. Sequential ART is now not preferred and integrating ART after 2–8 weeks of ATT is the current practice.

- CD4 count <50 cells/μL—start ART within 2 weeks of ATT; watch for immune reconstitution inflammatory syndrome (IRIS)
- CD4 count >50 cells/μL—start ART within 8 weeks of ATT
- CNS TB—irrespective of CD4 count, ART should be withheld for 8 weeks
- Consider prophylactic steroids for 4 weeks in patients with CD4 cell counts <100 cells/μL and starting ART within 30 days of starting ATT.

Further Reading

Panel on Opportunistic Infections in HIV-Infected Adults and Adolescents. Guidelines for the prevention and treatment of opportunistic infections in HIV-infected adults and adolescents: Recommendations from the Centers for Disease Control and Prevention, the National Institutes of Health, and the HIV Medicine Association of the Infectious Diseases Society of America.. [online] Available from http://aidsinfo.nih.gov/contentfiles/lvguidelines/adult_oi.pdf [Last accessed February, 2020].

World Health Organization. Guidelines for treatment of drug-susceptible tuberculosis and patient care, 2017 update. [online] Available from http://apps.who.int/iris/bitstream/10665/255052/1/9789241550000-eng.pdf?ua=1 [Last accessed February, 2020].

Ans. 61

- *Diagnosis*: Immune reconstitution inflammatory syndrome
- High risk in those with CD4 count < 50 cells/μL or those with CD4 count < 200 cells/μL and tuberculosis

- *Management*: Supportive care, rule out drug-resistant diseases (PTB and HIV), rule out other opportunistic/infectious diseases, addition of steroids—prednisolone 1 mg/kg with tapering once symptoms settle.

NEUROLOGY

Ans. 62

- T2 FLAIR MRI shows bilateral hyperintensities in thalamus and basal ganglia, bilateral parieto-occipital region suggestive of hypoxic ischemic encephalopathy (HIE).
- Diffusion image showing areas of diffusion restriction in cortex.
- A close differential will be hypoglycemia—in which thalamus will be spared.
- Mild-to-moderate hypoxia causes infarcts in water-shed areas. Severe HIE affects the cerebral cortex, basal ganglia, thalami, hippocampus, and cerebellum.
- Initially MRI may show restricted diffusion due to cytotoxic edema—a bright signal on diffusion weighted images (DWI) with a corresponding low signal on apparent diffusion coefficient (ADC) map that normalize (pseudonormalize) in a week.
- In acute stages, the T2WI/FLAIR images start showing hyperintense signals in the involved areas and in chronic longstanding cases, the cortical changes on T1W images become more prominent.

Further Reading

Maurya VK, Ravikumar R, Bhatia M, Rai R. Hypoxic-Ischemic brain injury in an adult: Magnetic resonance imaging findings. Med J Armed Forces India. 2016;72(1):75-7.

Ans. 63

T2 FLAIR images showing hyperintensity in pons suggestive of pontine myelinolysis/osmotic demyelination syndrome.

Chronic alcoholism, concurrent hypokalemia, and liver transplant are risk factors for central pontine myelinolysis.

Extrapontine sites for demyelination include splenium of corpus callosum, internal capsule, thalami, basal ganglia, caudate nuclei, etc.

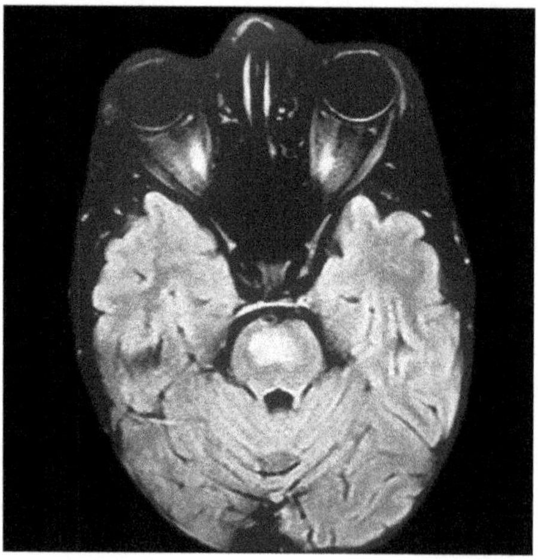

Further Reading

George JC, Zafar W, Bucaloiu ID, Chang AR. Risk factors and outcomes of rapid correction of severe hyponatremia. Clin J Am Soc Nephrol. 2018;13(7):984-92.

Ans. 64

T2 FLAIR image showing hyperintensity in temporal region suggestive of herpes encephalitis.

- Clinical features suggestive of HSV include an elderly presentation, acute presentation, history of preceding fever, other systems involvement like gastrointestinal symptoms, and absence of rash.

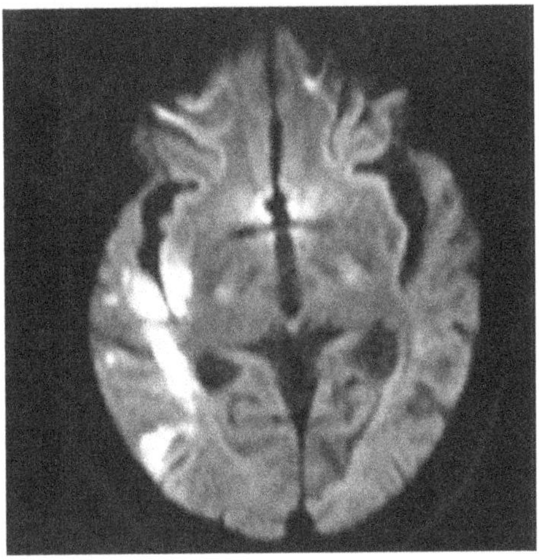

- Few patients have normal CSF while majority will have a lymphocytic pleocytosis, normal to mildly reduced glucose, and increased protein. Red blood cells in an atraumatic CSF tap also suggest HSV encephalitis, although not diagnostic.
- Recommended empirical treatment in adults is acyclovir 10 mg/kg tid for 14 days with a higher dose in children.
- Repeat lumbar puncture (LP) is suggested after 14 days and if CSF PCR is still positive for HSV, acyclovir should be continued for an additional week, with weekly LP until CSF is negative.
- Role of steroids—low quality evidence/no evidence.

Further Reading

Kennedy PG, Chaudhuri A. Herpes simplex encephalitis. J Neurol Neurosurg Psychiatry. 2002;73(3):237-8.

Meyfroidt G, Kurtz P, Sonneville R. Critical care management of infectious meningitis and encephalitis. Intensive Care Med. 2020;46(2):192-201.

Tyler KL. Acute viral encephalitis. New Engl J Med. 2018;379(6):557-66.

Ans. 65

- Laboratory results are positive for hyperchloremic metabolic acidosis (SID—34) with respiratory alkalosis, leukocytosis, hyperglycemia, deranged RFT, and urine analysis shows eosinophil cast, urinary ketones.
- Possible causes in this patient include diabetic ketoacidosis, interstitial nephritis due to acyclovir.

- Management: Slow administration of IV acyclovir, IV insulin, maintain a urinary output of 50 mL/h, and balanced crystalloid for maintenance and resuscitation.

Ans. 66

- CT is suggestive of occlusion of extra- and intracranial internal carotid artery (ICA) left side.
- Internal carotid artery occlusions are resistant to thrombolysis than middle cerebral artery occlusions as they harbor larger and longer clots. Moreover, these atherosclerotic thrombi are more resistant than fibrin rich thrombus.
- Currently mechanical thrombectomy is recommended over intra-arterial thrombolysis especially if they have a low pre-stroke modified Rankin score, age ≥18 years; NIHSS score of ≥6; ASPECTS of ≥6 and if groin puncture can be initiated within 6 hours of symptom onset.

Ans. 67

- Contrast-enhanced MRI showing multiple peripherally enhancing lesions in bilateral cerebral hemisphere.

Differential diagnosis:

- Tuberculoma
- Metastasis
- Neurocysticercosis

In patients with high clinical suspicion of neurocysticercosis, serology EITB (enzyme-linked immunoelectrotransfer blot) using glycoproteins should be done. Commercially available ELISA using unfractionated antigens are discouraged.

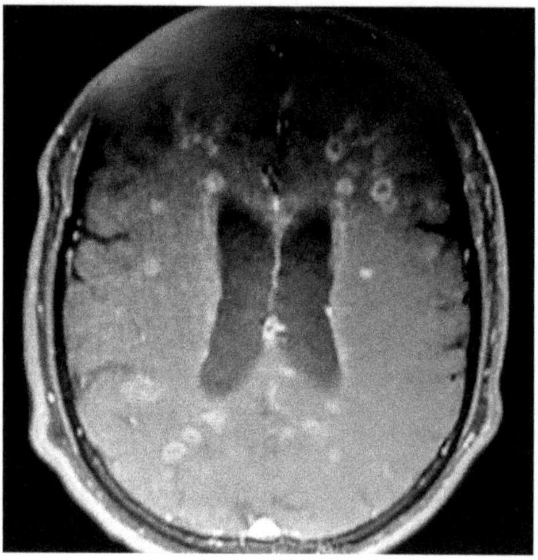

Ans. 68

CT showing acute on chronic subdural hematoma (SDH) in left frontotemporal region with mass effect causing effacement of the lateral ventricle on left side, midline shift.

Management: Neurosurgical reference for evacuation

Meanwhile:

- Rapid sequence intubation
- Avoid hypo or hypercapnia

- Avoid hypoxia or hypotension
- Urgent correction of coagulopathy
- Head in neutral position to permit venous drainage.

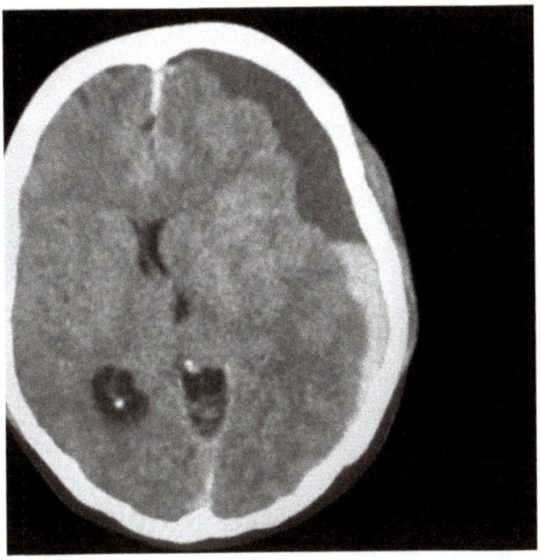

Ans. 69

CT brain showing diffuse cerebral edema, with mild pneumocephalus, partial effacement of right lateral ventricle, and midline shift. Head trauma needs to be ruled out on imaging.

Treatment depends on the etiology and unless tension pneumocephalus is present, the patient can be observed.

Tension pneumocephalus presents with nonspecific features including restlessness, worsening sensorium, focal neurological deficits, and can lead to cardiac arrest. It has a characteristic Mount Fuji appearance on CT due to frontal lobe compression.

Tension pneumocephalus requires urgent burr hole and surgical decompression and is a neurosurgical emergency. Mild cases require observation and increased FiO_2 only.

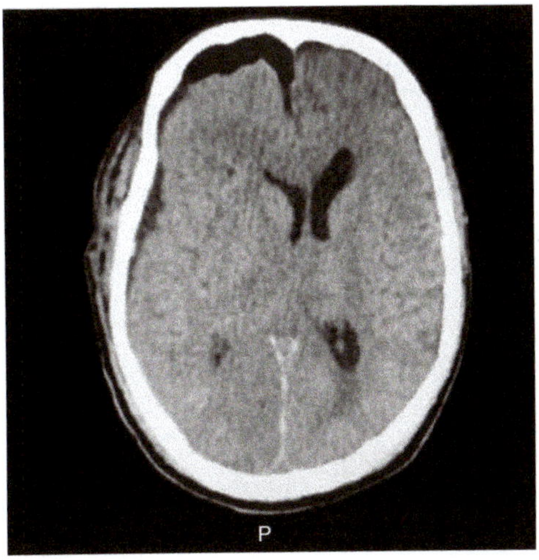

Ans. 70

CT showing acute SDH and mild subarachnoid hemorrhage (SAH), effacement of sulci, gyri, and lateral ventricle on right side, with midline shift and subfalcine herniation.

Transtentorial herniation compresses the motor fibers causing hemiparesis is a false localizing sign called Kernohan notch.

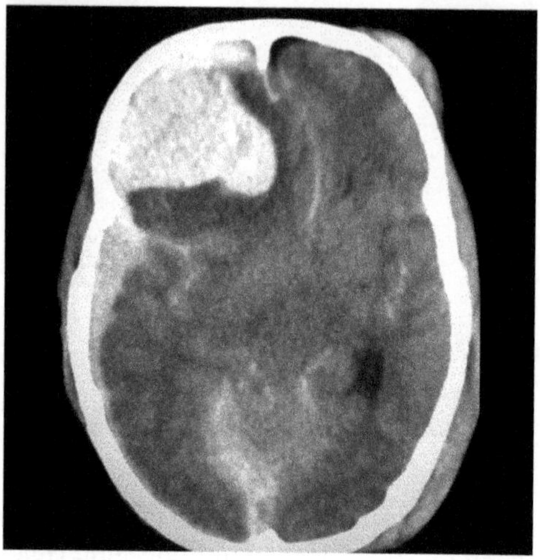

- Supratentorial herniation:
  - Transtentorial/Uncal
  - Central
  - Subfalcine (Cingulate/transfalcine)
  - Transcalvarial
  - Tectal (posterior)
- Infratentorial herniation:
  - Reverse herniation of cerebellum
  - Tonsillar herniation of cerebellum

Further Reading

Brain herniation. [online] Available from https://pdfs.semanticscholar.org/5e11/d914ae4d66ca 57f47a6672a27516f6a9c59d.pdf [Last accessed February, 2020].

Ans. 71

Indication for ICP monitoring in TBI include admission Glasgow Coma Scale (GCS) <8 and CT brain showing any of the following pathologies such as mass lesions, hematoma or contusion, swelling (edema), midline shift, and compressed basal cisterns;

Or

If two or more of the poor prognostic factors are present:

- Age > 40 years
- Unilateral or bilateral motor posturing
- Hypotension < 90 mm Hg

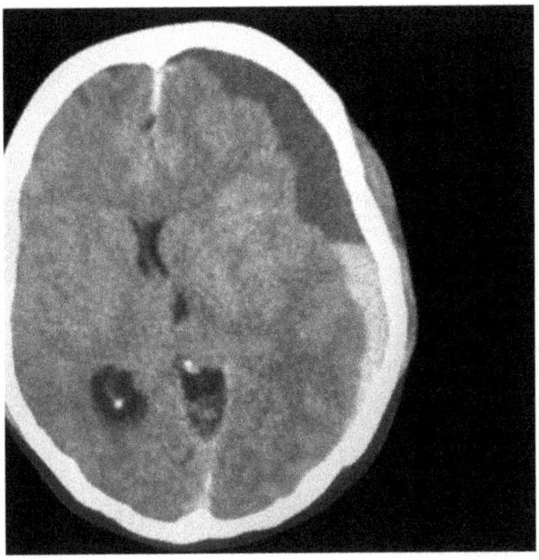

Further Reading

Le Roux P. Intracranial pressure monitoring and management. In: Laskowitz D, Grant G (Eds). Translational Research in Traumatic Brain Injury. Boca Raton (FL): CRC Press/Taylor and Francis Group; 2016.

Ans. 72

T2 FLAIR showing white matter intensity in right parietooccipital region suggestive of posterior reversible encephalopathy syndrome or PRES.

Management is supportive with addition of anticonvulsants, oxygen therapy, antihypertensives, etc. and has a good prognosis, usually with complete resolution if it is recognized early and appropriate treatment is initiated early.

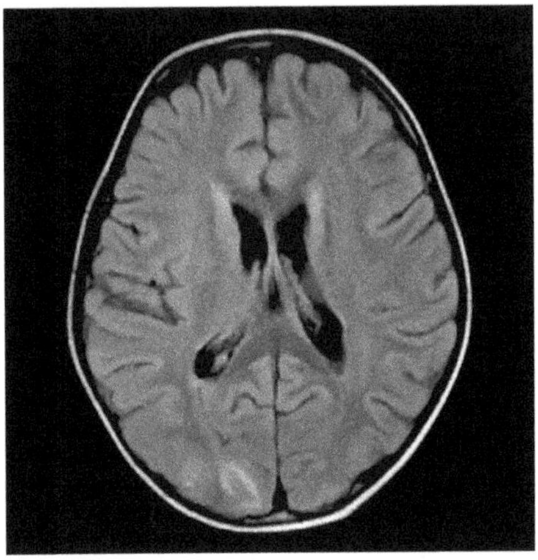

Further Reading

Fischer M, Schmutzhard E. Posterior reversible encephalopathy syndrome. J Neurol. 2017;264(8):1608-16.

Ans. 73

Clinical diagnosis—status epilepticus

CT showing diffuse cerebral edema with effacement of sulci and loss of gray-white differentiation suggestive of diffuse cerebral edema and raised ICP.

Management includes:
- Airway control
- IV benzodiazepines and algorithm for control of status epilepticus
- Control of sugar, fever, and blood pressure

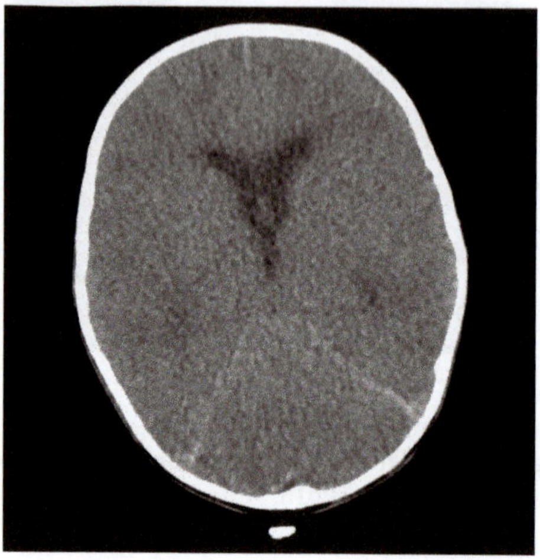

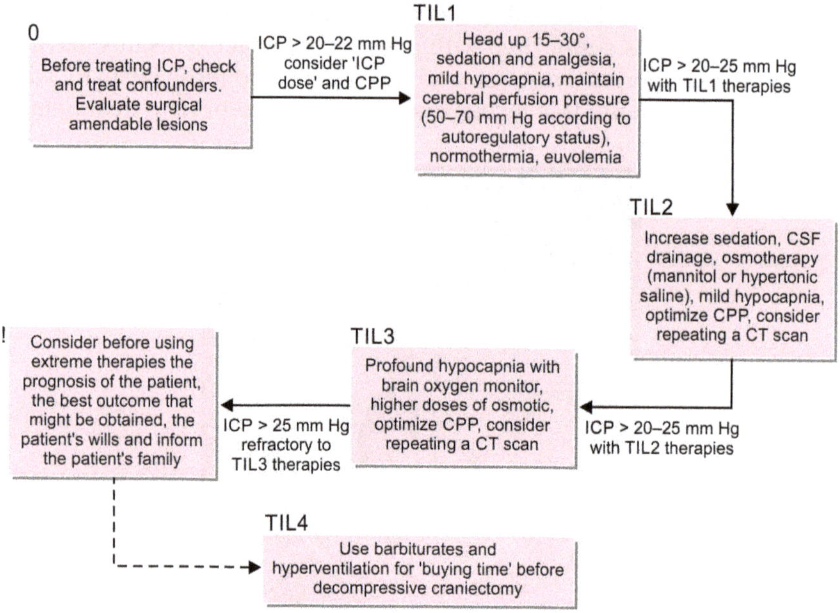

Further Reading

Robba C, Citerio G. How I manage intracranial hypertension. Crit Care. 2019;23:243.

Ans. 74

Contrast MRI showing multiple heterogeneously enhancing focal lesions in bilateral basal and suprasellar cisterns with mild prominence of temporal horn of lateral ventricle.

Persistence of dilated temporal horns are suggestive of hydrocephalus and tuberculous meningitis although other cuts are needed to confirm the diagnosis of hydrocephalus.

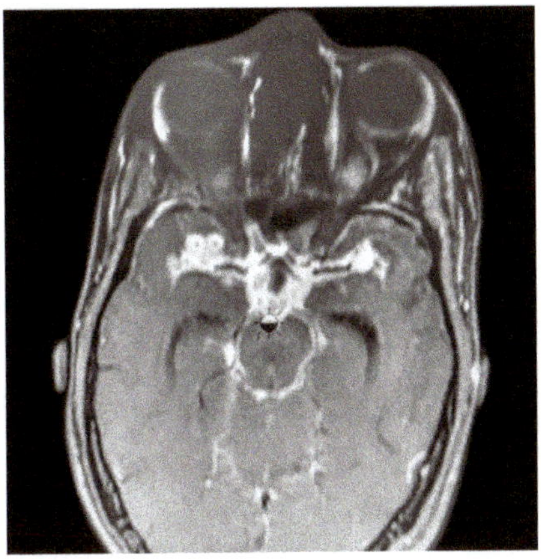

Management includes:

- Management of raised ICP and seizure
- Antitubercular treatment

Currently, WHO recommends a 2-month treatment with four first-line drugs in the intensive phase, followed by a continuation phase with at least rifampicin and isoniazid and ethambutol for 4–10 months.

- Corticosteroids
- Neurosurgery opinion for management of hydrocephalus if hydrocephalus is present.

Further Reading

Sharma SK, Ryan H, Khaparde S, Sachdeva KS, Singh AD, Mohan A, et al. Index-TB guidelines: Guidelines on extrapulmonary tuberculosis for India. Indian J Med Res. 2017;145(4):448-63.

World Health Organization. (2016). Index TB guidelines: Guidelines for extra-pulmonary tuberculosis for India. [online] Available from http://tbcindia.gov.in/showfile.php?lid=3245 [Last accessed February, 2020].

Ans. 75

Complete occlusion of basilar artery.

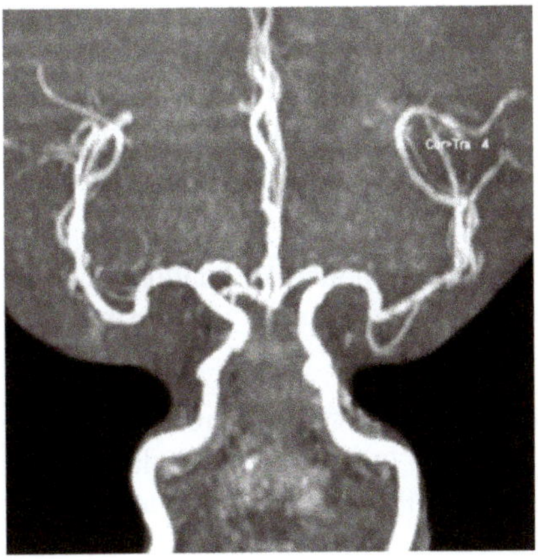

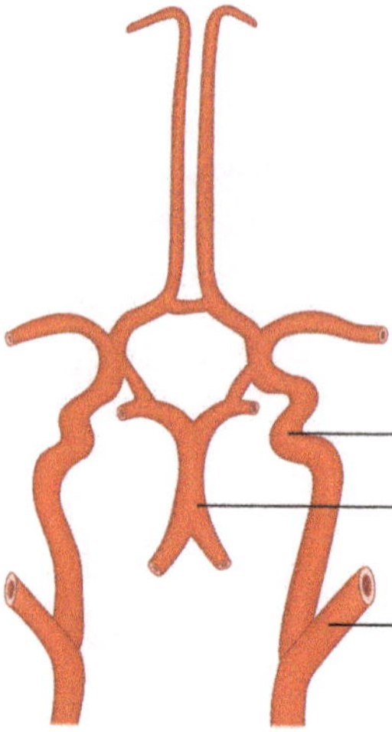

Normal anatomy of cerebral circulation. However in the given CT angiography image, there is complete occlusion of the basilar artery.

Ans. 76

CT brain showing tiny hyperdense hemorrhagic contusion in left thalamus and splenium of corpus callosum suggestive of diffuse axonal injury.

Diffuse axonal injury is classified as:

- *Grade I:* Involvement of the gray–white matter junction such as parasagittal regions of frontal lobes, periventricular temporal lobes, and occasionally involving the parietal and occipital lobes and cerebellum.
- *Grade II:* Involvement of the gray–white matter junction as grade I and also involvement of the corpus callosum, usually in the posterior aspect, i.e., posterior body and splenium.
- *Grade III:* Grade I and II locations along with involvement of the brainstem (midbrain, cerebellar peduncles, corticospinal tracts, etc.).

Further Reading

https://radiopaedia.org/articles/diffuse-axonal-injury-grading-1?lang=us

Ans. 77

- The child is a known case of CNS disease and has presented with features of raised ICP.
- Chest X-ray shows presence of a VP shunt.
- Shunt infection and blockage should be the first differential, in this child with the given history and the clinical picture of raised ICP.

Further Reading

Paff M, Alexandru-Abrams D, Muhonen M, Loudon W. Ventriculoperitoneal shunt complications: A review. Interdisciplinary Neurosurgery. 2018;13:66-70.

Ans. 78

- Hypertension-related intracranial hemorrhage frequently involves putamen (55%), cerebral cortex (15%), thalamus, pons, and cerebellum. Hypertension-related ICH in younger patients involves the basal ganglia.

- Elevated blood pressure is seen in 46–56% of patients with ICH. Elevated systolic, diastolic, and mean arterial pressures are associated with a poor outcome in ICH. It remains unclear if elevated blood pressure directly causes hematoma expansion.
- Scoring systems used to predict hematoma expansion include—BRAIN score, BAT score, and a 9-point prediction score.
- The 2015 update to the AHA/ASA Guidelines for the Management of Spontaneous ICH recommends acute lowering of SBP to 140 mm Hg for patients presenting with SBP between 150 and 200 mm Hg. This should be continued for 7 days. There *is no role for steroids, and hyperventilation may be harmful due to vasoconstriction in other areas.*
- The optimum target for patients presenting with SBP > 220 mm Hg is less clear. If there is clinical deterioration with aggressive blood pressure management, the target blood pressure should be actively reassessed.

Further Reading

Dastur CK, Yu W. Current management of spontaneous intracerebral haemorrhage. Stroke and Vascular Neurology. 2017;2.

Ans. 79

- Apart from routine neurologic scoring systems such as modified Rankin scores, Glasgow outcome scale, and extended Glasgow outcome scale, the ICH score and FUNC (Functional Outcome Risk Stratification) score are two clinical grading scales used to prognosticate patients with hemorrhagic stroke.
- The ICH score predicts 30-day mortality using factors including age, ICH volume, GCS score, and presence of intraventricular extension.
- In the FUNC score, the patient is assessed for risk of functional impairment at 90 days post-stroke. The FUNC scores range from 0 to 11 based on ICH volume, age, site of ICH, GCS score, and pre-ICH cognitive impairment. A greater score is associated with a greater chance of functional independence, defined as GCS ≥ 4 at 90 days.
- The limitation of the ICH score is that it is solely used to prognosticate survival at 30 days without accounting for functional outcome. The ICH score should thus be used in combination with the FUNC score to assess functional outcome.
- The limitation of FUNC score is that only scores at the extreme ends seem to be clinically useful as scores in the mid-range have little predictive value.

Further Reading

Dastur CK, Yu W. Current management of spontaneous intracerebral haemorrhage. Stroke and Vascular Neurology. 2017;2.

Hemphill JC III, Bonovich DC, Besmertis L, Manley GT, Johnston SC. The ICH score: a simple, reliable grading scale for intracerebral hemorrhage. Stroke. 200;32(4):891-7.

Rost NS, Smith EE, Chang Y, Snider RW, Chanderraj R, Schwab K, et al. Prediction of functional outcome in patients with primary intracerebral hemorrhage: the FUNC score. Stroke 2008;39(8):2304-9.

Ans. 80

- The CT shows acute subdural hematoma (SDH) with significant intracranial hypertension, mass effect, and midline shift with herniation.

- Care should be taken to assess the airway, breathing, and circulation of this patient and, if required, intubation should be carried out with rapid sequence protocol. Maintenance of euthermia, euglycemia, and eucapnia is important.
- Apart from sending routine laboratories and coagulation studies, urgent measures need to be taken to correct coagulopathy including withholding warfarin, administration of vitamin K, and administration of prothrombin concentrate complex or fresh frozen plasma (15–30 mL/kg).
- A neurosurgery opinion also needs to be taken for consideration of any surgical intervention.

Further Reading

Hull RD, Garcia DA. Management of warfarin-associated bleeding or supratherapeutic INR. [online] Available from https://www.uptodate.com/contents/management-of-warfarin-associated-bleeding-or-supratherapeutic-inr [Last accessed February, 2020].

Ans. 81

- Indications for surgical evacuation include an acute SDH > 10 mm thickness or the presence of a midline shift > 5 mm regardless of the patient's Glasgow Coma Scale (GCS) score.
- A comatose patient (GCS score < 9) with drop in GCS score by 2 or more points or patients with asymmetric or fixed and dilated pupils and/or the ICP exceeds 20 mm Hg.

Further Reading

Bullock MR, Chesnut R, Ghajar J, Gordon D, Hartl R, Newell DW, et al. Surgical management of acute subdural hematomas. Neurosurgery. 2006;58(3 Suppl):S16–24.

Ans. 82

- Extradural hematoma or epidural hematoma (EDH) where arterial bleeding from the middle meningeal artery or its branch is collected in the space between the duramater and the skull but limited by the sutures.
- It is a life-threatening condition and may require immediate intervention and has significant morbidity and mortality if left untreated.

It can be classified based on the radiographic progression into three types:

1. *Type I:* Acute unclotted blood
2. *Type II:* Subacute EDH which is usually solid (2–3 days)
3. *Type III:* Chronic EDH with mixed appearance (2–3 weeks)

EDH patients usually present with classic lucid interval although it is not pathognomonic.

Further Reading

Khairat A, Waseem M. Epidural Hematoma. Treasure Island (FL): StatPearls Publishing; 2020.

Ans. 83

- EDH is a neurosurgical emergency that requires urgent surgical evacuation within 1 to 2 hours of presentation. The priority is to stabilize the patient, including the airway, breathing, and circulation. Surgical intervention is recommended in patients with:

- Acute EDH
- Hematoma volume > 30 mL regardless of GCS
- GCS < 9 with pupillary abnormalities like anisocoria

- In experienced neurosurgical centers, a nonsurgical approach may be offered in a patient with acute EDH but mild symptoms and has all of the following—an EDH volume < 30 mL, clot diameter < 15 mm, midline shift < 5 mm, and GCS > 8, and on physical examination with no focal neurological deficits.

Further Reading

Khairat A, Waseem M. Epidural Hematoma. Treasure Island (FL): StatPearls Publishing; 2020.

Ans. 84

CT scan shows a patient with intracranial hemorrhage, brain edema, and probably raised ICP, status post decompressive craniectomy. This is the last step in management of intractable intracranial hypertension when all other measures fail.

Indications include: Traumatic brain injury (TBI) and ischemic stroke, subarachnoid hemorrhage, venous thrombosis, toxoplasmosis, Reye's syndrome, and encephalitis.

Complications include: Hemorrhage, postoperative collections in the subgaleal and subdural space, on the side of surgery, herniation of brain through the craniotomy causing venous infarcts, Sinking flap syndrome, worsening of brain injury, etc.

In middle cerebral artery (MCA) infarct patients, Decompressive craniectomy reduced the mortality by 50%, however in TBI patients, the mortality remained unchanged and had worse neurological outcome.

Indications	*Evidence*
Ischemic stroke	• Early craniectomy within 48 hours; In those with age <60 (DESTINY II TRIAL looked into age >60 and showed a significant benefit), improved mortality from 80% to 30% without any change in disability outcome • Trials: DECIMAL, HAMLET, DESTINY
Traumatic brain injury	• Early neuroprotective bifrontal decompressive craniectomy—similar mortality, (19% vs. 18%), but an unfavorable outcome (GOSE 70% vs. 51%; p = 0.02) • Late decompressive craniectomy had substantially lower mortality (26.9% vs. 48.9%) but worse disability • Trials: DECRA, RESCUE ICP

Further Reading

Beez T, Munoz-Bendix C, Steiger H, Beseoglu K. Decompressive craniectomy for acute ischemic stroke. Crit Care. 2019;23:209.

Cooper DJ, Rosenfeld JV, Murray L, Arabi YM, Davies AR, D'Urso P, et al. Decompressive craniectomy in diffuse traumatic brain injury. N Engl J Med. 2011;364(16):1493-502.

Kakar V, Nagaria J, Kirkpatrick J. The current status of decompressive craniectomy. Br J Neurosurg. 2009;23(2):147-57.

Kolias AG, Viaroli E, Rubiano AM, Adams H, Khan T, Gupta D, et al. The current status of decompressive craniectomy in traumatic brain injury. Curr Trauma Rep. 2018;4(4):326-32.

Ans. 85

- *Diagnosis:* Ischemic stroke

According to Dawn Study

- Signs and symptoms consistent with the diagnosis of an acute ischemic stroke, and the patient has either failed IV thrombolysis or not a candidate for IV thrombolysis, with age ≥18 years, with no significant pre-stroke disability (pre-stroke mRS must be 0 or 1), having a baseline NIHSS score ≥ 10 points, presenting within 6–24 hours after time last known well and having <1/3 MCA territory involved, as evidenced by CT or MRI and occlusion of the intracranial ICA and/or MCA-M1 as evidenced by MRA or CTA and a clinical core mismatch.
- Patients aged >80 years with NIHSS score of >10 and a core volume < 21 mL
- Patients younger than 80 years, NIHSS score of >10 and a core volume <31 mL
- Or an NIHSS score of >20 and a core volume < 51 mL.

According to Defuse 3 Study

Clinical inclusion criteria:

- Patients of age 18–90 years having a baseline NIHSS score ≥ 6 and signs and symptoms consistent with the diagnosis of an acute anterior circulation ischemic stroke in whom treatment can *be i*nitiated (femoral puncture) between 6 and 16 hours of the time the patient was last known to be at their neurologic baseline
- Modified Rankin Scale ≤ 2 prior to qualifying stroke
  1. ICA or MCA-M1 occlusion (carotid occlusions can be cervical or intracranial; with or without tandem MCA lesions) by MRA or CTA
  2. Target mismatch profile on CT perfusion or MRI (ischemic core volume < 70 mL, mismatch ratio ≥ 1.8, and mismatch volume ≥ 15 mL)

Further Reading

Albers GW, Lansberg MG, Kemp S, Tsai JP, Lavori P, Christensen S, et al. A multicenter randomized controlled trial of endovascular therapy following imaging evaluation for ischemic stroke (DEFUSE 3). Int J Stroke. 2017;12(8):896-905.

Nogueira RG, Jadhav AP, Haussen DC, Bonafe A, Budzik RF, Bhuva P, et al. Thrombectomy 6 to 24 hours after stroke with a mismatch between deficit and infarct. N Engl J Med. 2018;378(1):11-21.

Ans. 86

Inclusion criteria:

- Patients aged ≥18 years, with a clinical diagnosis of ischemic stroke and neurologic deficit and presenting to treatment facility where treatment can be started within 4.5 hours of onset of symptoms, and imaging showing no signs of acute bleed.
- If presenting after 4.5 hours, but within 6 hours, thrombolysis may still be considered unless age >80 years, use of oral anticoagulant, regardless of INR, NIHSS score > 25, or a past history of ischemic stroke and diabetes mellitus.

Indications for repeat imaging after thrombolysis:

- In case of worsening of clinical status and an intracranial bleed is suspected
- After 24 hours, prior to start of antiplatelet agents

Trial	*Population*	*Intervention*	*Result*
MAST-I. Lancet. 1995;346(8989): 1509-14.	Stroke within 6 hours	Streptokinase	• Increased mortality at 6 months, disability decreased at 6 months
ECASS. JAMA. 1995;274(13):1017-25.	Strokes within 6 hours	Alteplase 1.1 mg	• No difference in performance scores • Increase in mortality with treatment
NINDS 1. NEJM. 1995;333(24):1581-7.	Stroke within 3 hours	t-Pa (0.9 mg/kg; 10% given as a bolus and 90% over 60 minutes)	• No significant difference between the two groups at 24 hours
NINDS 2. NEJM. 1995;333(24):1581-7.	Stroke within 3 hours	t-Pa (0.9 mg/kg; 10% given as a bolus and 90% over 60 minutes)	• Favorable outcome at 3 months • An increase in symptomatic and fatal intracerebral hemorrhage in the tPA-treated group
MAST 2. *NEJM. 1996;335(3):145-50.*	Stroke within 6 hours	Streptokinase 1.5 million units over 1 hour	• No difference in the primary outcome of death or disability • Increased intracranial hemorrhage
ASK Trial. JAMA. 1996;276(12):961-6.	Stroke within 4 hours	1.5 million units of streptokinase over 1 hour	• Increased mortality with streptokinase • Increased intracranial hemorrhage
ECASS II. Lancet. 1998;352:1245-51.	Stroke within 6 hours	t-PA (0.9 mg/kg)	• No change in mortality, • an increase in major intracerebral hemorrhage
ECASS III. NEJM. 2008;359(13):1317-29.	Stroke patients, NIHSS <25, within 3 hours, select group within 3–4.5 hours	t-PA (0.9 mg/kg)	• Favorable Modified Rankin score in treatment versus placebo • Unchanged mortality • Significant hemorrhage in treatment group
IST-3. Lancet. 2012;379(9834): 2352-63.	Stroke within 6 hours	t-Pa (0.9 mg/kg)	• No difference in mortality • Increased intracranial hemorrhage

Further Reading

Powers WJ, Rabinstein AA, Ackerson T, Adeoye OM, Bambakidis NC, Becker K, et al. Guidelines for the Early Management of Patients With Acute Ischemic Stroke: 2019 Update to the 2018 Guidelines for the Early Management of Acute Ischemic Stroke: A Guideline for Healthcare Professionals From the American Heart Association/American Stroke Association. Stroke. 2019;50(12):e344.

Ans. 87

This is a case of acute ischemic stroke.

Immediate management requires:
- Urgent brain imaging to rule out a bleed
- Obtaining blood sugar values
- Baseline ECG and troponin.

Medical management includes thrombolysis, airway assistance, and breathing support in patients with saturation < 94%, management of blood pressure (euvolemia, management of hypo or hypertension), maintaining euglycemia (140–180), statins, avoiding hypoxia, and treating fever.

Role of Heparin in Ischemic Stroke

Unfractionated heparin:
- No role in immediate management of stroke
- Heparin may reduce the risk of early recurrent stroke, but cause an increased rate of bleeding complications
- There are certain subpopulation of ischemic stroke patients that may derive benefit from heparin when given acutely, including patients with symptomatic large artery stenosis >70%, nonocclusive intraluminal thrombus, and in patients with high-risk cardiac conditions including left ventricular thrombus, left ventricular assist devices, and mechanical heart valves.

Role of Dual Antiplatelets
- Aspirin (162–325 mg/day) monotherapy for patients with moderate or higher stroke severity defined by an NIHSS score > 3
- Dual antiplatelet therapy (DAPT) for 21 days using aspirin plus clopidogrel for most patients with minor ischemic stroke, defined by an NIHSS score ≤ 3
- DAPT for 90 days using aspirin plus clopidogrel for patients with stroke due to intracranial large artery atherosclerosis
- The duration of DAPT when employed for acute stroke is limited to 21 days for patients with minor ischemic stroke and 90 days for patients with stroke due to intracranial large artery atherosclerosis.

Further Reading

Powers WJ, Rabinstein AA, Ackerson T, Adeoye OM, Bambakidis NC, Becker K, et al. Guidelines for the Early Management of Patients With Acute Ischemic Stroke: 2019 Update to the 2018 Guidelines for the Early Management of Acute Ischemic Stroke: A Guideline for Healthcare Professionals From the American Heart Association/American Stroke Association. Stroke. 2019;50(12):e344.

Powers WJ, Rabinstein AA, Ackerson T, Adeoye OM, Bambakidis NC, Becker K, et al. 2018 Guidelines for the Early Management of Patients With Acute Ischemic Stroke: A Guideline for Healthcare Professionals From the American Heart Association/American Stroke Association. Stroke. 2018;49(3):e46-e110.

Ruff IM, Jindal JA. Use of heparin in acute ischemic stroke: Is there still a role? Curr Atheroscler Rep. 2015;17(9):51.

Ans. 88

- Lentiform fork sign—bilateral hyperintensities in the basal ganglia surrounded by a hyperintense rim delineating the lentiform nucleus.
- It is commonly seen in uremic encephalopathy, diabetes mellitus, acidosis due to toxins such as methanol and ethylene glycol.
- Methyl alcohol and ethylene glycol toxicity causes a high anion gap metabolic acidosis that do not usually respond to resuscitation with intravenous fluids, correction of hypoglycemia, and thiamine administration. Ethylene glycol usually causes lactate gap, hypocalcemia, and calcium oxalate crystals in urine.
- In the absence of the same, methanol poisoning should be suspected and fomepizole should be started.

NEPHROLOGY

Ans. 89

A. *Regular intermittent dialysis circuit, with regional anticoagulation*: Principle of solute removal is *diffusion* (semipermeable membrane separates dialysate and blood) and molecules diffuse across the membrane from a high concentration gradient to lower concentration gradient.

B. *A continuous venovenous hemodiafiltration circuit with regional anticoagulation*: Principle includes diffusion as described above and *convection* [Convection is the process whereby solutes pass through membrane pores, dragged by fluid movement (ultrafiltration) caused by a hydrostatic and/or osmotic transmembrane pressure gradient].

C. *A continuous venovenous hemofiltration or slow continuous ultrafiltration*: Principle includes *convection* for solute removal. The ultrafiltration rate is dependent on the hydrostatic pressure across the membrane.

Further Reading

Neri M, Villa G, Garzotto F, Bagshaw S, Bellomo R, Cerda J, et al. Nomenclature for renal replacement therapy in acute kidney injury: basic principles. Crit Care. 2016;20:318.

Ans. 90

	Maximum rate	*Commonly prescribed rates*
Blood flow in CRRT	250 mL/min	150 mL/min
Rate of fluid replacement in CRRT	Up to 2000 mL/hr	1000–1500 mL/hr
Rate of dialysate flow in CRRT	2000 mL/hr in IHD	1000 mL/hr
Maximal fluid removal from patient (Net ultrafiltration from patient in CRRT)	8 mL/min in IHD	2–4 mL/min

Further reading

Macedo E, Mehta RL. Continuous dialysis therapies: Core curriculum 2016. Am J Kidney Dis. 2016;68(4):645-57.

Ans. 91

	Dosing based on estimated urea clearance (K calc)
CVVH postdilution	$K = Q_{UF} = Q_R$
CVVH predilution	$K = Q_{UF}$
CVVHD	$K_{CALC} = \frac{Q_{UF}}{1+\frac{Q_R}{Q_B}}$
CVVHDF postdilution	$K = Q_R + Q_D$

(CVVH: continuous venovenous hemofiltration; CVVHD: continuous venovenous hemodialysis; CVVHDF: continuous venovenous hemodiafiltration; Q_{UF}: ultrafiltration rate, Q_R: infusion rate; Q_B: blood flow, Q_R: replacement flow; Q_D: dialysate flow)

Dose of CRRT: The dose of CRRT is the volume of blood "purified" per unit time. Practically it is the effluent flow rate (= ultrafiltrate + dialysate flow rate). More definitively, the dose is the clearance rate of a representative marker solute; usually indexed to body weight (K/wt = L/kg/h) where Clearance (K) = volume of blood cleared (L)/time (min).

Dose calculation in various CRRT types:

Q_{UF} = ultrafiltration rate, Q_R = replacement fluid rate, Q_B = blood flow rate

Optimal dose = 20–25 mL/kg/h

To increase efficiency:

- Increase filter lifespan with anticoagulation and predilution
- Reduce interruptions in CRRT—imaging, etc.
- Improve vascular access—good blood flow rate
- Increase the blood flow rate
- Increase the dose of dialysis—increase in ultrafiltration rates, replacement fluid rate.

Further Reading

Ricci Z, Romagnoli S, Ronco C. Continuous renal replacement therapy. F1000Res. 2016;5.

Ans. 92

A = Sodium citrate solution

B = Calcium gluconate solution

Complications of RCA:

- Citrate accumulation (common complication), especially in patients with liver disease
- Metabolic alkalosis related to buffer overload
- Metabolic acidosis—inadequate buffer supply
- Hypercalcemia/hypocalcemia
- Hypernatremia.

Clotting factors inhibited by RCA—Factors X and VII.

Further Reading

Morabito S, Pistolesi V, Tritapepe L, Fiaccadori E. Regional citrate anticoagulation for RRTs in critically ill patients with AKI. Clin J Am Soc Nephrol. 2014;9(12):2173-88.

Ans. 93

- High flow rate from the patient (limited catheter movement, avoiding kinks, and use of wide bore catheter)
- Predilution use of replacement fluid
- Use of RCA
- Use of heparin anticoagulation
- Use of warfarin and prostacyclins.

Further Reading

Morabito S, Guzzo I, Solazzo A, Muzi L, Luciani R, Pierucci A. Continuous renal replacement therapies: anticoagulation in the critically ill at high risk of bleeding. J Nephrol. 2003;16(4):566-71.

Tan HK, Baldwin I, Bellomo R. Continuous veno-venous hemofiltration without anticoagulation in high-risk patients. Intensive Care Med. 2000;26(11):1652-7.

Ans. 94

Low return pressure troubleshooting.

Causes: Low blood pump speed, line disconnection, presensor, and post-pump line is clamped (the reading is thus 0 mm Hg).

Troubleshooting:

- Check circuit and patient and, if no disconnection is present, override alarm
- De-clamp lines
- Evaluate for circuit change
- Increase set blood flow rate

Further Reading

Zaccaria R, Baldwin I, Ronco C. Alarms and troubleshooting. In: Kellum JA, Bellomo R, Ronco C. Continuous Renal Replacement Therapy. Oxford: Oxford University Press; 2016.

Ans. 95

Transmembrane pressure is the pressure gradient across the membranes. That is difference between pressure in blood compartment and dialysate compartment. It is calculated by the below formula:

Transmembrane pressure (TMP) = (Filter pressure + Return pressure)/2 – (Effluent pressure)

Filter pressure is a calculated value displayed on the screen used to determine the pressure conditions in the hollow fibers. It is calculated as filter pod pressure–return pod pressure (ΔP). Filter clogging increases filter pressure.

Causes of high TMP alarm: Clogging of filter, kinked or clamped dialysis line, and blood flow too slow for ultrafiltration setting.

Further Reading

Prisma system. Operator's manual. [online] Available from https://www.crrtonline.com/docs/OperatorsPrismaEng.pdf [Last accessed February, 2020].

Zaccaria R, Baldwin I, Ronco C. Alarms and troubleshooting. In: Kellum JA, Bellomo R, Ronco C. Continuous Renal Replacement Therapy. Oxford: Oxford University Press; 2016.

Ans. 96

Indications for RRT in ICU

- *Conventional indications:*
  - Fluid overload resistant to diuretic therapy
  - Metabolic acidosis (pH <7.15) refractory to medical management
  - Hyperkalemia (K >6.5 mEq/L) refractory to medical management
  - Uremic symptoms or signs (encephalopathy, pericarditis, and bleeding diathesis)
- *Other important indications:*
  - Poisoning with a dialyzable drug or toxin
  - Hyperthermia refractory to regular cooling techniques
  - Life-threatening electrolyte derangements in the setting of acute kidney injury.

Appraise the current evidence regarding timing of renal replacement therapy in ICU.

Evidence for timing of RRT: The timing of the RRT in the absence of absolute indications is challenging. The initiation of RRT can be early or delayed although there is no hard definition differentiating between early and late with investigators using a variety of parameters including blood urea nitrogen (BUN) and creatinine, clinical markers like urine output and fluid balance and the time from onset of developing AKI to define it.

Observational data: PICARD trial, a multicenter observational study of AKI, showed that in patients with no previous chronic kidney disease (CKD) and required RRT, initiation of RRT at a lower BUN ≤ 76 mg/dL compared to ≥76 mg/dL was associated with lower 14 and 28-day mortality.

Randomized control trial (RCTs): Three major RCT of timing of RRT in AKI were ELAIN trial, AKIKI and IDEAL ICU trial. ELAIN trial was a single center randomized trial of 231 critically ill-patients that tested whether early RRT compared to delayed RRT would reduce all-cause mortality at 90 days. The primary outcome showed an absolute reduction in 90-day mortality of 15.4% in the early RRT group (39.3%) compared to the delayed RRT (54.7%). Early RRT also led to a higher likelihood of dialysis independence, significantly shorter duration of RRT (9 vs. 25 days), and shortening of hospital stay (51 vs. 82 days). AKIKI trial was a large multicenter French randomized trial of 620 critically ill-patients that tested whether delayed RRT compared to early RRT would reduce all-cause 60-day mortality. The primary outcome showed no significant difference in 60-day mortality between early RRT (48.5%) versus delayed RRT (49.7%). There was no difference in key secondary outcomes including ventilator and vasopressor-free days through day 28, ICU length of stay, hospital length of stay, and dialysis dependence at day 60.

The ELAIN and AKIKI trials were underpowered to detect difference in mortality between the two groups. The delayed RRT intervention of ELAIN was similar to the early RRT of AKIKI. The ELAIN trial primarily had postoperative patients (94%) with AKI, compared to predominantly medical patients with septic shock in AKIKI. The mode of RRT differed as well with CVVHDF used in ELAIN compared to mainly IHD in AKIKI.

The recent IDEAL-ICU trial, a multicenter RCT involving 488 septic patients, found no significant difference in 90-day mortality between early and delayed RRT. The study supports the findings of AKIKI trial.

All the RCTs on timing of RRT had a high risk of bias for allocation concealment.

In conclusion, timing of RRT is still controversial and no evidence so far now is in favor of early RRT. The time of initiation should be based on patient profile and also on the indication of RRT.

Further Reading

Ahmed AR, Obilana A, Lappin D. Renal replacement therapy in the critical care setting. Crit Care Res Pract. 2019;2019:6948710. Published 2019 Jul 16.

Ans. 97

Sieving coefficient (SC): The ratio between the concentration of a drug in the ultrafiltrate to its concentration in prefilter plasma is called Sieving coefficient. This expresses the ability of the drug or solute to pass through a filter membrane. Drugs with SC of one, are readily filtered and require increased drug dosing or decreased time between dosing intervals.

Numerous variables affecting drug dosing in patients receiving RRT are:

1. *The CRRT technique*: Drug clearance is greatest with continuous venovenous hemodiafiltration followed by continuous venovenous hemodialysis, and then continuous venovenous hemofiltration.
2. *Filter properties*: Membrane permeability–CRRT filters have increased pore size and are effective in removing molecules up to 50,000 Da. This is important as protein binding with albumin significantly reduces clearance of drugs via CRRT. The unbound fraction of a drug diffuses freely across the filter membrane.
3. *Age of the CRRT filter*: With an increase in age of the filter, the filtration reduces.
4. *Flow rates*: Flow rate has the largest effect of all variables on drug clearance in patients on CRRT. Higher flow rates of blood, dialysate, or ultrafiltrate result in increased drug removal. Hence, for drugs removed by CRRT, increased flow rates result in a need to increase drug dosing or to decrease time between dosing intervals.
5. *Volume of distribution*: May be altered in critically ill-patients, with either an increase or decrease in volume of distribution resulting in alteration of clearance. Drugs with a low volume of distribution are removed more readily by CRRT and may require increased or more frequent dosing.

Dose adjustments in CRRT	*Pharmacokinetics*	*EG*	*Comments*
Drugs requiring no dose adjustment during CRRT	High volume of distribution	Moxifloxacin Moxifloxacin Itraconazole Clindamycin Liposomal amphotericin	These drugs have a large volume of distribution and the circulating free drug concentration is negligible. Hence, they are not eliminated by RRT and should be administered in same dose of normal patients

Contd...

Contd...

	Highly bound to protein or lipid	Ceftriaxone Colistin	Ceftriaxone is highly protein bound, colistin binds to both albumin and alpha 1 acid glycoprotein and during dialysis, additional 10% dose needs to be given
	Predominantly hepatic clearance	Linezolid Ceftriaxone	These drugs are cleared in the liver renal failure and CRRT will not affect their clearance
	CRRT clearance at par with renal clearance	β-lactams Carbapenems Aminoglycosides Most cephalosporins Aciclovir	These drugs are easily cleared from CRRT, similar to the glomerular filtration
Drugs with require a dose increase during CRRT	Increased clearance by CRRT	Fluconazole	Increased filter clearance, which requires increase in dose
Drugs which require a reduced dosing but an increased dosing interval during CRRT	Lack of active transport	Vancomycin Levofloxacin Daptomycin	These drugs are usually dependant on the renal function and an additional mechanism, such as exchange pump or active transport mechanism in the tubule which is absent with filter. Hence, the free concentration increases, requiring a decrease in dose or increased dosing interval

Further Reading

Ricci, Zaccaria, Baldwin I, Ronco C. Continuous renal replacement therapy. 2016;15.

Ans. 98

Replacement fluids for CRRT contain electrolytes and glucose with a concentration as follows: sodium 140 mmol/L; chloride 108–112 mmol/L; potassium 0–4 mmol/L; calcium 1.5–1.75 mmol/L; magnesium 0.5–0.75 mmol/L, and glucose 0–15.00 mg/L. Commonly bicarbonate or lactate are used as the buffering solution.

Electrolyte disturbances in CRRT: Hypophosphatemia, hypomagnesemia, hypocalcemia, hypokalemia, hypo- or hypernatremia.

Further Reading

Ronco C, Bellomo R, Kellum JA (Eds). Acute kidney injury. Contrib Nephrol. Basel, Karger. 2007;156:287-96.

Sigwalt F, Bouteleux A, Dambricourt F, Asselborn T, Moriceau F, Rimmelé T. Clinical complications of continuous renal replacement therapy. Contrib Nephrol. 2018;194:109-17.

Ans. 99

Blood leak alarm in the circuit A

Air alarm D.

Further Reading

Ricci, Zaccaria, Baldwin I, Ronco C. Continuous renal replacement therapy. 2016:15.

Ans. 100

Diagnosis: Dialysis disequilibrium syndrome.

Prevention: Initial dialysis should be slow with gradual reduction in urea, hemofiltration, instead of dialysis can used as a modality as the osmolarities of the body fluid compartments will not change as rapidly as they do during standard hemodialysis. Addition of an osmotic agent to the blood stream such as mannitol will help to prevent the development of a blood-brain osmotic gradient and consequently help to prevent cerebral edema. Similarly sodium modelling may be done, so that the sodium concentration of the dialysate remains at a higher concentration throughout the treatment.

Further Reading

Zepeda-Orozco D, Quigley R. Dialysis disequilibrium syndrome. Pediatr Nephrol. 2012;27(12):2205-11.

MICROBIOLOGY AND INFECTION CONTROL

Ans. 101

1. *Diagnosis:* Leptospirosis

Test: Enzyme-linked immune sorbent assay (ELISA) (preferably not card test), microscopic agglutination test (MAT), polymerase chain reaction (PCR), and culture.

2. *Criteria for diagnosis:* A presumptive diagnosis for leptospirosis can be made by:
   - A positive IgM-based immune-assays, or
   - A positive titer of 100/200/400 for MAT or
   - A positive direct staining.
3. *For confirmation of the diagnosis:*
   - Leptospires should be isolated from clinical specimen, or
   - Have a lab evidence of a fourfold or greater rise in the serial MAT titer between acute and convalescent phase serum or
   - By PCR test.

(PCR: Sensitivity 54 % for serum, 59% for buffy coat, and 45% for urine with a specificity of above 95%, MAT: 17–20% sensitivity)

Blood and CSF culture are positive in the initial 10 days with a sensitivity of 50–70%. Urine culture is positive after 2nd week and remains positive up to a month (culture is often opted for research purposes rather than as a diagnostic modality).

Further Reading

Budihal SV, Perwez K. Leptospirosis diagnosis: Competency of various laboratory tests. J Clin Diagn Res. 2014;8(1):199-202.

Ans. 102

1. *Community-acquired meningitis:* Commonly pathogens implicated are *Streptococcus pneumoniae, Neisseria meningitidis, Staphylococcus aureus, Haemophilus influenzae*, gram-negative bacilli, and *Listeria*.

2. The empirical therapy for community-acquired meningitis will be a third-generation cephalosporin such as ceftriaxone 2 g IV BD (twice a day) and vancomycin 500 mg IV q6h (every 6 hours).
   The history of immunocompromised status and lab picture is suggestive of meningitis caused by *Listeria monocytogenes*. If *Listeria* is suspected, treatment should be modified to ampicillin 2 g IV every 4th hourly and gentamicin 2 mg/kg loading dose followed by 1.7 mg/kg 8 hours as cephalosporins are not effective against *Listeria*.
3. In case of penicillin allergy, ampicillin may have to be replaced with co-trimoxazole/erythromycin/vancomycin/fluoroquinolones.

Further Reading

Temple ME, Nahata MC. Treatment of listeriosis. Ann Pharmacother. 2000;34(5):656-61.
Weisfelt M, de Gans J, van der Ende A, van de Beek D. Community-acquired bacterial meningitis in alcoholic patients. PLoS One. 2010;5:e9102.

Ans. 103

1. The clinical picture is suggestive of viral encephalitis more than aseptic meningitis, although the difference is marginal.
2. The common etiological agents are herpes simplex virus (HSV), Japanese encephalitis virus, measles, mumps, rubella, Hendra/Nipah, West Nile virus, Rabies, etc.

Cerebrospinal fluid PCR should be performed for the common viruses such as HSV-1 and 2, human immunodeficiency virus (HIV), and Enteroviruses. However, for diagnosis of arbovirus such as West Nile fever, immunoglobulin M (IgM) antibody-capture enzyme-linked immunosorbent assay (MAC-ELISA) is preferred over PCR and IgM antibodies appear by day 5–8 of the disease.

Further Reading

Kennedy PG. Viral encephalitis: Causes, differential diagnosis, and management. J Neurol Neurosurg Psychiatr. 2004;75:i10-i15.

Ans. 104

- Attached figure shows the lytic colonies of *S. pneumoniae* on blood agar, with typical carrom-coin appearance.
- The patient has CAP and has four points of the CURB-65 score suggesting a high risk with 27.8% 30-day mortality, necessitating inpatient treatment with possible intensive care admission.
- The Smart cop score of 8 also gives a fair prediction of requirement of IV vasopressors and respiratory support.
- The current *American Thoracic Society* (ATS) guidelines suggest sputum culture and blood culture in patients with severe disease and favor a combination of beta-lactam macrolide/fluoroquinolone such as ampicillin + sulbactam 1.5–3 g every 6 hours, cefotaxime 1–2 g every 8 hours, ceftriaxone 1–2 g daily, and azithromycin 500 mg daily or clarithromycin 500 mg twice daily or levofloxacin 750 mg daily in patients with no risk factors for methicillin-resistant *Staphylococcus aureus* (MRSA)/*Pseudomonas aeruginosa*.
- However, if the patient has not improved with empirical treatment, drug-resistant pneumococci needs to be considered and clindamycin or vancomycin needs to be added

- Risk factors for developing resistance in *S. pneumoniae* include elderly with age >65 years, previous treatment with similar antibiotics such as beta-lactam, macrolide, or fluoroquinolone therapy within the past 3–6 months, immunosuppression and other medical comorbidities, alcoholism, etc.
- This patient is at high risk for further pneumococcal disease and should be advised vaccination against pneumococci as per schedule.
- Based on the latest evidence, the Advisory Committee on Immunization Practices currently recommends only 23-valent pneumococcal polysaccharide vaccine (PPSV23) among adults aged ≥65 years, and to consider the need of PCV13-based individual clinical decisions with respect to the risk factors and prevalence and to administer PCV13, at least 1 year before PPSV23, if a decision to administer both are made.

Further Reading

Matanock A, Lee G, Gierke R, Kobayashi M, Leidner A, Pilishvili T. Use of 13-valent pneumococcal conjugate vaccine and 23-valent pneumococcal polysaccharide vaccine among adults aged ≥65 years: Updated Recommendations of the Advisory Committee on Immunization Practices. MMWR Morb Mortal Wkly Rep. 2019;68(46):1069.

Wang CY, Chen YH, Fang C, Zhou MM, Xu HM, Jing CM, et al. Antibiotic resistance profiles and multidrug resistance patterns of *Streptococcus pneumoniae* in pediatrics: A multicenter retrospective study in mainland China. Medicine. 2019;98(24):e15942.

Ans. 105

1. Film-array (real-time PCR that tests for multiple pathogens based upon the system involved).
   - This patient has B/L pneumonia, tachypnea, multilobar consolidation, and pF ratio (arterial pO_2 divided by the FiO_2) <250, suggestive of severe pneumonia.
2. In this patient, as there is probable involvement of multiple pathogens (probable primary viral with secondary bacterial infection), choice of film-array pneumonia screen would be more economical and time-efficient in diagnosis.

Note: Rapid influenza molecular assay with nucleic acid amplification tests (NAATs) are now advised as against antigen-based detection tests.

Further Reading

McLoughlin KS. Microarrays for pathogen detection and analysis. Brief Funct Genomics. 2011;10(6):342-53.

Ans. 106

1. Picture shows branching filamentous acid fast bacterium, *Nocardia*. Cotrimoxazole 15 mg/kg/d + amikacin (7.5 mg/kg IV every 12 hours) for 6 weeks have been the antimicrobial of choice to treat nocardiosis in mild-moderate presentation. However in severe cases, imipenem 500 mg q6h with amikacin or linezolid may be required.

Further Reading

Wilson JW. Nocardiosis: Updates and clinical overview. Mayo Clin Proc. 2012;87(4): 403-7.

Ans. 107

Thoracic tomography shows multiple discrete nodules with halo sign suggestive of angioinvasive aspergillosis. The culture shows fungal colonies on Sabouraud agar.

1. Voriconazole/echinocandin, voriconazole >> echinocandins
2. 1, 3 Beta D glucan (BDG) assay and galactomannan assay of serum and preferably a paired sample with BAL. The sensitivity and positive predictive value of galactomannan is found to be higher in BAL than in serum. 1,3 BDG is a nonspecific fungal marker that can help in the initial screening, while galactomannan assay is specific for *Aspergillus* species. False-positive reactions due to some cross-reactivity with *Histoplasma capsulatum* and *Penicillium* species can occur and also in those patients treated with antibiotics such as piperacillin-tazobactam.
3. The treatment for fungal infections can be classified as prophylactic, empirical, pre-emptive, and targeted treatment
   - High risk patients + no signs of infection: prophylactic
   - High risk patients + signs of infection: empirical
   - High risk patients + serological tests: pre-emptive
   - High risk patients + culture positive: targeted treatment

Further Reading

Kulkarni AP, Sengar M, Chinnaswamy G, Hegde A, Rodrigues C, Soman R, et al. Indian antimicrobial prescription guidelines in critically ill immunocompromised patients. Indian J Crit Care Med. 2019;23(Suppl 1):S64-S96.

Panackal AA, Bennett JE, Williamson PR. Treatment options in invasive aspergillosis. Curr Treat Options Infect Dis. 2014;6(3):309-25.

Park SY, Lee SO, Choi SH, Jeong JY, Sung H, Kim MN, et al. Serum and bronchoalveolar lavage fluid galactomannan assays in patients with pulmonary aspergilloma. Clin Infect Dis. 2011;52(7):e149-52.

Ans. 108

1.

Causes of infectious diarrhea in immunocompromised host	
Bacteria	Pathogenic *Escherichia coli, Salmonella, Shigella, Campylobacter, Clostridioides difficile, Chlamydia trachomatis, Mycobacterium avium* complex
Viruses	Rotavirus, cytomegalovirus, norovirus herpes simplex virus, adenovirus, human immunodeficiency virus
Parasites	*Entamoeba histolytica, Cryptosporidium, Cystoisospora belli* (previously called *Isospora belli*), *Giardia lamblia, Cyclospora, Strongyloides stercoralis*
Fungi	*Microsporidium, Histoplasmosis candida*
Noninfectious causes	AIDS enteropathy, lymphoma, Kaposi sarcoma, highly active antiretroviral therapy

(AIDS: acquired immunodeficiency syndrome)

2. Workup
   - Workup and evaluation of HIV-associated diarrhea includes assessment of disease status including CD4 count, HIV viral load, treatment history,

stool, microscopy for ova, cysts and parasites, special stains such as modified ZN (Ziehl-Neelsen) stain, stool culture, stool virology, and specific PCR or investigations targeting *C. difficile* such as glutamate dehydrogenase, toxin A and B screening assays need to be called for (antigen tests may be considered for confirmation of positive ZN report).
   - Endoscopic examination including biopsies may be needed if stool study is negative or idiopathic.
3. Treatment depends upon the etiology
   - *Nitazoxanide:* Nitazoxanide is the only proven antiparasitic treatment for *Cryptosporidium* infection. However, it is not effective in severely immunocompromised patients. Immune reconstitution or a decreased immunosuppression is critical to therapy in AIDS and transplant patients.
   - Ivermectin 200 mg/kg orally once a day for 1–2 days is the drug of choice in strongyloidiasis.
   - Cystoisosporiasis responds well to trimethoprim/sulfamethoxazole or as ciprofloxacin in case of allergy to sulfonamides.
   - Ganciclovir [5 mg/kg intravenously (IV) twice daily for at least 3 weeks] is the treatment of choice for cytomegalovirus (CMV) colitis.
   - Itraconazole may be tried for diarrhea of fungal etiology.

Further Reading

Kaiser L, Surawicz CM. Infectious causes of chronic diarrhoea. Best Pract Res Clin Gastroenterol. 2012;26(5):563-71.

Krones E, Högenauer C. Diarrhea in the immunocompromised patient. Gastroenterol Clin North Am. 2012;41(3):677-701.

Sparks H, Nair G, White CA. Treatment of cryptosporidium: What we know, gaps, and the way forward. Curr Trop Med Rep. 2015;2(3):181-7.

Ans. 109

1. With the typical travel history, endemic diseases which may be otherwise rare also needs to be added to the list of differential diagnosis, e.g., coccidioidomycosis, histoplasmosis, rickettsial diseases, typhoid, etc. Tularemia is a rare disease that is almost endemic to the northern hemisphere, e.g., Scandinavian nations, northern America, Japan, and Russia.
2. The investigations of choice would include real-time PCR, serologic assays of serial samples to demonstrate rise/fall of titer, and blood culture. Suspected cases require special culture media such as CHAB (cysteine heart agar supplemented with 9% heated sheep red blood cells) for isolation of species.
   Given the lack of risk of infection for laboratory staff, serological tests demonstrating the rise/fall of titer to *F. tularensis*, agglutination, or an ELISA at the end of 2 weeks are an attractive alternative to culture.
3. In suspected cases of tularemia, treatment should be initiated with streptomycin and doxycycline/chloramphenicol. Given the lack of evidence for patient-to-patient transmission, in suspected cases of tularemia, isolation is not required. However, standard aseptic precautions need to be carried out.

If clinical samples are being sent to the microbiological/molecular diagnosis laboratory, they need to be alerted of the tularemia differential. Higher biosafety level (level 3) and more stringent precautions are required for manipulating samples that might contain *Francisella*.

Geographical area	*Common*	*Occasional*	*Rare but important*
Sub-Saharan Africa	HIV-associated Pulmonary Infections TB	Katayama Syndrome, Tropical Pulmonary Eosinophilia (*Wuchereria Bancrofti*), Loeffler's Syndrome (Hookworm, Strongyloides) Hydatidosis	Histoplasmosis, Pneumonic Plague, Paragonimiasis
North Africa, Middle East and Mediterranean		Q Fever, Tropical Pulmonary Eosinophilia (*Wuchereria Bancrofti*), Loeffler's Syndrome (Hookworm, Ascariasis, Strongyloides) Hydatidosis, Toxocariasis	MERS
Eastern Europe and Scandinavia	Legionellosis	Pertussis, Toxocariasis	Hantavirus, Tularemia
South and Central Asia	Diphtheria, TB, Avian Flu	Melioidosis, Loeffler's Syndrome (Hookworm, Ascariasis, Strongyloides) Hydatidosis	Nipah Virus
Southeast Asia	Avian Flu	Melioidosis, Tropical Pulmonary Eosinophilia (*Brugia malayi*), Loeffler's Syndrome (Strongyloides, Hookworm), Leptospirosis, Diphtheria	SARS, Hantavirus, Nipah Virus, Dirofilariasis, Katayama Syndrome, Paragonmiasis
Northern Australia		Q Fever	Melioidosis, Dirofilarisis, Pertussis
Latin America and Caribbean		Coccidioidomycosis Histoplasmosis, Leptospirosis, Diphtheria, Tropical Pulmonary Eosinophilia (*Wuchereria Bancrofti*), Loeffler's Syndrome (Ascariasis, Strongyloides), Hydatidosis, Toxocariasis	Hantavirus, Dirofilariasis
North America	Legionellosis, Pertussis, Diphtheria	Coccidioidomycosis Histoplasmosis, Toxocariasis	Dirofilariasis, Q Fever

(HIV: human immunodeficiency virus; MERS: Middle Eastern respiratory syndrome; SARS: severe acute respiratory syndrome; TB: tuberculosis)

Further Reading

Ellis J, Oyston PC, Green M, Titball RW. Tularemia. Clin Microbiol Rev. 2002;15(4):631-46.

Trimble A, Moffat V, Collins AM. Pulmonary infections in the returned traveller. Pneumonia. 2017;9:1.

Ans. 110

1. The differential diagnosis includes lymphoproliferative disorders of the mediastinum, primary cardiac tumors, invasive fungal infections, sclerosing mediastinitis due to tuberculosis, histoplasmosis, and aspergillosis.
   Attached image shows the white cotton growth of mucor on the obverse of Sabouraud dextrose agar medium, obtained on day 7 of inoculation of a fine-needle aspirate from the mediastinal lymph node.
2. Pan fungal PCR can be done on the clinical specimen, which will yield the result, and has the added advantage of giving an optimal report when more than one fungal species is involved.

Further Reading

Trubiano JA, Dennison AM, Morrissey CO, Chua KY, Halliday CL, Chen SC, et al. Clinical utility of panfungal polymerase chain reaction for the diagnosis of invasive fungal disease: A single center experience. Med Mycol. 2016;54(2)138-46.

Ans. 111

1. *Diagnosis:* Diphtheria
2. *Definitive diagnosis:* Demonstration of toxigenic strain of *Corynebacterium diphtheriae* in culture from respiratory tract secretions/pseudomembranes, Elek test, or a positive PCR detection of Toxin A and B. Special stains may be required for staining and include Albert's stain/Neisser's stain/Ponder's stain.
3. Management includes providing respiratory droplet isolation, securing airway if compromised, assessment of other organ damage including cardiac, neurological evaluation, early administration of diphtheria antitoxin, administration of antibiotics such as macrolides, penicillin, and vancomycin or linezolid in drug-resistant cases, and to be quarantined till there are two negative cultures 24 hours apart. These patients should further be administered immunization with diphtheria toxoid during their convalescence since natural infection does not induce immunity.

Medical staff and close contacts exposed to oral or respiratory secretions of the case need to be identified, screened with appropriate cultures, and considered for prophylaxis with diphtheria toxoid and/or treated with oral erythromycin (500 mg four times daily for 7–10 days).

Further Reading

World Health Organization. Operational protocol for clinical management of Diphtheria Bangladesh, Cox's Bazar (Version 10th Dec 2017). [online] Available from https://www.who.int/health-cluster/resources/publications/WHO-operational-protocols-diphtheria.pdf?ua=1 [Last accessed February, 2020].

Ans. 112

1. Urine is showing growth of ESBL Enterobacteriaceae. Oral fosfomycin and nitrofurantoin have been used in pregnancy without safety concerns. In patients requiring intravenous antibiotics, beta lactam–beta lactamase inhibitor (BL-BLI) therapy would suffice and be optimal with close monitoring for risk of resistance.
2. However, in case of blood stream infections with ESBL organisms, use of BL-BLI is associated with poor outcome and carbapenems are to be opted for. The drug of choice would be meropenem even if in vitro susceptibility

to BL-BLI is documented. Efforts to find the resistance mechanism/enzyme needs to be done. Carbapenems except imipenem–cilastatin are safe in pregnancy. Imipenem cilastatin has shown fetal adverse effects and is included as type C category drugs in pregnancy.

Further Reading

Rodriguez-Bano J, Gutierrez-Gutierrez B, Machuca I, Pascual A. Treatment of infections caused by extended-spectrum-beta-lactamase-, Amp C-, and carbapenemase-producing enterobacteriaceae. Clin Microbiol Rev. 2018;31(2):e00079-17.

Schuetz AN, Reyes S, Tamma PD. Point-counterpoint: Piperacillin tazobactam should be used to treat infections with extended-spectrum-beta-lactamase positive organisms. J Clin Microbiol. 2018;56:e01917-17.

Ans. 113

1. *Diagnosis:* Staphylococcal-scalded skin syndrome. Management includes treatment with clindamycin + cloxacillin (beta-lactamase resistant penicillin), or linezolid, if strains are showing methicillin resistance.
2. The attached figure shows lawn culture of *Staphylococcus* strain demonstrating inducible clindamycin resistance as seen by the significant reduction of zone of clindamycin in the vicinity of macrolide antibiotic.
3. Staphylococcal-scalded skin syndrome is often witnessed and documented in children. When diagnosed in adults, immune workup of the patient may be considered, as SSSS is mostly documented in immunocompromised/immunosuppressed people, such as those with immunological deficiencies, renal failure, or other such chronic illnesses.

Further Reading

Bamberger DM, Boyd SE. Management of *Staphylococcus aureus* infections. Am Fam Physician. 2005;72(12):2474-81.

Cribier B, Bernard Y, Grosshans E. Staphylococcal scalded skin syndrome in adults. J Am Acad Dermatol. 1994;30(2):319-24.

Nedamanuru K, Dampetla AJ, Gopineni D. A case report on staphylococcal scalded skin syndrome. Indian J Pharma Prac. 2018;11(2):99-100.

Ans. 114

1. *The attached figure shows growth of Escherichia coli (yellow colonies) and growth of S. typhimurium [black colonies, due to hydrogen sulfide production, on* Xylose lysine deoxycholate *(XLD) medium].* Generally, antibiotics are not recommended in acute diarrheal disease with nontyphoidal *Salmonella,* due to its self-limiting nature of the disease and because it does not typically shorten the length of illness. Antibiotics are recommended only in high-risk population such as those with underlying medical history, young children, and in disseminated infection. Treatment consists of the following antibiotics: fluoroquinolones/azithromycin/trimethoprim-sulfamethoxazole.
2. Maintaining hand hygiene, and the prompt neutralizing and discard of patient-refuse.

Further Reading

American Society for Microbiology. [online] Available from https://www.asm.org/Case-Studies/Salmonella-gastroenteritis-Lab-Testing-and-Treatment (Last accessed March, 2020).

Ans. 115

1. Differential diagnosis would be that of community-acquired meningitis. Such rapid deterioration warrants consideration of meningococci. Diagnosis can be made by CSF/blood PCR—preferably multiplex PCR the sensitivity of cultures for CSF is 80–90% while that of blood is 50–60% and that of petechial culture (skin biopsy) is 30%. Loop-mediated isothermal amplification (LAMP), under evaluation, seems promising.
2. The empiric treatment is third-generation cephalosporins, e.g., ceftriaxone for 7 days or chloramphenicol.
3. *Droplet infection precautions:* Persons with prolonged close contact with patients' oral secretions needs to be administered chemoprophylaxis. Rifampin is administered twice daily for 2 days (600 mg every 12 hours for adults, 10 mg/kg of body weight every 12 hours for children ≥1 month of age, and 5 mg/kg every 12 hours for infants <1 month of age). Alternatively, a single 500 mg oral dose of ciprofloxacin or ceftriaxone in a single parenteral dose (an intramuscular dose of 125 mg for children and 250 mg for adults) may be considered. Healthcare workers do not have prolonged exposure, although they have brief intermittent exposure during suction and aspiration. Hence, chemoprophylaxis is not routinely indicated for healthcare workers.

Further Reading

Łyczko KŁ, Borger J. Meningococcal prophylaxis. In: StatPearls. Treasure Island (FL): StatPearls Publishing; 2019. [online] Available from https://www.ncbi.nlm.nih.gov/books/NBK537338/ [Last accessed February, 2020].

Ans. 116

1. Now that *Enterococcus* has grown in blood culture, echinocandins may be stopped and continued voriconazole prophylaxis as per protocol. In view of persistent fever, vancomycin may be replaced with teicoplanin.
2. Enterococci are a common source of healthcare-associated infections in high-risk patients such as hematology-oncology and bone marrow transplant. Commonly isolated species include *E. faecalis* and *E. faecium*. *E. faecalis* species are usually sensitive to ampicillin and are associated with high rates of endocarditis. *E. faecium* are ampicillin resistant and currently vancomycin, aminoglycosides, and beta-lactam resistance is also increasing.
3. *E. gallinarum* and *Enterococci casseliflavus* strains have intrinsic resistance to vancomycin but usually are ampicillin sensitive. Teicoplanin retains its activity against *E. gallinarum* and *E. casseliflavus,* and this might be a therapeutic option along with tigecycline, linezolid, and daptomycin.

Further Reading

Britt NS, Potter EM. Clinical epidemiology of vancomycin-resistant *Enterococcus gallinarum* and *Enterococcus casseliflavus* bloodstream infections. J Global Antimicrob Resis. 2016;5:57-61.

Ans. 117

1. At this juncture, it can only be labeled as probable CLABSI. For further confirmation, catheter-tip culture maybe requested for.

2. *CLABSI:* A primary blood stream infection in a patient with a central line within the previous 48-hour period before the development of a documented blood stream infection and is not related to an infection at another site.
   - Catheter-related bloodstream infection (CRBSI) is a bloodstream infection attributed to be caused by an intravascular catheter as demonstrated by recovering >15 colony-forming units from the culture of the catheter tip and the same organism from percutaneous blood culture, or isolation of the same organism from a peripheral and a catheter lumen blood culture, with growth detected 2 hours earlier in the catheter sample or same organism recovered from a quantitative peripheral and a catheter lumen blood culture, with three-fold greater colony count in the latter.
   - CRBSI is mostly used for research, and CLABSI used for surveillance. CLABSI may over report the incidence of true CRBSI.

Further Reading

Mermel LA, Allom M, Bouza E, Craven DE, Flynn P, O'Grady NP, et al. Clinical Practice Guidelines for the diagnosis and management of Intravascular catheter-related infection: 2009 Update by the Infectious Diseases Society of America. Clin Infect Dis. 2009;49(1):1-45.

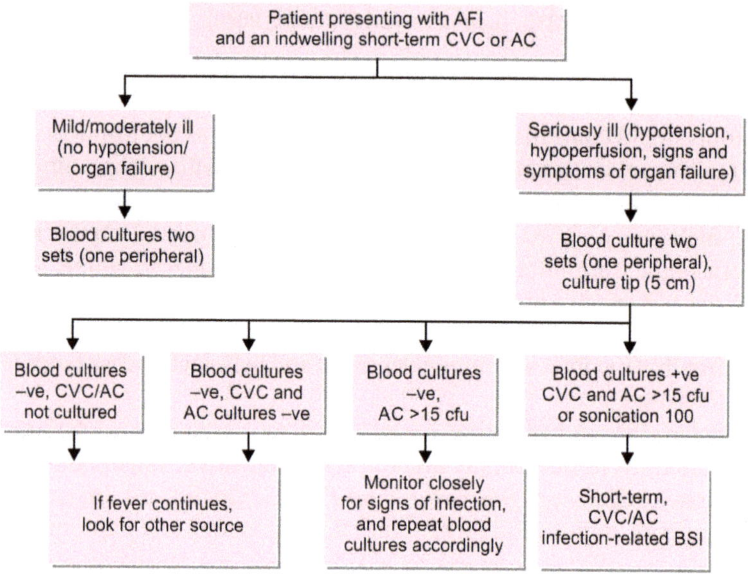

(AC: arterial catheter; AFI: amniotic fluid index; BSI: blood stream infection; cfu: colony forming units; CVC: central venous catheter)

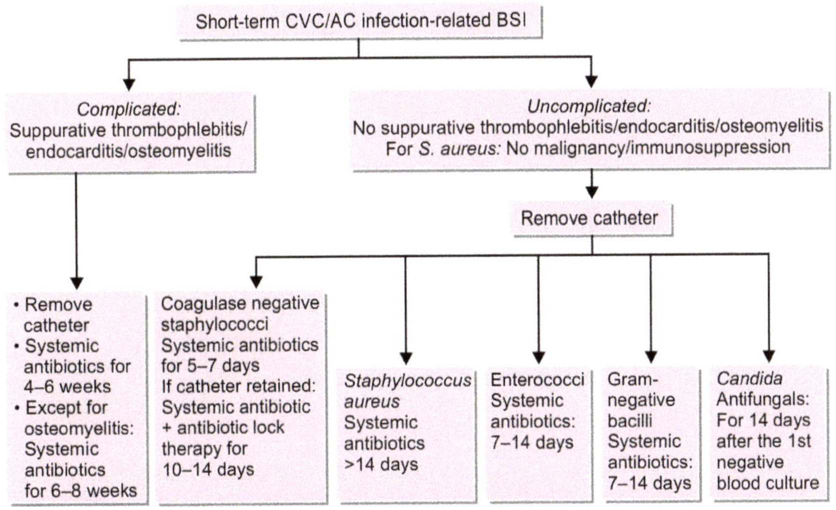

(AC: arterial catheter; BSI: blood stream infection; CVC: central venous catheter)

Ans. 118

1. This patient is hospitalized in for 10 days and has received multiple antibiotics, presumably surgical prophylaxis and then amoxicillin-clavulanate and clindamycin.

   Antibiotic-associated diarrhea is very common and has an incidence of approximately 5-30% of patients either during the course of antibiotic therapy or as late as up to 2 months after the end of the treatment.

   Antibiotics that act on anaerobes are particularly implicated in this and drugs belonging to aminopenicillins, aminopenicillins-clavulanate combination, cephalosporins, and clindamycin carry a higher incidence.

   The common host factors for antibiotic-associated diarrhea include elderly (age over 65 years), ICU stay, prolonged hospitalization, and immunosuppression. Some drugs such as erythromycin cause diarrhea due their action on motilin receptors per se. Clinical presentations range from mild diarrhea to fulminant pseudomembranous colitis, and complications such as toxic megacolon, perforation, and shock can happen.

2. Management includes stopping the offending agent, rehydration, and evaluation for *C. difficile* including antigen assays (immunoassays). Glutamate dehydrogenase is used as a screening test and assays for toxin A and toxin B.

   Nucleic acid amplification tests for *C. difficile* toxin genes should be performed only in patients with high suspicion for *C. difficile* infection and as a part of an algorithm approach as it can increase detection of asymptomatic colonization.

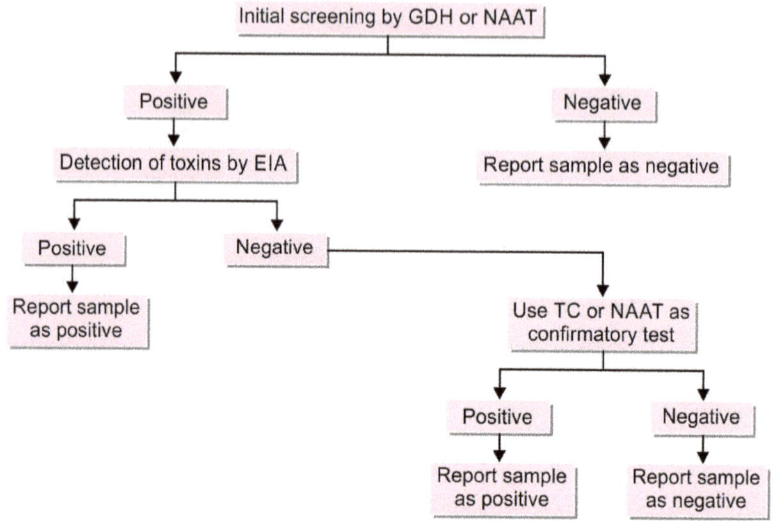

(GDH: glutamate dehydrogenase; NAAT: nucleic acid amplification test; TC: toxigenic culture)

Management of confirmed case of *C. difficile* is discontinuation of the inciting agent.

Treatment for *Clostridium difficile*

Vancomycin 125 mg orally four times per day or

Fidaxomicin 200 mg twice daily for 10 days or

If vancomycin/fidaxomicin is unavailable/contraindicated: Metronidazole 500 mg orally three times per day for 10 days.

- Fulminant *C. difficile* infection (CDI): Oral vancomycin 500 mg orally four times per day is the regimen of choice.
- In case of ileus, vancomycin 500 mg in approximately 100 mL normal saline per rectum every 6 hours as a retention enema may be tried.
- Metronidazole 500 mg may be administered together with oral or rectal vancomycin, particularly if ileus is present.

Further Reading

Barbut F, Meynard JL. Managing antibiotic associated diarrhoea. BMJ. 2002;324(7350):1345-6.

John S. *Clostridium difficile* associated diarrhoea: diagnosis and treatment. BMJ. 2005;331:498.

Martínez-Meléndez A, Camacho-Ortiz A, Morfin-Otero R, Maldonado-Garza HJ, Villarreal-Treviño L, Garza-González E. Current knowledge on the laboratory diagnosis of *Clostridium difficile* infection. World J Gastroenterol. 2017;23(9):1552-67.

McDonald LC, Gerding DN, Johnson S, Bakken JS, Carroll KC, Coffin SE, et al. Clinical Practice Guidelines for *Clostridium difficile* Infection in Adults and Children: 2017 Update by the Infectious Diseases Society of America (IDSA) and Society for Healthcare Epidemiology of America (SHEA). Clin Infect Dis. 2018;66(7):e1-e48.

Sartelli M, Di Bella S, McFarland LV, Khanna S, Furuya-Kanamori L, Abuzeid N, et al. 2019 update of the WSES guidelines for management of *Clostridioides* (*Clostridium*) *difficile* infection in surgical patients. World J Emerg Surg. 2019;14:8.

Ans. 119

1. Culture is showing *H. influenzae* Type B, a highly fastidious organism that requires both X factor and V factor for its growth; these may be supplied externally as discs (Fig. 1A) or by growing it alongside *S. aureus* strain (Fig. 1B).
2. It is associated more with late-onset VAP (>5 days of ventilation) than early-onset VAP. It is usually found in conjunct with gram-positive cocci, as a second pathogen. The main risk factor implicated for VAP by *H. influenzae* is the absence of prior antimicrobial therapy.

Further Reading

Rello J, Ricart M. Pneumonia due to *Haemophilus influenzae* among mechanically ventilated patients. Incidence, outcome, and risk factors. Chest. 1992;102(5):1562-5.

Restrepo MI, Peterson J, Fernandez JF, Qin Z, Fisher AC, Nicholson SC. Comparison of the bacterial etiology of early-onset and late-onset ventilator-associated pneumonia in subjects enrolled in 2 large clinical studies. Respir Care. 2013;58:1220-5.

Ans. 120

1. *B. cepacia* complex is often associated with multidrug resistance.
2. Screening of disinfectant solutions, mouth wash, intravenous solutions, and even moisturizing solutions and audit of infection control practices including hand wash and hand hygiene among healthcare workers in the ICU.

Further Reading

Antony B, Cherian EV, Boloor R, Shenoy KV. A sporadic outbreak of Burkholderis cepacia complex bacteremia in pediatric intensive care unit of a tertiary care hospital in coastal Karnataka, South India. Indian J Pathol Microbiol. 2016;59(2):197-9.

Ans. 121

1. Brucellosis may be diagnosed in cases of high clinical suspicion by culture of blood, body fluids, or bone marrow. Alternatively, a fourfold rise in serum titers of *Brucella* antibody between the acute phase and convalescent phase obtained more than 2 weeks apart is also diagnostic of brucellosis. The other methods for diagnosing brucellosis include a total antibody titer for *Brucella* in serum more than 160 by standard tube agglutination test (SAT) or detection of *Brucella* DNA by PCR, IgM ELISA and Rose Bengal Plate Agglutination test, lateral flow assay, complement fixation test.
2. Doxycycline + Rifampicin for 6 weeks.

Further Reading

Dias M, Dias E. Comparative evaluation of various serological tests in the laboratory diagnosis of Brucellosis. CHRISMED J Health Res. 2015;2(2):136-9.

Ans. 122

1. An assessment of both antigen and antibody is necessary to detect cases efficiently. There are three envelope polypeptides of particular importance:

HBsAg (hepatitis B surface antigen), HBeAg (hepatitis B e-antigen), and HBcAg (hepatitis B core antigen).
- Hepatitis B surface antigen appears first.
- After HBsAg is cleared from blood, antibody to that antigen can be detected (anti-HBsAg).
- There may be a time when neither the antigen nor the antibody is detectable. Measurement of antibody to core antigen (anti-HBc) is necessary to detect cases in the window period. Testing for anti-HBc also allows differentiation between immunity from HBV vaccination recovery from previous HBV infection.
- HBeAg correlates well with viral infectivity.
- Hepatitis B virus (HBV) quantitative DNA PCR: Method to confirm active infection.

2. All procedures and instrumentations are to be done following proper contact precautions, and biomedical waste are to be disposed off stringently following guidelines. This patient should be evaluated for infectivity, liver cirrhosis and liver fibrosis by measurement of HBV DNA, HbeAg, and ultrasound of the liver. Based on these results, if the patient has HBV DNA levels >2,000 IU/mL, and having transaminitis or fibrosis, or if he has evidence of cirrhosis and any detectable HBV DNA, or if he has a high HBV DNA levels more than 20,000 IU/mL with transaminitis, he should be referred for treatment.

   Patients aged more than 30, with only HBeAg-positivity, and no transaminitis, but have high HBV DNA levels, also may benefit from treatment and needs to be referred for the same.

Further Reading

Rotman Y, Brown TA, Hoofnagle JH. Evaluation of the patient with hepatitis B. Hepatology. 2009;49(5 Suppl):S22-S27.

EASL 2017 Clinical Practice Guidelines on the management of hepatitis B virus infection. J Hepat. 2017;67:370-98.

Ans. 123

1. *Pneumocystis jiroveci*
2. BAL sample: PCR/GMS (Grocott methenamine silver) stain
   In GMS stain, *P. jiroveci* is visible as typical "Copper-penny" appearance.
3. *HIV indicator infections:* These are infections that warrant the testing of the patient for HIV, if no other immunosuppressive conditions are present.

Bacterial
- *Mycobacterium tuberculosis*
- *Mycobacterium avium* complex/*Mycobacterium kansasii*
- Recurrent pneumonia (more than two episodes in 12 months)
- Recurrent *Salmonella* septicemia

Parasitic
- Cerebral toxoplasmosis
- Cryptosporidiosis diarrhea (>1 month)
- Isosporiasis (>1 month)
- Atypical disseminated leishmaniasis
- Reactivation of American trypanosomiasis

Viral
- CMV retinitis
- HCV ulcer (>1 month)/bronchitis/pneumonia
- Progressive multifocal leukoencephalopathy

Fungal
- *P. jirovecii* pneumonia
- Candidiasis esophageal/bronchial/tracheal
- Cryptococcosis (extrapulmonary)
- Histoplasmosis (disseminated/extrapulmonary)
- Penicilliosis, disseminated

Further Reading

Available from www.nice.org.uk/guidance/qs 157/chapter/Quality-statement-3-HIV-indicator-conditions.

Robert-Gangneux F, Belaz S, Revest M, Tattevin P, Jouneau S, Decaux O, et al. Diagnosis of *Pneumocystis jirovecii* pneumonia in immunocompromised patients by real-time PCR: a 4-year prospective study. J Clin Microbiol. 2014;52(9):3370-6.

Ans. 124

1. Beta D glucan may be considered superior to colonization indices and *Candida* score for the diagnosis of intra-abdominal candidiasis. Sensitivity of two consecutive positive tests of BDG was 65% and the specificity 78%.

A positive BDG test predicted the diagnosis of intra-abdominal candidiasis by a median of 5 days.

Of note, galactomannan assays are often performed together with BDG.

A positive BDG and a negative galactomannan suggest candidiasis, whereas the reverse suggests of aspergillosis/other mold such as fungi.

2. A *Candida* score > 2.5: Patient would benefit from antifungal treatment.

Candida score
0.908 (total parenteral nutrition)
+
0.997 (surgery)
+
1.112 (multifocal *Candida* species colonization)
+
2.038 (severe sepsis)

3. *Colonization index*: The ration of number of distinct nonblood body sites colonized by *Candida* species, to the total number of body sites culture (only *Candida* with same genetic identity are included in the calculation). It is an important method to characterize the dynamics of colonization, which increases early in patients who develop invasive candidiasis.

Further Reading

Eggiimann P, Pittet D. Candida colonisation index and subsequent infection in critically ill surgical patients: 20 years later. Intensive Care Med. 2014;40(10):1429-48.

Leroy G, Lambiotte F, Thévenin D, Lemaire C, Parmentier E, Devos P, et al. Evaluation of "Candida score" in critically ill patients: a prospective, multicenter, observational, cohort study. Ann Intens Care. 2011;1(1):50.

Tissot F, Lamoth F, Hauser PM, Orasch C, Flückiger U, Siegemund M, et al. Beta-glucan antigenemia anticipates diagnosis of blood culture-negative intra-abdominal candidiasis. Am J Respir Crit Care Med. 2013;188(9):1100-9.

Ans. 125

1. In cases of subacute or protracted meningitis, cryptococcal meningitis should be considered as a differential. Diagnosis is usually made from lumbar puncture and cryptococcal antigen. During lumbar puncture, very high opening pressures may be noticed. The CSF will be cellular with mononuclear cells predominance.
2. Cultures take 3–5 days and the yield increases with the amount of CSF cultured, while a paired sample of both serum and CSF for cryptococcal antigen assay gives result rapidly with sensitivity of 93–100% and specificity of 93–98%. However, the yield of cryptococcal antigen from serum in non-HIV patients is less.
3. Nonpulmonary Cryptococcoses are seen associated with primary or secondary immunodeficiencies. They should be treated with liposomal amphotericin B 3–4 mg/kg IV per day + flucytosine 100 mg/kg/d orally in four divided doses for minimum 2 weeks.

Further Reading

Abassi M, Boulware DR, Rhein J. Cryptococcal meningitis: Diagnosis and management update. Curr Trop Med Rep. 2015;2(2):90-9.

Ans. 126

- In suspected cases of candidemia, the indwelling central lines should be removed as early as possible in all patients, especially in those patients with septic shock.
- A differential time to positivity cut off of >2 hours is not useful in these cases and a positive peripheral blood culture within 48 hours is associated with a higher risk of central line infection with *C. glabrata.*
- *C. glabrata* is associated with pan-azole resistance. In cases of suspected/ confirmed cases of *C. glabrata,* echinocandins are preferred; although there is an increase in the documented echinocandin resistant strains of *C. glabrata.*
- Fluconazole may be considered only in cases where the candidemia is caused by susceptible species, candidemia has been cleared with echinocandin or amphotericin B formulation, and the patient is clinically stable with all possible infected foci addressed and fluconazole is used at maximal dose of 2 mg/kg.

Further Reading

Ben-Ami R. Treatment of invasive candidiasis: A narrative review. J Fungi (Basel). 2018;4(3):97.

Stempel JM, Farmakiotis D, Tarrand JJ, Kontoyiannis DP. Time-to-reporting of blood culture positivity and central venous catheter-associated Candida glabrata fungemia in cancer patients. Diagn Microbiol Infect Dis. 2016;85(3):391-3.

Ans. 127

1. Bronchoscopy, lavage, and lung biopsy should be sent for fungal culture.
2. An elevated 1,3 beta D glucan level along with clinical presentation may point toward the requirement of opting for a fungal culture of the biopsy sample. Infection is usually self-limited in immunocompetent hosts and requires no treatment; while in immunosuppressed hosts, it can cause life-threatening disease. In patients with moderate or severe symptoms

or in those with symptoms for > 4 weeks, initial treatment with 0.7–1 mg/kg amphotericin B, or 3–5 mg/kg liposomal amphotericin B, may be considered and later switched to itraconazole, 400 mg/day for 12 weeks.

Further Reading

Kauffman CA. Histoplasmosis: a clinical and laboratory update. Clin Microbiol Rev. 2007;20(1):115-32.

Wheat LJ, Freifeld AG, Kleiman MB, Baddley JW, McKinsey DS, Loyd JE, et al. Clinical practice guidelines for the management of patients with histoplasmosis: 2007 update by the Infectious Diseases Society of America. Clin Infect Dis. 2007;45:807-25.

Ans. 128

1. Presumptive diagnosis: Rabies

Confirmation of diagnosis:

- No single test is sufficient for the antemortem confirmatory diagnosis of rabies.
- Saliva can be tested for reverse transcription followed by polymerase chain reaction (*RT-PCR*) or isolation of the virus by *culture*.
- Serum and spinal fluid are screened for *antirabies antibodies*.
- Skin biopsies of hair follicles at the nape of the neck need to be examined for rabies antigen in the cutaneous nerves at the base of hair follicles.
- General donning of personal protective equipment (PPE) is advised, especially if there is a risk of body fluid exposure.
- Rabies postexposure prophylaxis (PEP) for the attending staff is indicated only if and when there is exposure of mucous membrane/nonintact skin, to secretions (including saliva) of the patient.
- Postexposure prophylaxis: Immediate thorough cleansing of wounds with soap and water. Povidone-iodine solution irrigation is recommended. If exposure is to mucous membranes, it should be flushed with water.
- The combination of human rabies immunoglobulin (HRIG) and vaccine is recommended for both bite and nonbite exposures, regardless of the interval between exposure and initiation of treatment.
- In previously immunized persons, HRIG should not be administered. Only two doses vaccine is indicated: 0 and 3
- Postexposure prophylaxis, for previously unimmunized cases, consists of:
  - A dose of HRIG, first dose of rabies vaccine given on the day of the rabies exposure (referred to as day 0) and tetanus toxoid. HRIG has to be infiltrated locally at the site of wound, as much as possible and the rest administered as IM at a distant site RM vaccine. The vaccine doses needs to be given further on days 3, 7, and 14.

2. Therapeutic coma (midazolam and phenobarbital), ketamine, and antiviral therapies.
3. The Milwaukee Protocol was developed by Rodney Willoughby Jr.
   - It involves chemically inducing the patient into a coma, administration of antiviral drugs combined with ketamine and amantadine on the notion that rabies pathology stems from the central nervous system's neurotransmitter dysfunction.

- It assumes that with suppressed brain activity, the damage and spread can be minimized while the patient's immune system fights off the infection.

Further Reading

Center for Disease Control and Prevention. Rabies. Postexposure prophylaxis. [online] https://www.cdc.gov/rabies/medical_care/index.html [Last accessed February, 2020].

Jackson AC. Rabies in the critical care unit: Diagnostic and therapeutic approaches. Can J Neurol Sci. 2011;38(5):689-95.

Ans. 129

- The culture and sensitivity report suggests that the presence of an extensively drug-resistant *Acinetobacter* As *Acinetobacter* is a colonizer of the urinary tract, particularly in catheterized patients, treatment needs to be initiated only when there is pyuria and systemic signs or symptoms in the absence of another source of infection. The urinary catheter should be changed and antibiotics should be administered for 14 days.
- Treatment options for multidrug resistant (MDR) *A. baumannii* include polymyxins, and tetracyclines such as tigecycline and minocycline. However, both tigecycline and polymyxin B may not reach adequate levels in the urinary tract to successfully treat infections. Hence, treatment options are limited to colistin, minocycline, or high-dose tigecycline along with other measures such as high-dose carbapenems given as extended infusion according to pharmacokinetic/pharmacodynamic (PK/PD) properties.
- Plazomicin is a novel aminoglycoside derivative of sisomicin approved by the Food and Drug Administration (FDA) for the treatment of complicated urinary tract infection (cUTI) due to *A. baumannii.*
- Cefiderocol a novel siderophore antibiotic Eravacycline, a novel synthetic fluorocycline are new drugs in pipeline for drug resistant *A. baumannii.*

Further Reading

Bassetti M, Peghin M, Vena A, Giacobbe DR. Treatment of infections due to MDR gram-negative bacteria. Front Med (Lausanne). 2019;6:74.

Hooton TM, Bradley SF, Cardenas DD, Colgan R, Geerlings SE, Rice JC, et al. Diagnosis, prevention, and treatment of catheter-associated urinary tract infection in adults: 2009 International Clinical Practice Guidelines from the Infectious Diseases Society of America. Clin Infect Dis. 2010;50(5):625-63.

Ans. 130

- *Step 1* would be to assess the protection status against Varicella virus, especially if there is history of Varicella vaccination. Varicella immunoglobulin G (IgG) level in serum is to be requested for. If protective levels are present, no further steps maybe required.
- *Step 2* would be in cases negative for Varicella IgG; immunoglobulin maybe indicated. VZIG (varicella zoster immune globulin) is effective when given up to 10 days after contact (in the case of continuous exposures, this is defined as 10 days from the appearance of the rash in the index case).
- *Step 3:* Postdelivery vaccination. Varicella vaccine two doses 28 days apart.

Further Reading

Chickenpox in pregnancy. (2015) Royal College of Obstetricians and Gynecologists. [online] https://www.rcog.org.uk/globalassets/documents/guidelines/gtg13.pdf [Last accessed February, 2020].

Ans. 131

- *Neisseria* spp
- *Moraxella catarrhalis*
- *Helicobacter pylori*
- *Proteus* species
- *Serratia* species
- *Morganella morganii*
- *Chromobacterium*
- *Brucella* species
- *Burkholderia* species

Further Reading

Olaitan AO, Morand S, Rolain JM. Mechanisms of polymyxin resistance: Acquired and intrinsic resistance in bacteria. Front Microbiol. 2014;5:643.

Ans. 132

- Fluid exposure that are considered as high risk are blood, semen, vaginal secretions, CSF, amniotic fluid, synovial, pleural, pericardial, ascitic fluid, and any other body fluids that contain blood. Fluids that are considered low risk are tears, sweat, saliva, urine, and feces (unless blood tinged).
- Immediately wash the wound (if present) and surrounding skin with water and soap, and rinse. Do not scrub; do not use antiseptics or skin washes (bleach, chlorine, alcohol, Betadine). Mucosal exposure should be rinsed with water/saline.
- He must be asked to immediately report to Nodal officer and also document the incident of sharp injury
- The decision to start PEP is made on the basis of degree of exposure to HIV and the HIV status of the source.
- *It should begin as soon as possible preferably within 2 hours, and before 72 hours.*

2. There are two regimens: basic regimen and expanded regimen.

Regimen	*Preferred*	*Alternative*
Basic regimen	Zidovudine + lamivudine	Stavudine + lamivudine
Expanded regimen	Basic regimen + protease inhibitor (lopinavir/ritonavir or nelfinavir or indinavir)	

- *Zidovudine:* 330 mg twice daily
- *Lamivudine:* 150 mg twice daily
- *Stavudine:* 30 mg twice daily
- *Lopinavir/ritonavir:* 400/100 mg twice daily
- *Nelfinavir:* 1,250 twice a day
- *Indinavir:* 750 thrice a day

Further Reading

Postexposure prophylaxis. NACO guidelines. [online] Available from http://www.upsacs.in/pdf/GUIDELINES/PEP.pdf [Last accessed February, 2020].

U.S. Department of Health and Human Services. (2019) HIV prevention. Post exposure prophylaxis (PEP). [online] https://aidsinfo.nih.gov/understanding-hiv-aids/fact-sheets/20/87/post-exposure-prophylaxis--pep- [Last accessed February, 2020].

Ans. 133

- Vancomycin is the drug of choice for most MRSA infections, while teicoplanin and daptomycin are alternatives if vancomycin is not available or not being tolerated. Daptomycin is not recommended for treating lung infections as it is rapidly inactivated in the lung.

Other drugs active against MRSA include:

- Ceftaroline is a fifth-generation cephalosporin.
- Telavancin, dalbavancin, and oritavancin—lipoglycopeptide
- Linezolid and tedizolid—oxazolidinone group—bacteriostatic, effective in lung infections (caution for thrombocytopenia, lactic acidosis, serotonin syndrome)
- *Other options:* Trimethoprim-sulfamethoxazole, minocycline, doxycycline, clindamycin, fosfomycin, rifampicin, tigecycline, quinupristin-dalfopristin

Infection	*Treatment*
Skin and soft tissue	*CA-MRSA* • Clindamycin, cotrimoxazole, tetracycline, linezolid (oral agents) • Children: Mupirocin 2% should be given preference, if possible
	HA-MRSA • Vancomycin/teicoplanin (IV), linezolid (oral/IV) • Daptomycin (IV), telavancin (IV)
Bacteremia	*Uncomplicated* Vancomycin/teicoplanin/daptomycin (IV) 2 weeks
	Complicated Vancomycin/teicoplanin/daptomycin (IV) 4–6 weeks
Infective endocarditis	*Native valve* Vancomycin/teicoplanin/daptomycin (IV) 6 weeks (Adding gentamicin/rifampin to vancomycin is not recommended in patients with bacteremia or native valve infective endocarditis)
	Prosthetic valve Vancomycin and rifampin (at least 6 weeks) + gentamicin 2 weeks
	Children Vancomycin IV 2–6 weeks (data regarding safety and effectiveness of alternatives in children are limited)
Pneumonia	*Adults* Vancomycin/teicoplanin/linezolid/clindamycin (if susceptible): 7–21 days (in patients with MRSA pneumonia complicated by empyema, antimicrobial therapy should be used with drainage procedures)
	Children Vancomycin/linezolid IV. Can be transitioned to susceptible oral agents

Contd...

Contd...

Infection	*Treatment*
Bone and joint infections	*Osteomyelitis* IV Vancomycin/daptomycin: Minimum 8 weeks *Oral:* Cotrimoxazole + rifampin/linezolid/clindamycin: Minimum 8 weeks *Septic arthritis* • Drainage + debridement. Followed by antibiotic regimen: • IV: Vancomycin/daptomycin: Minimum 8 weeks • Oral: Cotrimoxazole + rifampin/linezolid/clindamycin: Minimum 8 weeks

(CA-MRSA: community-associated methicillin-resistant *Staphylococcus aureus*; HA-MRSA: hospital-associated methicillin-resistant *Staphylococcus aureus;* IV: intravenous)

Further Reading

Lambert M. IDSA Guidelines on the treatment of MRSA infections in adults and children. Am Fam Physician. 2011;84(4):455-63.

Ans. 134

1. World Health Organization (WHO) Classification of Severe Malaria: Presence of one or more of the following:
   - *General examination:* Presence of prostration (generalized weakness so that the person is unable to sit, stand, or walk without assistance)
   - *CNS:* Impaired mental status (a Glasgow coma score <11 in adults or a Blantyre coma score <3 in children), seizures (more than two episodes/day)
   - *Respiratory system:* Acute respiratory distress syndrome (ARDS)/ respiratory distress/pulmonary edema
   - CVS: Circulatory collapse
   - *Hematology:* Severe anemia, Hb <7 g/dL, and hematocrit (HCT) <20%, in adults with a parasite count >10,000/μL, coagulopathy
   - *Liver function:* Jaundice, hemoglobinuria
   - *Renal:* Plasma or serum creatinine >3 mg/dL or blood urea >20 mmol/L
   - *Acidosis*: A base deficit of >8 mEq/L or a plasma bicarbonate level of < 15 mmol/L or venous plasma lactate ≥5 mmol/L.
   - *Hypoglycemia:* Blood or plasma glucose <40 mg/dL
   - High parasite titer
2. In the laboratory, malaria is diagnosed using different techniques:
   - Conventional microscopic diagnosis by staining thin and thick peripheral blood smears (Giemsa, Wright's, Field's):

Sensitivity: 50–100 parasites/μL

- Other concentration techniques, e.g. quantitative buffy coat

Quantative buffy coat (QBC) method: It is highly sensitive in case of *P. falciparum*, but notably low sensitivity in case of non-Falciparum species

- Rapid diagnostic tests (RDTs)

Most products target a *P. falciparum*-specific protein, e.g. histidine-rich protein II (HRP-II) or lactate dehydrogenase (LDH).

Some tests detect *P. falciparum* specific and pan-specific antigens [aldolase or pan-malaria Parasite lactate dehydrogenase (pLDH)], and distinguish non-*P. falciparum* infections from mixed malaria infections.

- Immunofluorescence antibody testing (IFA)

Although IFA is time-consuming and subjective, it is highly sensitive and specific.

- Molecular diagnostic method

Polymerase chain reaction, LAMP, microarray, mass spectrometry (MS), and flow cytometric (FCM) assay techniques

3. *Treatment of malaria:* Preferably by artemisinin derivatives, for 3 days, with at least 24 hour of parenteral therapy. Dose 2.4 mg/kg/dose with higher doses in children
   - *Regimens suggested include:*
     - Artesunate + amodiaquine, Artesunate + sulfadoxine-pyrimethamine, artemether-lumefantrine, dihydroartemisinin plus piperaquine
   - Second-line alternatives
     - Artesunate plus doxycycline or clindamycin, quinine plus doxycycline or clindamycin
     - Empirical broad-spectrum antibiotic to cover for concomitant gram-negative sepsis
     - Quinine may be tried in cases of nonavailability of artesunate
   - Total duration of 7 days.
   - Doxycycline is added to nonpregnant adults.
   - If pregnant, then add clindamycin.

Further Reading

Guidelines for the Treatment of Malaria, 3rd edition. Geneva: World Health Organization; 2015. 7. Treatment of severe malaria. [online] Available from https://www.ncbi.nlm.nih.gov/books/NBK294445/ [Last accessed February, 2020].

Tangpukdee N, Duangdee C, Wilairatana P, Krudsood S. Malaria diagnosis: A brief review. Korean J Parasitol. 2009;47(2):93-102.

Ans. 135

1. Amebic meningoencephalitis (*Naegleria, Acanthamoeba*):
   - The two free-living amoebae that are often associated with warm, stagnant, fresh-water ponds are *Naegleria* and *Acanthamoeba.* Following bathing/swimming in such protozoan-infested ponds, these parasites gain entry into the CNS, resulting in meningoencephalitis. They will be missed unless there is a suggestive history, or routine wet mount screening of CSF is done.
2. *CSF wet mount/PCR:* Differentiation between the various species, though only of epidemiological value is possible only by PCR.
   - Treatment options are unclear, and a combination of conventional amphotericin B, rifampicin, fluconazole, miltefosine, and azithromycin (500 mg IV or orally) can be considered. A close differential will be *Acanthamoeba,* which may not be inhibited by amphotericin B.
   - Steroids need to be continued in view of cerebral edema.

Ans. 136

1. Clinical diagnosis could be dengue or any similar tropical infection causing thrombocytopenia. During the early stage of disease, after the initial 3rd

day, NS1 antigen is to be looked for. IgM gains value only later on in the course of the disease.

Laboratory confirmation can be made from serum obtained early (≤*7 days* after fever onset) in the illness by detecting viral genomic sequences with *rRT-PCR*, or *dengue NS1* antigen by immunoassay.

Later in the illness (≥4 days after fever onset), IgM against dengue virus can be detected with ELISA. For patients presenting *during the 1st week after fever onset*, diagnostic testing should include a test for dengue virus (*rRT-PCR or NS1*) and *IgM*.

Immunoglobulin G detection by ELISA in a single serum sample is not useful for diagnostic testing because it remains detectable for life after a dengue virus infection.

2. The differential diagnosis includes tropical fevers such as Leptospirosis, Malaria, Rickettsia Infection, Hantavirus Scrub Typhus, Meningococci, etc.

Further Reading

Centers for Disease Control and Prevention. (2019) Dengue Diagnosis. Key facts. [online] https://www.cdc.gov/dengue/healthcare-providers/diagnosis.html [Last accessed February, 2020].

Ans. 137

1. Eschar-Scrub typhus, also known as bush typhus, is caused by *Orientia tsutsugamushi*. Scrub typhus is spread to people through bites of infected chiggers. The most common symptoms of scrub typhus include fever, headache, body aches, and sometimes rash.
2. *Diagnosis:*
   - *Serology:* Weil felix (tube agglutination method)/Scrub Elisa (IgM)/ immunofluorescence/RDTs

Specificity: Scrub ELISA > IFA > Weil Felix > RDT

- Biopsy of the eschar
- PCR

Further Reading

Pote K, Narang R, Deshmukh P. Diagnostic performance of serological tests to detect antibodies against acute scrub typhus infection in central India. Indian J Med Microbiol. 2018;36:108-12.

Ans. 138

- Ticarcillin, piperacillin
- Cefoperazone, ceftazidime, ceftazidime/avibactam
- Cefepime
- Ceftolozane/tazobactam
- Aztreonam, imipenem, meropenem

Further Reading

Pandey N, Cascella M. Beta lactam antibiotics. In: StatPearls. Treasure Island (FL): StatPearls Publishing; 2020. [online] Available from https://www.ncbi.nlm.nih.gov/books/NBK545311/ [Last accessed February, 2020].

Ans. 139

1. *CMV RNA/DNA detection methods:* PCR. This is the preferred method for diagnosis of CMV infection in solid organ transplant recipients (SOTR). CMV RNA is more specific of recent/acute infection than CMV DNA.
   Antigenemia assay: Semiquantitative assay that detects pp65 antigen in CMV-infected peripheral blood leukocytes. Specificity is comparable to that of nucleic acid *testing* (NAT), and therefore is a good alternative.
   Viral culture: Highly specific, but diagnostic utility is restricted because of the slow turn-around-time.
2. *Treatment:* Intravenous ganciclovir is the treatment of choice and the duration of treatment is continued up to complete CMV viral eradication in atleast two assays and clinical response. Foscarnet can be used for ganciclovir-resistant CMV with monitoring of nephrotoxicity.

Further Reading

Cannon MJ, Schmid DS, Hyde TB. Review of cytomegalovirus seroprevalence and demographic characteristics associated with infection. Rev Med Virol. 2010;20:202-13.

Ans. 140

1. The pathogen is likely to be lipophilic fungus of the genus *Malassezia*. Species confirmation can be done either manually based on a panel of complicated biochemical analysis or by MALDI-TOF (matrix-assisted laser desorption ionization-time of flight). Identification of this particular genus by automated systems is often highly challenging.
2. Liposomal amphotericin B

Further Reading

Iatta R, Cafarchia C, Cuna T, Montagna O, Laforgia N, Gentile O, et al. Bloodstream infections by *Malassezia* and *Candida* species in critical care patients. Med Mycol. 2014;52(3):264-9.

Ans. 141

1.

Ambler Class	*Substrate*	*Enzyme*	*Examples*
A	Penicillin	Narrow-spectrum beta-lactams	TEM-1, TEM-2, SHV-1
	Extended-spectrum beta-lactams (ESBL)	ESBL	SHV-2, CTX-M-15, PER-1, VEB-1
	Carbapenems	Serine Carbapenemases	KPC-1, IMI-1, SME-1
B	Carbapenems	Metallo beta-lactamases	Vim-1, IMP-1, NDM-1
C	Cephalosporins (Cephamycins)	Cephalosporinases (Inducible)	AmpC, P99, ACT-1, CMY-2, FOX-1, MIR-1
D	Oxacillin, oxyimino beta-lactams, carbapenems	OXA-type enzyme (*Pseudomonas* and *Acinetobacter*)	OXA enzymes

Stability of various beta-lactams: *Enterobacteriaceae*

	Temocillin	*Piperacillin*	*Ceftazidime*	*Mero/ Imi-penem*	*Ertapenem*	*Aztreonam*	*Mecillinam*
AmpC	+	–	–	+	Moderately +	–	+
TEM-ESBL	+	–	–	+	+	–	Moderately +
SHV-ESBL	+	–	–	+	+	–	–
CTX-M ESBL	+	–	–	+	+	–	Moderately +
OXA-1	+	–	+	+	+	+	+
OXA-48	–	–	+	–	–	–	–
KPC	Moderately +	–	–	–	–	–	–
IMP/ VIM/ NDM	–	–	–	–	–	+	–

(ESBL: extended-spectrum beta-lactamase; KPC: *Klebsiella pneumoniae* carbapenemase)

Stability of various beta-lactams: *nonfermenters*

Acinetobacter native	*Inherent-*	*–*	*–*	*+*	*Inherent-*	*Inherent-*	*Inherent-*
Acinetobacter OXA 23/24/58	Inherent-	–	–	–	Inherent-	Inherent-	Inherent-
Burkholderia native	v	v	v	v	Inherent-	Inherent-	Inherent-
Pseudomonas	Inherent-	+	+	+	Inherent-	+	Inherent-

Activity of various inhibitors against Enterobacteriaceae beta-lactamases

	Clavulanate	*Sulbactam*	*Tazobactam*	*Avibactam*
AmpC	–	–	–	+
TEM-ESBL	+	+	+	+
SHV-ESBL	+	+	+	+
CTX-M ESBL	+	+	+	+
OXA-1	Weak+	Weak+	Weak+	?
OXA-48	–	–	–	+
KPC	–	–	–	+
IMP/VIM/NDM	–	–	–	–

2.

- *Time-kill assay (TKA)*: The standard reference method for antimicrobial synergy testing. TKA looks at the actual reduction in the viable count of the organism after exposure to the drug combination as compared to the most active single agent, at different time intervals.

- *Checkerboard assay*: This is performed by using panel of antimicrobial combinations at different concentrations.
- *E*-test strips may be used to determine the synergistic combinations.

E-test cross method or *E*-test fixed ratio method or *E*-test agar method or *E*-test MIC: MIC method.

Further Reading

Brennan-Krohn T, Kirby JE. Antimicrobial synergy testing by the inkjet printer-assisted automated checkerboard array and the manual time-kill method. J Vis Exp. 2019;146:e58636.

Ans. 142

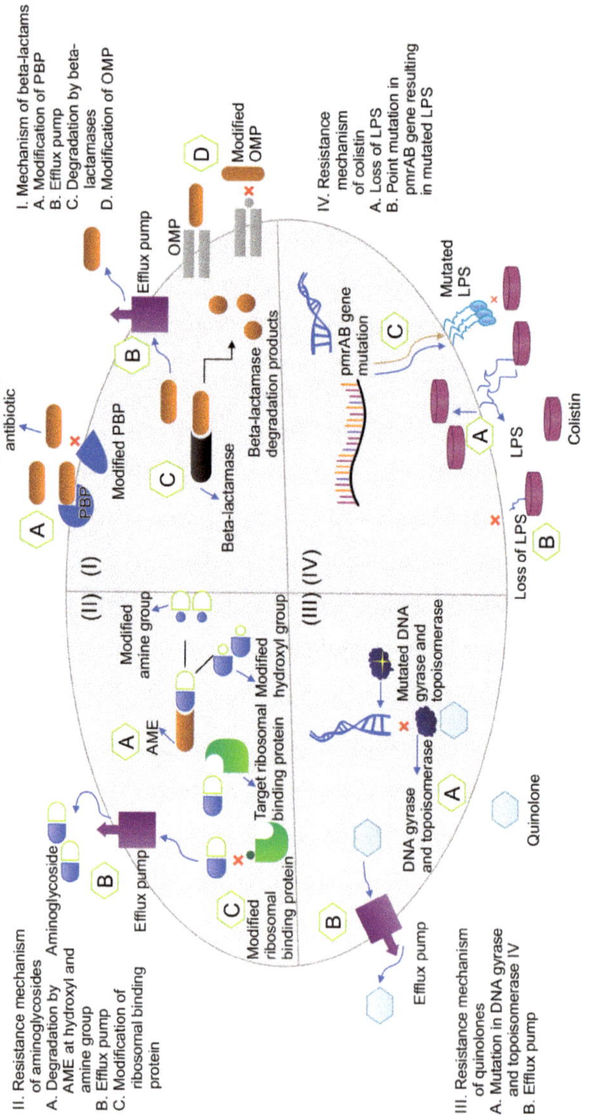

(AME: aminoglycoside-modifying enzyme; DNA: deoxyribose nucleic acid; IV: intravenous; LPS: lipopolysaccharides; OMP: outer membrane protein; PBP: penicillin-binding *protein*)

Further Reading

Asif M, Alvi IA, Rehman SU. Insight into *Acinetobacter baumannii*: pathogenesis, global resistance, mechanisms of resistance, treatment options, and alternative modalities. Infect Drug Resist. 2018;11:1249-60.

Ans. 143

1. All the staff involved in handling of biomedical waste in the health care facility must be immunized against the communicable diseases, especially against hepatitis B and tetanus. Other recommended vaccines for health care workers include yearly influenza vaccine and MMR vaccine with varicella vaccine if there is no previous history of infection.
2. Sharps should be collected in white translucent, puncture-proof, leak-proof, and tamper-proof break resistant container with a narrow opening so that someone cannot reach into it.

Further Reading

Central Pollution Control Board. Ministry of Environment, Forest & Climate Change. (2016) Guidelines for Management of Healthcare Waste as per Biomedical Waste Management Rules, 2016. [online] Available from http://www.hp.gov.in/dhsrhp/Guidelines_healthcare_June_2018.pdf [Last accessed February, 2020].

Ans. 144

1. Common antimicrobial agents for hand washing [including alcohols, chlorhexidine, hexachlorophene, iodophors, PCMX (para-chloro-meta-xylenol), and triclosan] are not active against spores; however, soap and water hand washing removes *C. difficile* spores from hands of volunteers when compared to alcohol-based hand rubs (ABHRs).
2. The occurrence of two or more epidemiologically related infections caused by an organism of the same type relating to place and time is defined as an outbreak.

Further Reading

Guide to preventing *Clostridium difficile* infections. APIC Implementation Guide. (2013) APIC. [online] Available from https://apic.org/wp-content/uploads/2019/07/2013CDiffFinal.pdf [Last accessed February, 2020].

Ans. 145

- Water
- Plain (nonantimicrobial) soap
- Alcohols (ethanol, isopropanol or n-propanol, or a combination of two of these products)
- Chlorhexidine
- Chloroxylenol
- Hexachlorophene
- Quaternary ammonium compounds
- Triclosan.

Further Reading

World Health Organization. (2007) WHO Guidelines for Hand Hygiene in Health Care (Advanced Draft.) [online] Available from https://www.who.int/patientsafety/information_centre/Last_April_versionHH_Guidelines%5B3%5D.pdf [Last accessed February, 2020].

Ans. 146

1. Pressure meter to detect the pressure difference between negative/positive pressure rooms.
2. *Airborne precautions*: Airborne precautions prevent transmission of infectious agents that remain infectious over long distances when suspended in the air [e.g., Rubeola virus (measles), varicella virus (chickenpox), *M. tuberculosis*, and possibly severe acute respiratory syndrome-associated *coronavirus* (SARS-CoV)]:
   - *Airborne infection isolation room (AIIR):* Formerly, negative pressure isolation room.
   - Protective environment refers to isolation practices designed to decrease the risk of exposure to environmental fungal agents in allogeneic hematopoietic stem cell transplantation (HSCT).

Further Reading

Center for Disease Control and Prevention. (2019) 2007 Guideline for Isolation Precautions: Preventing Transmission of Infectious Agents in Healthcare Settings. [online] Available from https://www.cdc.gov/infectioncontrol/pdf/guidelines/isolation-guidelines-H.pdf [Last accessed February, 2020].

Ans. 147

1. Eye wash station
2. Flush for the exposed eyes.

After exposure of the eye:

- Irrigate exposed eye immediately with water or normal saline.
- Sit in a chair, tilt the head back and ask a person to gently pour water or normal saline over the eye, gently pulling the eyelids up and down to make sure the eye is cleaned thoroughly.
- If wearing contact lenses, leave them in place while irrigating, as they form a barrier over the eye and will help protect it. Once the eye has been cleaned, remove the contact lenses and clean them in the normal manner. This will make them safe to wear again.
- Do not use soap or disinfectant on the eye.

Further Reading

World Health Organization. (2009) Exposure to blood or other body fluids. [online] Available from https://www.who.int/ith/ITH2009Chapter8.pdf [Last accessed February, 2020].

Ans. 148

1. Biomedical waste (BMW) is any waste produced during the diagnosis, treatment, or immunization of human or animal research activities pertaining thereto or in the production or testing of biological or in health camps.
2. The basic principle of good BMW practice is based on the concept of three Rs, namely, reduce, recycle, and reuse.

Ans. 149

Cleaning methods for blood spills and body substances:

- Clean spills with a 0.5–1.0% chlorine solution.
- Clean spills of blood, body fluids, and other potentially infectious fluids immediately.

- Cover the area immediately with any absorbent material such as tissue paper, old newspaper, and gauze piece.
- *For small spills:* While wearing utility or examination gloves, remove visible material using a cloth soaked in a 0.5–1.0% chlorine solution, then wipe clean with a disinfectant cleaning solution.
- *For large spills:* While wearing gloves, flood the area with a 0.5–1.0% chlorine solution, mop up the solution, and then clean as usual with detergent and water.
- Wait for a few minutes, preferably 15 minutes after pouring chlorine solution. After disinfection, thorough cleaning of the floor with soap and water is necessary.

Further Reading

Hospital infection control manual for small healthcare organizations. [online] Available from https://nabh.co/Images/PDF/HIC_Guidebook.pdf [Last accessed February, 2020].

Ans. 150

1. *Five moments for hand hygiene*:
   - *Before touching a patient:*
     - When? Clean your hands before touching a patient.
     - Why? To protect the patient against harmful germs carried on your hands.
   - *Before clean or aseptic procedure:*
     - When? Clean your hands immediately before performing a clean or aseptic procedure.
     - Why? To protect the patient against harmful germs, including the patient's own.
   - *After body fluid exposure risk:*
     - When? Clean your hands immediately after an exposure risk to body fluids (and after glove removal).
     - Why? To protect yourself and the healthcare environment from harmful germs of the patient.
   - *After touching a patient:*
     - When? Clean your hands after touching a patient and patient's immediate surroundings.
     - Why? To protect yourself and the healthcare environment from harmful germs from the patient.
   - *After touching patient surroundings:*
     - When? Clean your hands after touching any object or furniture in the patient's immediate surroundings—even if the patient has not been touched.
     - Why? To protect yourself and the healthcare environment from harmful germs from the patient.
2. Disinfection is a process where most microbes are removed from a defined object or surface, except bacterial endospores:
   - Disinfectants may be classified according to their ability to destroy different categories of microorganisms. The agent which destroys only vegetative bacteria is termed a low-level disinfectant. If the agent

is capable of rendering mycobacteria nonviable, it is termed as an intermediate-level disinfectant. It is safe to assume that all the other categories of microbes which are classified more susceptible are also destroyed if efficacy against mycobacteria can be demonstrated. High-level disinfection is in other words sterilization wherein all microbial life is destroyed inclusive of endospores.

- *High-level disinfectants:* Glutaraldehyde 2%, ethylene oxide.
- *Intermediate-level disinfectants:* Alcohols, chlorine compounds, hydrogen peroxide, chlorhexidine, glutaraldehyde (short-term exposure).
- *Low-level disinfectants:* Benzalkonium chloride, some soaps.

Further Reading

Hospital infection control manual for small healthcare organizations. [online] Available from https://nabh.co/Images/PDF/HIC_Guidebook.pdf [Last accessed February, 2020].

Ans. 151

- Blood culture is a crucial investigation for sepsis management.
- For bacteremia, depending on the number of cultures sent, the yield ranges from 73% to 100%, while for candidemia, it is only 50%.
- For adults, collect 10–20 cc for each blood culture set; divide blood into two blood culture bottles, one for aerobes and one for anaerobes; two or three blood cultures (by separate stick) per septic episode is sufficient.
- The yield of culture positivity increases by approximately 3% for every mL of blood cultured.
- For one-paired sample, the yield is approximately 73–80%, 80–90% for two-paired cultures, and 95% and 98% with three-paired cultures.

Further Reading

Centers for Disease Control and Prevention. Antibiotic prescribing and use in hospitals and long-term care. [online] Available from https://www.cdc.gov/antibiotic-use/core-elements/collecting-cultures.html/last accessed on 21st January 2020 [Last accessed February, 2020].

Ans. 152

1. Droplet precaution:
   - Confine patient to a single room
   - Enforce cough etiquette
   - *Use appropriate PPE:* for patient a mask, and for staff—mask, gown, and gloves (note a N-95 respirator is advocated for airborne isolation and not for droplet isolation)
   - Limit patient movement in hospital
   - Prioritize daily cleaning of room.
2. *Remove PPEs in the following sequence:* (1) gloves, (2) goggles or face shield, (3) gown, and (4) mask or respirator.

Further Reading

Centers for Disease Control and Prevention. Infection control. Transmission-based precautions. [online] Available from https://www.cdc.gov/infectioncontrol/basics/transmission-based-precautions.html [Last accessed February, 2020]

HEMODYNAMICS

Ans. 153

- The patient is having complete heart block (CHB).
- Management is divided into resuscitation, stabilization, and identification and management of the cause. Usually, patient with CHB will present with hemodynamic instability.
- *Resuscitation*: The first quick response should be to initiate pharmacological therapy, injection atropine bolus to see the response. As it acts at AV node, the response is not always good. Usually, patient may require inotrope infusion, preferably with epinephrine. In patient who presents with severe hemodynamic instability, rapid pacing is needed. Transcutaneous pacing or transvenous pacing is done.
- *Causes*: Acute myocardial ischemia, idiopathic fibrosis, drugs (antiarrhythmic drugs class 4, digoxin).
- *Evaluation*: Follow-up electrocardiography (ECGs), troponins, digoxin levels if toxicity suspected, electrolytes, and hemogram.

Further Reading

Knabben V, Chhabra L, Slane M. Third-degree atrioventricular block. In: StatPearls. StatPearls Publishing; 2019.

Ans. 154

Indications of pacemaker:

- *Acquired atrioventricular (AV) block:* CHB, symptomatic second-degree block
- *Sinus node dysfunction:* Frequent symptomatic sinus bradycardia
- *After acute phase of myocardial infarction:* With CHB, advanced second-degree block
- Cardiac resynchronization therapy in patients with severe systolic heart failure
- Chronic bifascicular block
- Patients with congenital heart disease
- Neurocardiogenic syncope and hypersensitive carotid sinus syndrome
- Post cardiac transplantation
- Hypertrophic cardiomyopathy
- Pacing to detect and terminate tachycardia.

Ans. 155

- Common ECG abnormality is ventricular premature complex, bradycardia:
  - Digoxin overdose or toxicity is also associated with other ECG abnormalities such as bidirectional ventricular tachycardia, ventricular arrhythmias, atrial fibrillation, and AV and SA node block.
- *Digoxin toxicity:*
  - *Clinical diagnosis:* Combination of clinical suspicion, signs and symptoms, ECG abnormality, and high serum levels. Mere presence of elevated serum levels will suggest exposure and not toxicity.

Further Reading

Rehman R, Hai O. Digitalis toxicity. In: StatPearls. StatPearls Publishing; 2019.

Ans. 156

- Left anterior descending
- Lateral circumflex
- Right coronary artery

Ans. 157

The patient is having STEMI, inferoseptal. He has come after 24 hours duration.

Management:

- Oxygen (O_2) if hypoxic, pain relief
- Aspirin, clopidogrel, statins, anticoagulation
- Angiogram and percutaneous coronary intervention (PCI) at later date.

Ans. 158

- ECG shows STEMI, inferoseptal.
- Management:
  - O_2 if hypoxic, pain relief
  - Aspirin, clopidogrel , statins, anticoagulation
  - Send troponin, echocardiogram (ECHO)
  - Revascularization—primary PCI.

Ans. 159

Indications for PCI after thrombolysis:

- *Routine PCI:* 2–24 hours after thrombolysis, PCI to ischemia-related artery .
- *Rescue PCI:*
  - Nonresolution of ST change
  - Persistent chest pain and symptoms of myocardial ischemia
  - Cardiogenic shock.
- *Urgent PCI:*
  - Recurrent ST elevation/ischemia after successful thrombolysis

Further Reading

Ibanez B, James S, Agewall S, Antunes MJ, Bucciarelli-Ducci C, Bueno H, et al. 2017 ESC Guidelines for the management of acute myocardial infarction in patients presenting with ST-segment elevation: The Task Force for the management of acute myocardial infarction in patients presenting with ST-segment elevation of the European Society of Cardiology (ESC). Eur Heart J. 2018;39(2):119-77.

Ans. 160

- Causes of RBBB:
  - When there is delay in conduction system or increase in the distance travelled, there may be RBBB particularly when the abnormality happens in right heart
  - Hyperkalemia
  - Right ventricular hypertrophy
  - Idiopathic, fibrosis
  - Injury to right bundle branch:
    - Ischemia
    - Surgery
    - Increased intraventricular pressure—cor pulmonale
    - Infiltrative process.

Further Reading

Harkness WT, Hicks M. Right bundle branch block (RBBB). StatPearls. Treasure Island (FL): StatPearls Publishing; 2020-2019.

Ans. 161

- Axis of heart is determined by many methods:
  - Look at lead 1 and aVF (both are 90° to each other); if lead 1 is positive and lead aVF is negative, then left-axis deviation.
  - See the smallest amplitude; the heart axis will be 90° to it.

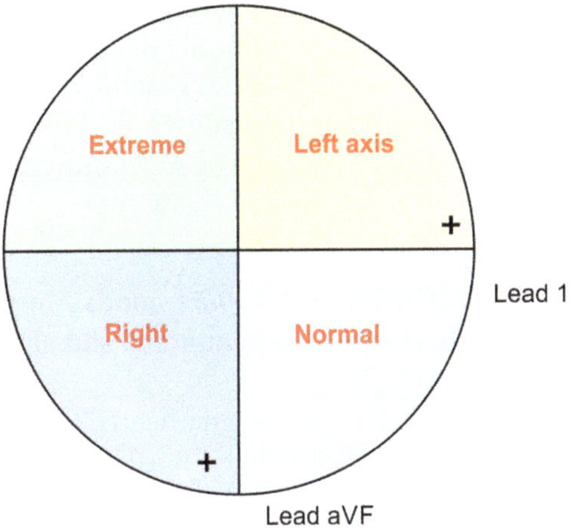

Ans. 162

Management:

- Immediate to stabilize the myocardium—calcium gluconate slow intravenous (IV).
- *Reduce potassium levels:*
  - Dextrose insulin infusion
  - Nebulization with 10 to 20 mg of salbutamol over 10 minutes
  - Intravenous isotonic soda bicarbonate if associated with metabolic acidosis.

Ans. 163

- Both hyperkalemia and hypokalemia affect repolarization phase and alter T wave and ST segment. In severe stage, affect QRS complex.
- *Hypokalemia:*
  - The changes are not always related with potassium levels.
  - ST changes, T-wave amplitude reduction, T-wave flattening, U-wave prominence, and T-U waves are seen commonly.
  - QRS prolongation may be seen with increasing severity.
- *Hyperkalemia:*
  - Tall T wave is the first change.
  - With increasing severity of hyperkalemia, there will be progressive slowing of conduction leading to prolong PR and QRS duration followed by sine wave.
  - ST elevation is also seen, particularly common in lead V1, V2.

Ans. 164

- Patients presenting to the ER with conditions that may cause palpitations are quite variable ranging from sinus tachycardia to arrythmias such as SVT, PSVT, AFib, a flutter or heart failure.
- It mostly depends on structural or electrical abnormality in the heart, or electrolyte disturbances.
- Treatment depends upon the symptoms and the hemodynamic status of the patients.

Ans. 165

- Supraventricular tachycardia is commonly divided into atrioventricular nodal re-entrant tachycardia (AVNRT), atrioventricular re-entrant tachycardia (AVRT), and atrial tachycardia (AT).
- The most common is AVNRT, followed by AVRT and AT.

Further classification depends on presence of AV block.

Ans. 166

- First-degree AV block, if PR interval is >0.2 seconds. Mostly asymptomatic.
- If PR > 0.3 seconds, this may cause symptoms and altered coordination between atrium and ventricle.
- Pacemaker is rarely indicated for first-degree heart block, but if symptomatic, pacemaker is advised particularly when PR > 0.3 seconds.
- Other indications for pacemaker with first-degree heart bock are coexisting neuromuscular disease or a prolonged QRS interval.

Further Reading

Oldroyd SH, Makaryus AN. First degree heart block. In: StatPearls. StatPearls Publishing; 2019.

Tracy CM, Epstein AE, Darbar D, DiMarco JP, Dunbar SB, EstesIII NA, et al. 2012 ACCF/AHA/HRS focused update of the 2008 guidelines for device-based therapy of cardiac rhythm abnormalities: a report of the American College of Cardiology Foundation/American Heart Association Task Force on Practice Guidelines and the Heart Rhythm Society. Circulation. 2012;126:1784-800.

Ans. 167

- Broad- or wide-complex tachycardia (QRS > 0.1 ms) recused by any cause which increases duration of electrical impulse to traverse such as conduction bock (bundle branch block), ventricular hypertrophy also ventricular arrhythmias (commonly hyper/hypokalemia, hypoxia, etc.).
- *Management:* Perform echocardiography if stable and evaluate for electrolyte imbalance, myocardial ischemia if hemodynamically unstable, perform urgent cardioversion. Medical management may be done with antiarrhythmics such as amiodarone.

Ans. 168

- Second-degree heart block
- *Management:*
  - To stop nebivolol, replace with other antihypertensive.
  - Atropine IV bolus
  - Prepare for temporary pacing if persistently symptomatic

Ans. 169

Complete heart block with VVI mode of pacemaker in situ. The pacemaker spikes senses ventricular activity, and if no native activity is sensed then ventricular pacing is initiated. VVI mode is used in patients with chronic atrial impairment, e.g. atrial fibrillation or flutter.

Ans. 170

- Management of symptomatic ventricular tachycardia:
  - *Stabilization:*
    - Quickly assess airway breathing circulation and start appropriate treatment.
  - Management:
    - Cardioversion with 100 J and see for improving symptoms
    - Identify the cause:
      - Perform ECG, ECHO, and cardiac enzymes
      - Electrolytes
      - Look for hypoxia, hypovlemia, hypothermia, hyperkalemia/ hypokalemia and increased hydrogen ion concentration (acidosis), tension pneumothorax, tamponade (cardiac), toxins, thrombosis (cardiac and pulmonary).

Ans. 171

- Ventricular tachycardia with unrecordable vitals
  - Nonpalpable pulse, so cardiac arrest with shockable rhythm
  - Start cardiopulmonary resuscitation
  - Rapid defibrillation once defibrillator become available
  - Defibrillation twice then epinephrine followed by defibrillation and amiodarone
  - Simultaneously assess for causes hypoxia, hypovelemia, hypothermia, hyperkalemia/hypokalemia and increased hydrogen ion concentration (acidosis), tension pneumothorax, tamponade (cardiac), toxins, thrombosis (cardiac and pulmonary).

Ans. 172

Inferior wall STEMI:

- Heart rate 60 beats/min, regular rhythm, P waves not clear? Junctional
- ST elevation in II, III, avF, with Q wave in III and reciprocal changes in I avL
- Probable RCA occlusion as suggested by the greater ST elevation in lead III more than ST elevation in lead II and presence of reciprocal ST depression in lead I.

Ans. 173

Diagnosis: Atrial flutter with variable block with capture beats:

- Ventricular rate 80/minute
- Irregular rhythm
- Normal axis
- Positive flutter waves in V1 anticlockwise re-entry circuit
- Comment on this ECG of a patient admitted to ICU with acute promyelocytic leukemia and differentiation.

Ans. 174

- *Causes of a prolonged QTc (>440 ms).*

Electrolyte abnormalities: Hypokalemia, hypomagnesemia, hypocalcemia

- *Medications/drugs:* Arsenic, terfenadine, astemizole, haloperidol, risperidone, citalopram, amitriptyline, quinolones, macrolide, quinine, etc.

Further Reading

Nachimuthu S, Assar MD, Schussler JM. Drug-induced QT interval prolongation: mechanisms and clinical management. Ther Adv Drug Saf. 2012;3(5):241-53.

Ans. 175

1. Pulmonary artery catheters range from 4 Fr to 8 Fr and 60–110 cm in length. It comes with ports, balloon tipped catheter, thermistor at tip to measure temperature and in combo with a heating coil proximally to measure cardiac output continuously.
2. Right atrial pressure, right ventricular pressure, pulmonary artery pressure, pulmonary artery occlusion pressure, mixed venous oxygen saturation, and cardiac output can be measured.
3. Pulmonary artery catheter has multiple ports:
   - Blue port is right atria port used to measure central venous pressure.
   - White lumen is used to infuse fluids and drugs; it opens proximal to blue lumen.
   - The yellow lumen is the distal port, pulmonary artery lumen. It is used to measure pulmonary artery pressure and mixed venous oxygen saturation.
   - The red lumen is the balloon port to inflate air.

Further Reading

Rodriguez Ziccardi M, Khalid N. Pulmonary artery catheterization. In: StatPearls. Treasure Island (FL): StatPearls Publishing; 2020. [online] Available from https://www.ncbi.nlm.nih.gov/books/NBK482170/ [Last accessed February, 2020].

Ans. 176

1. $ScVO_2$ is measured from superior vena cave, so it contains blood from upper body which will have lower value (due to high O_2 extraction at tissues) compared to SVO_2 which is measured at pulmonary artery (have mixed venous blood):
   - In shock states, the $ScVO_2$ is more than SVO_2 due to increased O_2 utilization by tissues and diversion of blood from splanchnic circulation; therefore, inferior *vena cava* (IVC) saturation is low.
2. PADP is always higher that PAOP so that forward flow is maintained. PADP-PAOP is 5–8 mm Hg in normal state.
3. The cardiac output is measured based on "conservation of indicator principle"—Stewart-Hamilton equation:
   - Cardiac output = Volume of injectate $(T_B - T_I)k_1/k_2$ (change in blood temperature over time)

     T_B = blood temperature, T_I = injectate temperature, k = constant

Further Reading

van Beest P, Wietasch G, Scheeren T, Spronk P, Kuiper M. Clinical review: use of venous oxygen saturations as a goal—a yet unfinished puzzle. Crit Care. 2011;15(5):232.

Ans. 177

1. PA catheter was widely used in critically ill-patients for hemodynamic assessments. In 1996, the support investigators conducted an observational study in critically ill-patients and found that the PA catheter was associated with a 24% increased mortality in ICU patients. In a group of high risk surgical patients, the Canadian critical care trial group randomized patients to a goal directed therapy guided by a PAC versus standard care without a PAC and found a higher incdence of pulmonary embolism with no benefits from PAC use similarly the FACTT, PACMAN or ESCAPE trials did not show any benefit from use of PA catheter in critically ill-patients with ARDS or heart failure. Currently, PA catheter is used for diagnosis and classification of PAH, assessing the severity of pulmonary hypertension and to assess vasoreactivity of the pulmonary circulation. in some cases, it may also help in accurately diagnosing between cardiogenic and noncardiogenic pulmonary edema, although the latest BERLIN criteria does not warrant the use for the same.
2. *Complications of PA catheter:*

During insertion and use	*During measurements*
• Vascular complications • Pneumothorax • Valve injury • Arrhythmias • Injury to heart • Migration • Pulmonary infarct • Infection	• Balloon rupture • Rupture of pulmonary artery • Pulmonary infarction • Wrong interpretation

Further Reading

Cecconi M, De Backer D, Antonelli M, Beale R, Bakker J, Hofer C, et al. Consensus on circulatory shock and hemodynamic monitoring. Task force of the European Society of Intensive Care Medicine. Intens Care Med. 2014;40(12):1795-815.

Ziccardi MR, Khalid N. Pulmonary artery catheterization. In: StatPearls. Treasure Island (FL): StatPearls Publishing; 2020. [online] Available from https://www.ncbi.nlm.nih.gov/books/NBK482170/ [Last accessed February, 2020].

Ans. 178

Principles of pulmonary artery catheter (PAC): Proper positioning—West zone:

- *West zone:* Theoretical (influence of gravity)
- Functional division rather anatomical.

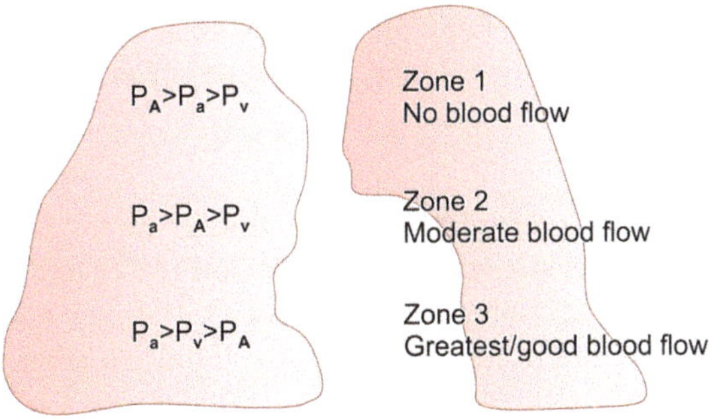

Our interest: Vascular pressure.
Principles of PAC: Identification of correct positioning:

- *Chest X-ray:* Catheter tip location below the level of the left atrium and not more than 4 cm from the midline
- PADP > PAOP (forward flow)
- Visible A and V waves within trace
- *When you change positive end-expiratory pressure (PEEP) (PEEP trial):* Change in PAOP less than half the change in PEEP

Ans. 179

Current application:

- Severe shock states associated with ARDS with pulmonary hypertension
- Shock with right ventricular dysfunction
- Cardiac transplantation
- Weaning failures
- Research settings.

Further Reading

Cecconi M, De Backer D, Antonelli M, Beale R, Bakker J, Hofer C, et al. Consensus on circulatory shock and hemodynamic monitoring. Task force of the European Society of Intensive Care Medicine. Intens Care Med. 2014;40(12):1795-815.

Ans. 180

1. The cardiac output is measured based on "conservation of indicator principle"—Stewart-Hamilton equation:

Cardiac output = Volume of injectate ($T_B - T_I$) k_1/k_2 (change in blood temperature over time)

T_B = blood temperature, T_I = injectate temperature, k = constant.

2. Compared to pulmonary thermodilution, the cold saline is injected into superior vena cava and thermistor is in femoral artery. The injectate mixes with blood in all the cardiac chambers before making its way into the arterial circulation to give the temperature over time curve.
3. *Limitations:*
   - When the cardiac output is very low, e.g., <2 L/min, the values are not accurate.
   - In case of pneumonectomy or lobectomy, tricuspid regurgitation the values are affected.

Ans. 181

The calibration is not valid. Only one reading is taken instead of average of three (accepted number). The values may not be correct to interpret.

Comments:

- Calibrate again.
- Values that depend on running thermodilution are not reliable but other parameters such as stroke volume variation (SVV) and *central venous pressure* (CVP) values may be relied upon.
- Low SVV favors fluid nonresponsive state, if prerequisites for measuring SVV are met.

Ans. 182

Pulmonary edema is commonly due to two mechanisms:

1. Increased hydrostatic pressure (more blood volume).
2. Increased permeability:

   First scenario: Increase in preload, i.e., the blood volume intern pulmonary blood volume (PBV) will increase the pulmonary edema, identified by extravascular lung water (EVLW).

   Second scenario: Despite volume status, increase in preload will increase pulmonary edema due to increased permeability.

   This is identified by a ratio—pulmonary vascular permeability index (PVPI):

   - PVPI = EVLW/PBV < 3 indicate hydrostatic mechanism
   - PVPI = EVLW/PBV > 3 indicate increased permeability.

   Our patient has PVPI 2.7, favoring hydrostatic mechanism, i.e., infusing fluids will worsen lung edema. The actual use is that it guides to take decision to remove fluid by diuretics or ultrafiltration which will ultimately improve lung condition.

Ans. 183

Using the given cardiac output monitor, the possible options for fluid responsiveness are:

- Stroke volume variation
- Tidal volume challenge with SVV, if patient is ventilated with low tidal volume of 6 mL/kg
- Passive leg raise test
- Fluid challenge test and following change in stroke volume (though not favored).

The given cardiac output monitor is:

- Noncalibrated device
- Does not represent beat-to-beat variations in stroke volume
- Does not give additional parameters as compared to thermodilution-based devices
- No safety parameters.

Ans. 184

Possible explanations for changes in SVV are:

Reduction in SVV:

- Fluid responsive to nonresponsive state.
- High SVV due to arrhythmia, spontaneous breathing, and lower values may be at conditions with corrected arrhythmias and with paralytic agents.
- Reduction in tidal volume will lead to reduction in SVV at same hemodynamic condition.

Ans. 185

- Subcostal image showing a huge clot in left atrial (LA), almost completely occluding LA.
- Differential includes LA tumors such as myxoma.

The left atrial appendage (LAA) is the most common location for atrial thrombus formation and is usually missed on transthoracic echocardiography. LAA clots are preferably diagnosed on transesophageal echo while left ventricular clots are diagnosed on transthoracic echocardiography (TTE).

Ans. 186

1. Parasternal long-axis view.
2. *Findings:*
   - Pericardial effusion
   - Pleural effusion.

Possible left ventricular hypertrophy—need more assessment to conclude.

Ans. 187

- *This is subcostal four-chamber view, showing:*
  - Dilated right atrium and ventricle
  - Clot in right atrium.

Possible cause of cardiac arrest may be pulmonary embolism.

Ans. 188

- In case of cardiac arrest due to pulmonary embolism, the prime management will be:
  - Continue cardiopulmonary resuscitation (CPCR)
  - Initiate vasopressors that may maintain perfusion to coronary arteries and systemic arteries
  - Thrombolysis with TPA and continue CPCR, rtPA (recombinant human tissue-type plasminogen activator) 0.6 mg/kg over 15 minutes, maximum dose of 50 mg.

Consider venoarterial extracorporeal membrane oxygenation, if severe hemodynamic instability.

Ans. 189

Thrombolysis dose pulmonary embolism:

Drugs	*Dose*
rtPA	100 mg over 2 hours
Streptokinase	250,000 IU over 30 minutes as loading dose followed by 100,000 IU/h over 12–24 hours
Urokinase	4,400 IU/kg as a loading dose over 10 minutes, followed by 4,400 IU/kg/h over 12 to 24 hours

(rtPA: recombinant human tissue-type plasminogen activator)

Ans. 190

1. The CT image shows clot in division of pulmonary artery and on both right and left main pulmonary trunk.
2. Management if patient is hemodynamically stable:
   - Initiate anticoagulation.
   - Avoid factors that increase pulmonary artery resistance, such as acidosis and hypercapnia.
   - Avoid positive pressure ventilation, if possible.
   - Avoid rapid fluid boluses unless the central venous pressure is low.

Ans. 191

1. In patient with pregnancy having pulmonary embolism, the diagnostic modality will be:
   - Perfusion scintigraphy
   - CT pulmonary angiogram (low-radiation dosing protocol)
   - Both are considered as choice
   - If initial chest X-ray is abnormal, then CTPA is preferred modality.

Ans. 192

1. The fast flush test reveals an overdamped arterial waveform.
2. Overdamping can be identified by the loss of normal shape of the arterial tracing waveform and approximation of the systolic blood pressure, diastolic blood pressure, and mean arterial blood pressure together. This leads to underestimation of systolic blood pressure and overestimation of diastolic blood pressure, although the mean arterial pressure is not affected.
3. *Causes of over damping:* Air bubbles, clot, overly compliant tubing or kinked tubing, stopcocks, low flush pressure, and/or impingement against the vessel wall.

Further Reading

McGhee BH, Bridges EJ. Monitoring arterial blood pressure: What you may not know. Crit Care Nurse. 2002;22:60-79.

Ans. 193

1. Stroke volume variation is the phasic variation in stroke volume due to heart-lung interactions.
   Stroke volume variation is accentuated on controlled mechanical ventilation and a 10% cut off is used to differentiate patients who will respond to fluid bolus (responders—those with SVV > 10%) compared to those who will not respond to fluid bolus (nonresponders).
2. Stroke volume variation becomes unreliable in patients with spontaneous breathing, cardiac arrhythmias, right ventricular failure, low HR/RR ratio (heart rate: respiratory rate) < 3.6, low tidal volume ventilation [<8 mL/kg predicted body weight (PBW)], and in conditions with poor lung compliance such as ARDS or open thorax.

Further Reading

Monnet X, Marik PE, Teboul JL. Prediction of fluid responsiveness: an update. Ann Intensive Care. 2016;6:111.

Ans. 194

- *Optic nerve sheath diameter:* It is used as a surrogate measure of intracranial pressure. It is measured as the widest diameter, 3 mm from the eyeball. Normally, the value range from 4.8 mm to 5.9 mm.
- The measurements are prone for interobserver variability but still can be utilized as a more reliable bedside measurement of intracranial hypertension than clinical judgment, especially in patients having altered sensorium or under sedation.

Further Reading

Chacko J. Optic nerve sheath diameter: an ultrasonographic window to view raised intracranial pressure? Indian J Crit Care Med. 2014;18:707-8.

Ans. 195

1. This is intra-aortic balloon pump (IABP).
2. IABP-SHOCK II (Intra-aortic Balloon Pump in Cardiogenic Shock *II*) trial (2012) showed that there was no 30-day and 1-year mortality benefit, and no secondary outcomes benefit (e.g. stroke or functional capacity) from IABP insertion for cardiogenic shock following MI when early revascularization was planned.
3. Cochrane review 2015 (that included seven eligible studies and a total of 790 patients) concluded that the IABP may have a beneficial effect on some hemodynamic parameters which does not seem to translate into a mortality benefit in cardiogenic shock.

Absolute contraindications:

- Aortic regurgitation
- Aortic aneurysm
- Aortic dissection
- Severe sepsis
- Uncontrolled coagulopathy.

Further Reading

Ranucci M, Castelvecchio S, Biondi A, de Vincentiis C, Ballotta A, Varrica A, et al. Surgical and Clinical Outcome Research (SCORE) Group. A randomized controlled trial of preoperative intra-aortic balloon pump in coronary patients with poor left ventricular function undergoing coronary artery bypass surgery*. Crit Care Med. 2013;41(11):2476-83.

Thiele H, Zeymer U, Neumann FJ, Ferenc M, Olbrich HG, Hausleiter J, et al. Intra-aortic balloon support for myocardial infarction with cardiogenic shock. N Engl J Med. 2012;367(14):1287-96.

Zeymer U, Prondzinsky R, Unverzagt S, Buerke M, de Waha A, Haerting J, et al. Intra-aortic balloon pump counterpulsation (IABP) for myocardial infarction complicated by cardiogenic shock (Review). Cochrane Database Syst Rev. 2015;27(3):CD007398.

Ans. 196

1. Balloon should be positioned so that the tip is about 1 cm distal to the origin of the left subclavian artery.
2. The lower end of the balloon should lie cephalad to the renal arteries. Incorrect placement causes vascular occlusion of renal vessels and compromises renal perfusion and drop in urine output.

Ans. 197

Image shows:

- A clear dicrotic notch with inflation starting after the dicrotic notch, suggestive of late IABP balloon inflation.

Pathophysiology: There is no diastolic augmentation, although the mean diastolic pressure is still higher than the previous readings. The coronaries may still be better perfused than without an IABP and the end-diastolic pressure is lower than the baseline suggestive of a reduced afterload of LV in the next beat.

Ans. 198

Image shows: Diastolic augmentation at the dicrotic notch with a prolonged inflation extending into the next beat, with a rise in end-diastolic pressure in aorta.

Suggestive of *late deflation of IABP balloon.*

Pathophysiology: At the initiation of the ventricular contraction, the aortic balloon is still inflated, the aortic pressure is higher than the baseline—resulting in significantly increased afterload and increased oxygen consumption—worsening the clinical situation.

Ans. 199

Image shows an early inflation of the IABP before the dicrotic notch occurs—the inflation occurs in systole.

Suggestive of—*early balloon inflation.*

Pathophysiology: As the balloon inflates in systole, the aortic pressure overshoots the LV pressure, causing premature closing of aortic valve and the systole is cut short resulting in reduced LV output. This causes an increased left ventricular afterload and can worsen myocardial oxygen demand.

Ans. 200

Image shows a rapid drop in pressures after the diastolic augmentation.

Suggestive of early deflation: The full effect of diastolic augmentation is not attained. Before the next contraction, the end-diastolic aortic pressure reached the baseline, resulting in a suboptimal reduction of afterload and a suboptimal reduction in myocardial oxygen demand.

Ans. 201

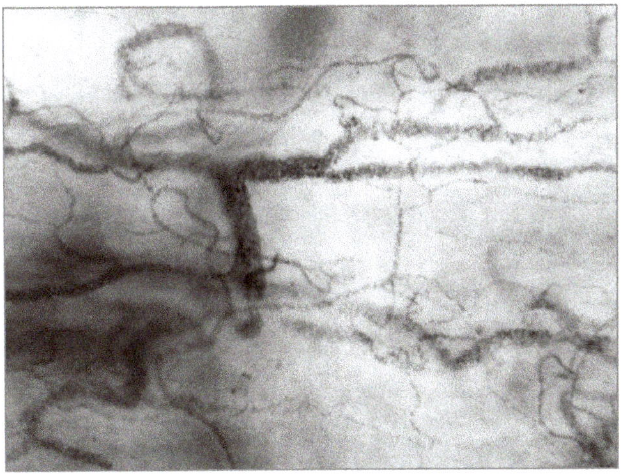

1. Sublingual microcirculation seen with either side-stream dark field imaging (SDFI) or orthogonal polarization spectral imaging (OPSI).
2. The terms used to describe the microcirculation are:
   - *PPV:* Proportion of perfused small vessels
   - *MFI:* Microvascular flow index
   - *hPPV:* Heterogeneity of proportion of perfused small vessels.

Ans. 202

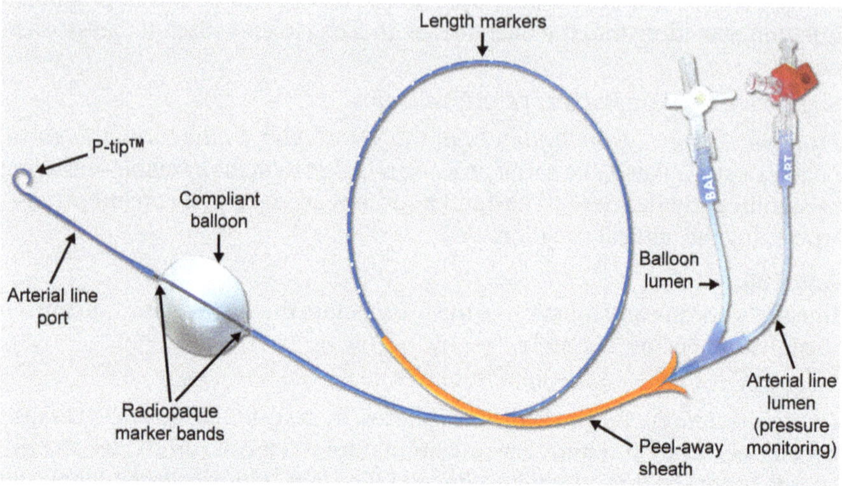

Source: www.prytimemedical.com

It is called the ER-REBOA™ catheter. It is used for balloon occlusion of the aorta in the ER when there is massive abdominal bleeding, with likely exsanguination in trauma.

Further Reading

PRYTIME MEDICAL. ER-REBOA™ Catheter. [online] Available from https://prytimemedical.com/product/er-reboa/ [Last accessed February, 2020].

Ans. 203

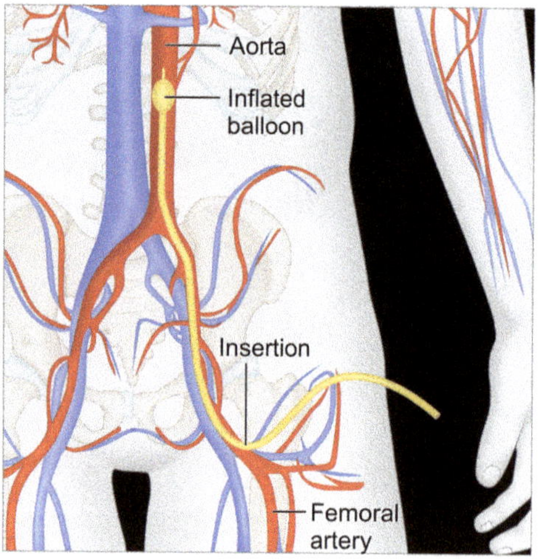

1. Insertion of REBOA catheter in trauma.
2. *Indications*:
   - Noncompressible hemorrhage below the diaphragm in the abdomen, pelvis or retroperitoneum
   - Positive FAST
   - Pelvic fracture with negative FAST

- Traumatic cardiac arrest without aortic dissection or pericardial tamponade
- Suspected traumatic abdominal hemorrhage
- Blunt pelvic injury or groin junctional hemorrhage.

Contraindications:
- Age ≤ 18 years or ≥ 70 years
- Atraumatic cardiac arrest
- Proximal traumatic aortic dissection
- Proximal aortic dissection
- Cardiac tamponade.

Further Reading

Resuscitative endovascular balloon occlusion of the aorta. [online] Available from https://wikem.org/wiki/Resuscitative_endovascular_balloon_occlusion_of_the_aorta [Last accessed February, 2020].

Ans. 204
- Subcostal transthoracic ECHO view of the heart showing inferior vena cava (IVC).
- The sensitivity of IVC index was 76% and specificity was 86% in a recent meta-analysis. Respiratory variations of IVC have been less studied than other dynamic index like pulse pressure variation (PPV) and stroke volume variation (SVV). Main limitations of use are patients on spontaneous respiration and the need to use a tidal volume of at least 7 mL/kg. Superior venae cava indices are more sensitive to assess fluid responsiveness, which require a transesophageal ECHO.

Further Reading

Pinsky MR, Teboul JL, Vincent JL. Hemodynamic Monitoring (Lessons from the ICU), 1st edition. Germany: Springer; 2019.

Ans. 205
- Velocity time integral (VTI) with a PLR maneuver.
- Velocity time integral is the flow of blood through the left ventricular outflow tract (LVOT), measured in five-chamber echocardiographic view using Doppler cardiography.
- In the absence of advanced invasive hemodynamic monitoring such as cardiac output monitoring, measurement of VTI with PLR maneuver is a simple noninvasive method to assess fluid responsiveness at the bedside.
- A change in VTI > 10% with PLR is indicative of fluid responsiveness.
- Velocity time integral is measured on a patient and again measured after 1–2 minutes of passive leg rise.

Ans. 206
- Transthoracic echo with measurement of transmitral velocity (E wave), and tissue Doppler image of measurement of lateral mitral valve annulus velocity (e').
- Measurement of left ventricular (LV) filling pressures can be used to distinguish between acute respiratory distress syndrome (ARDS) and hydrostatic pulmonary edema. Invasive measurement of pulmonary

artery occlusion pressure (PAOP) is the surrogate for measurement LV filling pressures. ECHO is a simple noninvasive method to measure LV filling pressures at the bedside. The e′ is a relatively preload independent parameter. E/e′ > 8 at the lateral mitral valve annulus has correlated with PAOP > 13 mm Hg.

- In this patient with breathlessness, a high-filling pressure was suggestive of cardiogenic hydrostatic pulmonary edema; hence, measures should be taken to reduce afterload.

Further Reading

In: de Backer D, Cholley BP, Slama M, Vieillard-Baron A, Vignon P (Eds). Hemodynamic Monitoring Using Echocardiography in the Critically Ill. Berlin, Heidelberg: Springer Verlag; 2011.

Ans. 207

- Measurement of transmitral Doppler flow velocity in apical four-chamber view echocardiography. Measurement of E wave velocity and A wave velocity.
- Diastolic heart failure is common in ICU patients. It is important to assess diastolic function in the ICU.
- Diastolic dysfunction is important in patient with sepsis and septic shock; septic cardiomyopathy can affect diastolic function. Septic patients have a reduced preload, tachycardia which may worsen diastolic dysfunction. It is important to maintain adequate preload and these septic patients may develop pulmonary edema due to high LV filling pressures and diastolic dysfunction.
- Patients with diastolic dysfunction may fail extubation due to weaning-induced pulmonary edema; hence, it is important to address diastolic function before extubation by reducing the LV afterload.

Further Reading

In: de Backer D, Cholley BP, Slama M, Vieillard-Baron A, Vignon P (Eds). Hemodynamic Monitoring Using Echocardiography in the Critically Ill. Berlin, Heidelberg: Springer Verlag; 2011.

Ans. 208

- This is a parasternal short-axis view showing vegetations in the aortic valve.
- The initial management is empirical antibiotics and supportive care.
- The indications for surgical management are refractory pulmonary edema or cardiogenic shock as a result of aortic or mitral *infective endocarditis* (IE) causing severe acute valve regurgitation; IE complicated by heart block, annular, or aortic abscess or destructive penetrating lesions; IE with persisting fever and positive blood cultures > 7–10 days; and IE caused by fungi or multiresistant organisms.
- Prevention of embolism.

Further Reading

Keynan Y, Singal R, Kumar K, Arora RC, Rubinstein E. Infective endocarditis in the intensive care unit. Crit Care Clin. 2013;29(4):923-51.

Ans. 209

- Measurement of right ventricular (RV) systolic function with M mode: tricuspid annulus plane systolic excursion (TAPSE).
- The measurement is obtained in longitudinal plane in apical four-chamber view, and M-mode cursor is placed at the lateral annulus. The excursion of the tricuspid annulus is measured as shown in the Figure.
- The American Society of Echocardiography recommends using the TAPSE routinely as a simple method to estimate the RV systolic function.
- TAPSE > 16 mm is suggestive of normal RV function; TAPSE < 16 mm strongly correlates with abnormal RV function.
- TAPSE is a simple, easy-to-measure method to evaluate RV systolic function in cases such as suspected pulmonary thromboembolism.

Further Reading

In: de Backer D, Cholley BP, Slama M, Vieillard-Baron A, Vignon P (Eds). Hemodynamic Monitoring Using Echocardiography in the Critically Ill. Berlin, Heidelberg: Springer Verlag; 2011.

Ans. 210

- Image shows ECHO assessment of measurement of tricuspid regurgitant (TR) jet velocity in this patient with RV dysfunction.
- Tricuspid regurgitant jet velocity is measured in continuous wave Doppler and finally pulmonary artery systolic pressure (PASP) is estimated using the Bernoulli's equation.
- In patients with pulmonary artery hypertension admitted to ICU, measurement of TR jet velocity and quantification of severity of pulmonary artery hypertension is useful.
- In this patient who had COPD and cor pulmonale, monitoring the severity of pulmonary artery hypertension over the course of illness in the ICU can help to target therapies to improve pulmonary hypertension [prostacyclin, phosphodiesterase (PDE)].

Further Reading

Parasuraman S, Walker S, Loudon BL, Gollop ND, Wilson AM, Lowery C, et al. Assessment of pulmonary artery pressure by echocardiography: a comprehensive review. Int J Cardiol Heart Vasc. 2016;12:45-51.

Ans. 211

- Image shows parasternal short-axis ECHO window with pericardial effusion.
- Pericardial effusion can be present in some of the patients admitted to the ICU. It is important to evaluate for tamponade effect by looking for diastolic collapse of the RV free wall/RVOT (left ventricular outflow tract). The pericardial effusion can be graded according to the thickness of the effusion: < 0.5 cm (mild), 0.5–2 cm (moderate), and > 2 cm (severe).
- Pericardial effusion present in diastole is abnormal.
- Pleural effusion must be differentiated from pericardial effusion. In parasternal long-axis view, a left-sided pleural effusion is seen posterior to the descending aorta; whereas, pericardial effusion is seen anterior to the descending aorta.

- If patient has tamponade effect, it should be drained using ECHO and it is safer than fluoroscopic guidance.

Further Reading

In: de Backer D, Cholley BP, Slama M, Vieillard-Baron A, Vignon P (Eds). Hemodynamic Monitoring Using Echocardiography in the Critically Ill. Berlin, Heidelberg: Springer Verlag; 2011.

Ans. 212

- The lung ultrasound finding shows a lung point.
- Lung point is a highly specific sign for pneumothorax.
- It is the junction between the sliding lung and the absent sliding lung, as seen the appearance of sea shore sign in M-mode in the background of stratosphere sign.
- Visualization of lung point in M-mode makes diagnosis of pneumothorax highly likely.

Further Reading

Lichtenstein D, Mezière G, Biderman P, Gepner A. The "lung point": an ultrasound sign specific to pneumothorax. Intensive Care Med. 2000;26(10):1434-40.

Ans. 213

- The figure shows pleural effusion seen in lung ultrasound.
- Presence of pleural effusion is common in ICU patients; mostly the effusions are managed conservatively.
- It requires therapeutic drainage in massive effusions causing hypoxemia and in cases of exudative effusion (septations).
- Effusion can be quantified using Balik's formula, but usually it is a semiquantitative quantification into mild, moderate, and massive effusion.
- Balik's formula: Patient is placed in supine position; transducer is kept perpendicular to the dorsolateral chest wall. Measurements are taken at maximum inspiration. The maximum distance (in millimeters) between the visceral pleura and parietal pleura was measured.
- Pleural effusion volume (mL) = (measured distance) × 20.
- Studies in mechanical-ventilated adults with therapeutic drainage have shown improvement in oxygenation but data on clinical outcomes is limited.

Further Reading

Maslove DM, Chen BT, Wang H, Kuschner WG. The diagnosis and management of pleural effusions in the ICU. J Intensive Care Med. 2013;28(1):24-36.

Ans. 214

- The image shows measurement of diaphragmatic excursion using lung ultrasound in M mode.
- Tidal excursion < 1.4 cm is abnormal and indicates diaphragmatic dysfunction.
- Other parameter that can be assessed using ultrasound of diaphragm is thickness, i.e., thickness fraction during tidal respiration.

- Diaphragm ultrasound can be used to assess patients with difficult weaning and to assess patient ventilator interaction including dyssynchrony.

Further Reading

Tuinman PR, Jonkman AH, Dres M, Shi ZH, Goligher EC, Goffi A, et al. Respiratory muscle ultrasonography: Methodology, basic and advanced principles and clinical applications in ICU and ED patients-a narrative review. Intensive Care Med. 2020;10.1007/s00134-019-05892-8.

Ans. 215

- The image shows comet tail artefacts or B lines s/o alveolar interstitial syndrome.
- Ultrasound differences between ARDS and cardiogenic pulmonary edema are shown in the table.

	ARDS	*Pulmonary edema*
B lines	Heterogeneous	Diffuse
Pleural line	Thickening	Normal
Lung side	May be absent or reduced	Present
Subpleural	Shreds	Normal
Consolidation	Usually present	Usually absent

(ARDS: acute respiratory distress syndrome)

Further Reading

Baston C, West TE. Lung ultrasound in acute respiratory distress syndrome and beyond. J Thorac Dis. 2016;8(12):E1763-E1766.

Ans. 216

- Recruitment in ARDS is usually guided by measurement of oxygenation, compliance, esophageal pressures, etc. Ultrasound is a simple, noninvasive bedside tool to assess and monitor recruitment maneuver.
- A lung aeration score can be used by dividing each hemithorax into six areas for exploration (6 + 6 = 12 areas in total). Each area is given a lung aeration score and change in ultrasound score can be checked after recruitment maneuver.

Score	*Ultrasound appearance*
0—normal lung	A-lines, maximum two B lines
1—moderate loss of aeration	More than three noncoalescent B lines
2—severe loss of aeration	Coalescent B lines
3—complete loss of aeration	Lung consolidation

- A reduction in lung ultrasound score (LUS) of > 5 has correlated with recruitment in ARDS in studies.

Further Reading

Bello G, Blanco P. Lung ultrasonography for assessing lung aeration in acute respiratory distress syndrome: A narrative review. J Ultrasound Med. 2019;38(1):27-37.

Ans. 217

- *Based on previous question:*
  - LUS in image A: 1
  - LUS in image B: 0
  - LUS in image C: 3

Ans. 218

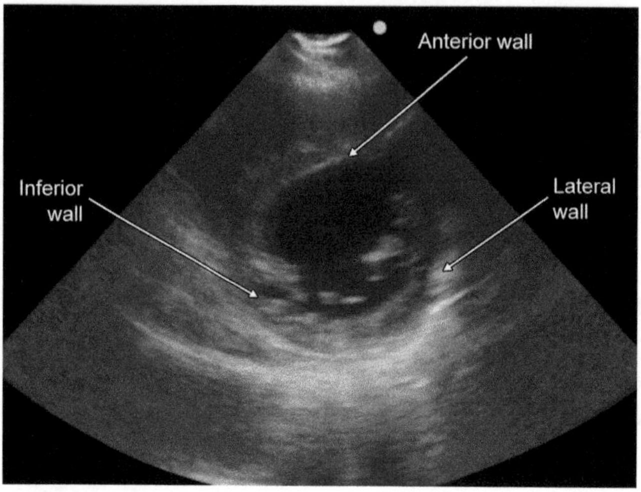

- Parasternal short-axis view.
- *Uses*: To assess the contractility by eye balling, to look for regional wall motion abnormalities as described in the image above, and to assess septal dyskinesia.

Further Reading

In: de Backer D, Cholley BP, Slama M, Vieillard-Baron A, Vignon P (Eds). Hemodynamic Monitoring Using Echocardiography in the Critically Ill. Berlin, Heidelberg: Springer Verlag; 2011.

Ans. 219

- Passive leg raise test (PLRT):
  - Start from 45° semirecumbent position
  - Move the bed and not the patient
  - Measure the time interval of 60 – 9 seconds after which the change in stroke volume needs to be measured in real time 60–90 seconds
  - Measure change in stroke volume—real time
  - Remeasure the stroke volume after PLR
- Real-time cardiac output monitoring for PLRT:
  - Cardiac output monitor
  - Echocardiography [velocity time integral (VTI)]
  - Esophageal Doppler
  - On invasive cardiac output monitors
  - Alternate or surrogate to cardiac output
    - End-tidal carbon dioxide ($ETCO_2$).

Ans. 220

- Utility of $ETCO_2$—hemodynamic:
  - *PLRT:* To monitor change in stroke volume
  - Cardiac arrest (CA): To know return of spontaneous circulation (ROSC)
  - Track change in cardiac output: Volume loss/volume repletion.

Ans. 221

1. *Skin perfusion using laser Doppler:*
   - Identification of perfusion problems even in dark-skin people.
   - It is a reflection of skin mottling.
   - It can give information on either improving or worsening tissue perfusion.

Ans. 222

Peripheral perfusion index PI is a noninvasive method of measuring peripheral perfusion.

It is calculated by means of pulse oximetry by expressing the pulsatile signal during arterial inflow as a percentage of nonpulsatile signal, both of which are derived from the amount of infrared light absorbed.

It indirectly reflects changes in cardiac output and oxygen supply to critical organs during anesthesia and critical illness.

- Peripheral perfusion index is the ratio of pulsatile blood flow to nonpulsatile blood flow derived from plethysmography trace.
- The pulsatile component correlates with the changes in the arterial blood volume and arterial flow, while the nonpulsatile component correlates with the venous blood.
- Values < 1.4 were predictive of poor tissue perfusion while values > 3.5 were suggestive of severe vasodilatation and could predict the development of hypotension following spinal anesthesia.

Ans. 223

1. Twelve trials involving 11,162 patients found no difference in cerebral performance category score, survival to hospital admission, and survival to discharge between manual CPR and mechanical CPR for out-of-hospital CA (OHCA) patients.
2. The ability to achieve ROSC with mechanical device was found to be inferior to manual chest compression during resuscitation. The use of mechanical chest compression cannot be recommended as a replacement for manual CPR, but rather a supplemental treatment in an overall strategy for treating CA patients.

Further Reading

Li H, Wang D, Yu Y, Zhao X, Jing X. Mechanical versus manual chest compressions for cardiac arrest : A systematic review and meta-analysis. Scand J Trauma Resusc Emerg Med. 2016;24:1-10.

Ans. 224

- Head-up position CPR has found to improve cerebral perfusion pressure. This simple maneuver has the potential to improve neurological outcomes after CA as per study conducted on pigs in 2016.

- The primary mechanism of benefit behind head-up CPR is the use of gravity to enhance venous drainage from brain and cerebral venous sinuses, and also the paravertebral venous plexus, thereby decreasing intracranial pressure (ICP) and creating potential for the forward flow of blood by decreasing the pressure transmitted to the brain via both the venous and arterial vasculatures, which effectively reduces a concussive injury with compression. Also, this position involves the redistributing blood flow through the lungs.
- Another study done on pigs in 2018 has shown that HUP as compared to standard supine position (SUP) has not improved cerebral oxygenation or metabolism.

Further Reading

Putzer G, Braun P, Martini J, Niederstätter I, Abram J, Katharina A, et al. Experimental paper effects of head-up vs. supine CPR on cerebral oxygenation and cerebral metabolism – a prospective, randomized porcine study. Resuscitation. 2018;128(January):51-5.

Ryu HH, Moore JC, Yannopoulos D, Lick M, McKnite S, Shin SD, et al. The effect of head up cardiopulmonary resuscitation on cerebral and systemic hemodynamics. Resuscitation. 2016;102:29-34.

Ans. 225

Classification of shock: The focused assessment with sonography for trauma (FAST) examination, although easily available and useful, can miss blunt mesenteric injuries, injuries to bowel, diaphragm, retroperitoneal injuries as well as isolated penetrating injury to the peritoneum. In case the blood is clotted, free fluid may not be visualized again leading to a false-negative FAST scan.

Parameter	*Class I*	*Class II (Mild)*	*Class III (Moderate)*	*Class IV (Severe)*
Approximate blood loss	<15%	15–30%	31–40%	>40%
Heart rate	↔	↔/↑	↑	↑/↑↑
Blood pressure	↔	↔	↔/↓	↓
Pulse pressure	↔	↓	↓	↓
Respiratory rate	↔	↔	↔/↑	↑
Urine output	↔	↔	↓	↓↓
Glasgow Coma Scale score	↔	↔	↓	↓
Base deficit*	0 to –2 mEq/L	–2 to –6 mEq/L	–6 to –10 mEq/L	–10 mEq/L or less
Need for blood products	Monitor	Possible	Yes	Massive Transfusion Protocol

*Base excess is the quantity of base (HCO_3^-, in mEq/L) that is a above or below the normal range in the body. A negative number is called a base deficit and indicates metabolic acidosis.

Source: Mutschler A, Nienaber U, Brockamp T, Wafaisade A, Wyen H, Peiniger S, et al. A critical reappraisal of the ATLS classification of hypovolaemic shock does it really reflect clinical reality? Resuscitation. 2013;84:309-13.

Ans. 226

1. Airway pressure release ventilation (APRV) mode of ventilation.
2. Aim is to maintain a high mean airway pressure to improve oxygenation by increasing Ti max or increasing P high or both or even prone position ventilation with APRV.
3. For improving ventilation, the "P high" should be increased and "T high" should be reduced simultaneously, thereby increasing minute ventilation while keeping the mean airway pressure stable or increase the "T low" by 0.05–0.1 second increments.
4. Airway pressure release ventilation is a spontaneous mode of ventilation and we should not paralyze a patient on APRV. Paralysis on APRV changes the mode similar to inverse pressure ventilation and places serious risk of rapid development of severe respiratory acidosis.

   In case of worsening oxygenation despite optimizing ventilation strategies, other rescue methods such as prone ventilation or extracorporeal membrane oxygenation (ECMO) may be tried.

   Similarly, APRV should not be used in patients who require deep sedation, e.g. cerebral edema with raised intracranial pressure.

Further Reading

Daoud EG. Airway pressure release ventilation. Ann Thorac Med. 2007;2(4):176-9.

DRUGS

Ans. 227

The three main principles of the WHO analgesic ladder are:

1. Administering medicines round the clock as opposed to on demand.
2. Preferring oral route of administration or least invasive route.
3. Use of the analgesic ladder, i.e., nonopioids (e.g., acetaminophen) followed by as and when necessary, mild opioids (e.g., codeine), and if pain is not yet controlled to add the strong opioids (e.g., morphine or hydromorphone) until the patient is free of pain.

"Adjuvants" may be added along with any stage of analgesia medications, e.g., antidepressants (e.g., amitriptyline), anticonvulsants (e.g., gabapentin), corticosteroids (e.g., dexamethasone), and anxiolytics (e.g., diazepam).

Ans. 228

HEAT Investigators and the Australian and New Zealand Intensive Care Society Clinical Trials Group 2015:

- Prospective, parallel-group, blinded, randomized, controlled trial.
- Seven hundred patients (medical or surgical patients) underwent randomization.
- 1:1 ratio in two groups, one an infusion containing 1 g of intravenous (IV) acetaminophen compared with an infusion of 5% dextrose in water, every 6 hours.
- Early administration of acetaminophen to treat fever due to probable infection has no effect on the number of ICU-free days, no significant difference in 28-day mortality, 90-day mortality, or survival time to day 90.

Further Reading

Young P, Saxena M, Bellomo R, Freebairn R, Hammond N, van Haren F, et al. Acetaminophen for fever in critically ill patients with suspected infection. N Engl J Med. 2015;373(23):2215-24.

Ans. 229

- Metabolic acidosis with pH < 7.10 and hemodynamic instability.
- Normal anion gap metabolic acidosis [especially renal tubular acidosis (RTA)].
- Alkalinization of urine to enhance the elimination of acidic drugs such as tricyclic antidepressants (TCAs) poisoning, carbamazepine overdose: TCAs are weak bases and therefore increasing serum pH will increase the proportion of nonionized drug thus causing a greater proportion of drug to be distributed throughout the body away from the heart. Increased serum sodium also overcomes the sodium receptor blockade. Alkalinization also accelerates recovery of sodium channels by neutralizing the protonation of the drug-receptor complex.
- Salicylate and phenobarbitone as an antidote to drugs that impair fast sodium channel function and as an alkalinizing agent to manipulate drug distribution and excretion.
- It is also used in profound metabolic acidosis with cyanide, isoniazid, and toxic alcohol toxicity.

Ans. 230

- The current data for the use of sodium bicarbonate in hyperkalemia is controversial.
- Isotonic soda bicarbonate reduces serum potassium although the effect may be negligible in stable hemodialysis patients with its effects mainly in acidotic patients. This was shown in the recent BICAR-ICU (sodium bicarbonate therapy for patients with severe metabolic acidemia in the intensive care unit) trial which used 4.2% sodium bicarbonate resulting in significantly lower potassium concentrations compared to the control group.
- The strength and mechanism of sodium bicarbonate that effectively reduces serum potassium needs further evaluation.
- In hyperkalemia with electrocardiogram (ECG) changes in acidotic patients with pH < 7.2, or in patients with preexisting hypercalcemia and/or patients with digoxin toxicity—as a membrane stabilizing agent (anticipating no reduction in potassium levels) 8.4% sodium bicarbonate may be considered.
- Isotonic soda-bicarbonate infusions may benefit patients with hyperkalemia and pre-existing metabolic acidosis by facilitating direct cellular entry, increased renal excretion, and hemodilution. However, these mechanisms need to be proven scientifically.

Further Reading

Dépret F, Peacock WF, Liu KD, Rafique Z, Rossignol P, Legrand M. Management of hyperkalemia in the acutely ill patient. Ann Intensive Care. 2019;9(1):32.
Weisberg LS. Management of severe hyperkalemia. Crit Care Med. 2008;36(12):3246-51.

Blumberg A, Weidmann P, Ferrari P. Effect of prolonged bicarbonate administration on plasma potassium in terminal renal failure. Kidney Int. 1992;41(2):369-74.

Gutierrez R, Schlessinger F, Oster JR, Rietberg B, Perez GO. Effect of hypertonic versus isotonic sodium bicarbonate on plasma potassium concentration in patients with end-stage renal disease. Miner Electrolyte Metab. 1991;17(5):297-302.

Ans. 231

- Kidney disease improving Global Outcomes (KDIGO) are clinical practice guidelines for acute kidney injury 2012.
- Kidney disease improving Global Outcomes recommended IV volume expansion with either isotonic sodium chloride or sodium bicarbonate solutions, rather than no IV volume expansion, in patients at increased risk for contrast-induced acute kidney injury (CI-AKI).
- *Evidence:* (1A).
- Sodium bicarbonate has volume expanding effects, may decrease generation of free radicals mediated by the Haber-Weiss reaction by increasing tubular pH, it may also scavenge the potent oxidant peroxynitrate, produced via a nitric oxide-mediated pathway as reactive oxygen species activate cytokine-induced inflammatory mediators, resulting in damage to proximal tubular cells and it is likely that the activation of these mediators is influenced by tissue hypoxia and intracellular medullary acidosis.

Further Reading

Kidney Disease Improving Global Outcomes (KDIGO) Acute Kidney Injury Work Group. KDIGO Clinical Practice Guideline for Acute Kidney Injury. Kidney Int Suppl. 2012;2:1-138.

Ans. 232

- Noradrenaline predominantly acts on alpha 1 (α1) receptors with α-agonists. At high doses, it also acts on beta-1 and beta-2 receptors.
- Activation of α-adrenergic receptors augment tumor necrosis factor alpha (TNF-α), interleukin-1 beta (IL-1β), and IL-6 favoring inflammation.
- At low concentrations norepinephrine's immunologic effects are β-adrenergic receptors-dependent potent anti-inflammatory effects such as attenuation of TNF-α and IL-6 and increase IL-10 production and reduced natural killer (NK) cell cytotoxicity.
- Norepinephrine may skew the immune response from a T-helper 1 (Th1) toward a Th2 cell phenotype favoring sepsis-induced immunoparalysis.

Further Reading

Stolk RF, van der Poll T, Angus DC, van der Hoeven JG, Pickkers P, Kox M. Potentially inadvertent immunomodulation: Norepinephrine use in sepsis. Am J Respir Crit Care Med. 2016;194(5):550-8.

Ans. 233

- Frequent premature ventricular complexes (PVCs; the most common abnormality).
- Digoxin can cause a multitude of dysrhythmias due to either increased automaticity (increased intracellular calcium) or decreased AV conduction (increased vagal effects at the AV node).
- The classic digoxin toxic dysrhythmia combines supraventricular tachycardia and slow ventricular response.

- Other common dysrhythmias associated with digoxin toxicity include: Ventricular bigeminy and trigeminy, sinus bradycardia, slow atrial fibrillation, any type of AV block (1st degree, 2nd degree, and 3rd degree), regularized AF = AF with complete heart block and a junctional or ventricular escape rhythm, ventricular tachycardia (VT) including polymorphic and bidirectional VT.

Ans. 234

Indication: Reversal of unfractionated heparin-induced anticoagulation, biologically, protamine binds to positively charged groups such as phosphate groups and may have important properties in angiogenesis and immune function, protamines are simple proteins of low-molecular weight that are rich in arginine and strongly basic, present in the sperm of salmon and certain other species of fish, the anticoagulant effect of protamine also may be caused by inhibition of platelet aggregation, alteration in the platelet surface membrane, or depression of the platelet response to various agonists, the recommended dose of protamine for heparin reversal is 1-1.3 mg protamine per 100 IU heparin; however, this dose often results in a protamine excess, protamine injection causes adverse hemodynamic effects, protamine reactions have been classified into three types, the most common is the type I reaction, characterized by hypotension, type II (immunologic) reactions are categorized as IIA (anaphylaxis), IIB (anaphylactoid), and IIC (noncardiogenic pulmonary edema), type III reactions are heralded by hypotension and catastrophic pulmonary hypertension leading to right-sided heart failure, protamine neutralization of heparin can be associated with "protamine reactions," which include vasodilatory hypotension, anaphylactoid reactions, and pulmonary hypertensive crises, thrombocytopenia, the phenomenon referred to as heparin rebound describes the re-establishment of a heparinized state after heparin has been neutralized with protamine.

Ans. 235

- Decoy drug for factor Xa inhibitors in the blood, and prevents drug inhibition of native factor Xa.
- Apixaban or rivaroxaban exposure within 24 hours of life-threatening bleed.
- Acute intracranial hemorrhage (approval from stroke neurologist/ neurointensivist/neurosurgeon).
- Spinal or epidural hemorrhage (approval from site medical director).
- Intraocular hemorrhage with vision compromise (approval from site medical director).
- Airway or pulmonary hemorrhage (approval from site medical director).
- Hemopericardium (approval from site medical director).
- Aortic rupture, dissection or hemorrhage (approval from site medical director).
- Closed-space hemorrhage—compartment syndrome risk (approval from site medical director).

Andexanet dose based on apixaban or rivaroxaban use			
Factor Xa inhibitor	*Dose of factor Xa inhibitor*	*Timing of FXa inhinitor last dose before andexanet initiation*	
		< 8 hours or Unknown	*≥ 8 hours*
Rivaroxaban	≤10 mg	Low dose	Low dose
Rivaroxaban	>10 mg or Unknown	High dose	
Apixaban	≤5 mg	Low dose	
Apixaban	>5 mg or Unknown	High dose	

*Dose**	*Initial IV bolus*	*Follow-up IV infusion*
Low dose	400 mg (~30 mg/min)	480 mg at rate of 4 mg/min for 120 min
High dose	800 mg (~30 mg/min)	960 mg at rate of 8 mg/min for 120 min

(IV: intravenous)

*Not indicated for bleeding from all other sites.

Ans. 236

- The most common method of administration is the IV route with rapid bolus followed by saline flush.
- It is frequently used for the termination of AV node-dependent tachycardias and for the attainment of hyperemia in noninvasive stress testing.

Contraindications

- Second and third-degree AV block
- Care with asthma and chronic obstructive pulmonary disease (COPD).
- Allergy.

Ans. 237

- Dexmedetomidine is a highly selective α2-adrenoceptor agonist eight times more selective for the α2-adrenoceptor than clonidine.
- *Sedation*: Mediated via agonism of α2-adrenoceptors primarily in the locus coeruleus of the pons where it results in dose-dependent inhibition of norepinephrine release. This sedation is characterized by preserved muscle tone and ventilation, by spontaneous and evoked movements, and by awakening by external stimuli.
- *Analgesia*: It acts mainly on posterior horns of the spinal cord where stimulation of α2 receptors in the substantia gelatinosa of the dorsal horn reduces the release of nociceptive neurotransmitters such as substance P.
- The cardiovascular effects of the drug are biphasic. At higher rates of infusion predominant effect is hypertension due to activation of α2B receptors on vascular smooth muscle. This is superseded by hypotension and bradycardia as a result of the centrally mediated inhibition of sympathetic outflow.
- It suppresses stress response to surgery and other noxious stimuli.

Uses

- As a bridge to extubation.
- Alternative to sedative-drug withdrawal by α2-agonist property.
- *Patients at particular risk of critical care delirium*: SEDCOM (Safety and Efficacy of Dexmedetomidine Compared with Midazolam), a phase IV trial comparing dexmedetomidine and midazolam for light sedation. They found a reduction in the prevalence and duration of delirium in the dexmedetomidine group. Society of Critical Care Medicine recommend dexmedetomine to be used for sedation of patients with delirium not related to benzodiazepine or alcohol withdrawal in preference to benzodiazepines.
- *Whenever sedation is required to tolerate noninvasive ventilation in the ICU*: Lack of respiratory depression and provision of "rousable sedation" might make it particularly suitable for such patients. Small trial evidence of its efficacy in this situation is available.
- There is early interest in a possible benefit of dexmedetomidine sedation in patients with sepsis via attenuation of immunosuppression.
- Perioperative use.
- *Sedative premedication*: Its anxiolytic, sedative, sympatholytic, and antisialagogue properties, along with a lack of respiratory depression make dexmedetomidine suitable for premedication.
- 0.2-0.7 μg/kg/h infusion.

Side effects

- Bradycardia and hypotension
- Nausea
- Dry mouth
- Initial transient hypertension with reflex bradycardia (stimulation of α2B subtypes of receptors present in vascular smooth muscles)
- *Discontinuation syndrome*: Tachycardia, nervousness, agitation, headaches, and hypertensive crisis (e.g. if prolonged use due to upregulation of α2 receptors).

Further Reading

Scott-Warren VL, Sebastian J. Dexmedetomidine : its use in intensive care medicine and anaesthesia. BJA Educ. 2016;16(7):242-6.

Ans. 238

Cardiac Arrest

- During advanced cardiac life support (ACLS), epinephrine can be given three ways: IV; intraosseous (IO), and endotracheal tube (ET).
- *Dosing*:
  - *Intravenous push/IO*: 1 mg epinephrine is diluted in 10 mL saline and is given IV every 3-5 minutes.
  - *IV infusion for bradycardia*: 1 mg epinephrine is mixed with 500 mL of normal saline (NS) or 5% dextrose in water (D5W). The infusion should run at 2-10 μg/min (titrated to effect).
  - *Intravenous infusion for postcardiac arrest hypotension*: The dosing is 0.1-0.5 μg/kg/min (for example a 70 kg adult: 7-35 μg/min would be given).

  - *Endotracheal tube*: 2-2.5 mg epinephrine is diluted in 10 cc NS and given directly into the ET tube.
- Epinephrine should be used with caution in patients suffering from myocardial infarction since epinephrine increases heart rate (HR) and raises blood pressure (BP). This increase in HR and BP can increase myocardial oxygen demand and worsen ischemia.

Status Asthmaticus
- It is not routinely indicated for other asthma exacerbations.
- Intramuscular (IM) epinephrine (adrenaline) is indicated in addition to standard therapy for acute asthma associated with anaphylaxis and angioedema.
- Patients who have a confirmed food allergy that puts them at risk for anaphylaxis must be trained and have an epinephrine autoinjector available at all times.

Anaphylaxis
- Intramuscular injection is the preferred route for initial administration of epinephrine for anaphylaxis.
- Recommended dose of epinephrine for patients of any age is 0.01 mg/kg (maximum dose of 0.5 mg) per single dose, injected IM into the mid-outer thigh (vastus lateralis muscle). The dose should be drawn up using a 1 mL syringe using the 1 mg/mL formulation of epinephrine.
- Intramuscular epinephrine may be repeated at 5-15 minutes intervals if there is no response or an inadequate response or even sooner if clinically indicated.
- Intravenous bolus epinephrine is associated with significantly more dosing errors and cardiovascular complications than IM epinephrine and should be avoided when possible.
- Slow administration of a 50–100 μg (0.05–0.1 mg) IV bolus of epinephrine, ideally with hemodynamic monitoring. This is best administered by slow push of 0.5–1 mL of 0.1 mg/mL (1:10,000) epinephrine solution. It is preferred when a patient is suffering cardiovascular collapse or impending cardiovascular collapse that is refractory to IM epinephrine and volume resuscitation, and an epinephrine infusion is not available.
- Slow, continuous infusion is preferred if patients have not responded to IM injections symptoms and signs suggestive of impending shock.
- *Intravenous epinephrine continuous infusion and indications*: Patients who do not respond to several IM injections of epinephrine and aggressive fluid resuscitation.

BIOCHEMISTRY

Ans. 239

Ionized calcium at the time of seizure: The most common cause for seizure in this patient will be development of hypocalcemia due to calcium chelation with citrate which is used as the anticoagulant. As the ionized calcium level falls, the neurons depolarize spontaneously resulting in symptoms of tetany.

Moderate hypocalcemia causes symptoms such as nausea, vomiting, perioral numbness, paresthesia of the extremities, chills, abdominal cramping, light headedness, or hypotension.

Severe symptoms include muscle cramps, tetany, blurred or double vision, loss of consciousness, cardiac arrhythmia, and seizures.

Ans. 240

- The patient has presented with spontaneous bleed (epistaxis).
- He is having a high anion gap metabolic acidosis—probably lactic acidosis and uremia, and prolonged coagulation profile.
- Management includes hemodynamic optimization, assess the cause of lactic acidosis (drugs, hypoperfusion, and address the coagulopathy).
- In view of history of anticoagulation and drug automatism, it can be assumed that the coagulopathy is because of anticoagulant overdose. Dabigatran is a nonvitamin K antagonist oral anticoagulant (NOAC), which can present with picture of raised thrombin time and its toxicity is potentiated in presence of renal failure.
- *Management*: Usual half-life of dabigatran is 12–17 hours and the dose would be completely eliminated by 2.5 days. For patients with prolonged thrombin time and cannot be managed on conservative lines, such as imminent surgery, neurosurgical bleed, or those in whom the half-life cannot be estimated (renal failure) 5 g of idarucizumab may be administered. Dabigatran is a dialyzable drug and as an emergency, renal replacement therapy (RRT), prothrombin complex concentrates may also be tried.

Drug	*T1/2*	*Major mechanism of elimination*	*Coagulation profile*	*Antidote*
Dabigatran	12–17 hours	Renal (80%)	Prolonged thrombin time PT, INR, aPTT can be increased	Idarucizumab
Rivaroxaban	7–13 hours	67% renal	• PT, INR, aPTT can be increased • Factor Xa assay	Andexanet alfa
Apixaban	8–13 hours	25% renal	• PT, INR, aPTT can be increased • Factor Xa assay	Andexanet alfa

Ans. 241

- The given patient is having a high anion gap metabolic acidosis.
- Common causes for high anion gap metabolic acidosis include ketoacidosis, lactic acidosis, uremia, toxins, drugs such as salicylates and paracetamol.
- In a patient with extensive small bowel resection, due to short bowel syndrome, the carbohydrates are metabolized into D-lactic acid which cannot be metabolized by the body. These patients can present with high anion gap metabolic acidosis and central nervous system (CNS) symptoms, which are often precipitated by a high carbohydrate diet, diabetic ketoacidosis or drugs that contain propylene glycol. The diagnosis

requires chromatographic assay of lactate which measures both D- and L-isomer of lactate. Urinary anion gap also may be positive.
- Management includes hydration, stopping offending agent (enteral carbohydrate in this case), soda bicarbonate in severe acidosis, and oral antibiotics such as metronidazole, neomycin, or vancomycin.

Ans. 242
- Any patient coming with pulmonary embolism needs to be evaluated for hemodynamic instability and also ventricular strain. Apart from vital sign monitoring, this patient should be evaluated in detail.
- Suggested laboratory workup include—complete blood count (CBC) with platelet count, coagulation studies, urine pregnancy test, serum biochemistry including renal and liver function, arterial blood gas, troponin, brain natriuretic peptide. D-dimer need not be done in this case as there is documented DVT and high-probability Wells score.
- For the first episode of a thromboembolism, a detailed evaluation for inheritable thrombophilia and antiphospholipid syndrome is not warranted except in those with a family history of thromboembolism, those with age <45 years, patient with recurrent thrombosis, patient with arterial thrombosis, those with warfarin-induced skin necrosis. In such patients, additional tests including protein C and protein S deficiency, antithrombin, factor V Leiden mutation, prothrombin gene mutation, antiphospholipid antigen.
- Acute thrombosis, heparin, warfarin, NOAC, factor Xa inhibitors affect the anticoagulant factors. It is recommended for testing after a minimum 2 weeks of discontinuation of anticoagulation [antithrombin, factor VIII, lupus anticoagulant (warfarin), protein C and protein S].
- Antiphospholipid antibodies (aPLA), factor V Leiden mutation, and prothrombin gene mutation are unaffected by thrombosis or warfarin and heparin treatment and may be sent immediately.

Ans. 243
- This patient is having high anion gap metabolic acidosis and high osmolar gap. In the background of alcoholism, the possible diagnosis includes poisoning with methyl alcohol or ethylene glycol. The other differentials include septic shock, acute tubular necrosis, liver failure, etc.
- In patients with ethylene glycol poisoning, urine analysis will show calcium oxalate crystals and the patient may have low-serum calcium levels.
- The point of care analyzers such as ABG machines measure lactate levels using lactate oxidase method. This may misinterpret glycolate or glyoxalate (metabolites of ethylene glycol) as lactate and report very high values.
- The laboratory analyzers on the contrary use lactate dehydrogenase method and accurately identify serum lactate level. The difference between the two lactate levels (lactate gap) can be presumed to be due to the presence of glyoxalate, and early initiation of fomepizole, hemodialysis may be needed apart from other general critical care measures, such as rewarming, assessment of airway, breathing and circulation, assessment of need for intubation, etc.

Ans. 244

- The presentation is of an elderly female with hypothermia, bradycardia, bradypnea, and diminished sensorium. In the absence of toxins or a cerebrovascular insult, the possibility of hypothyroidism and myxedema coma should be considered.
- The other clues for myxedema coma are history of amiodarone ingestion, presence of pericardial effusion, hypercholesterolemia.
- Workup will include samples for thyroid function test TSH, free thyroxine (T4), and serum cortisol.
- Treatment consists of administration of combined T4 and T3, glucocorticoids (until the possibility of coexisting adrenal insufficiency has been excluded), continuation of other supportive measures, and management of the acute stressors.

Ans. 245

- The patient is having symptomatic hyponatremia, high anion gap metabolic acidosis probably due to lactic acidosis immediately after a seizure.
- The patient needs to be protected from further seizures and requires immediate correction of hyponatremia.
- The immediate laboratory investigations that need to be done are serum osmolarity, urine spot sodium, and serum sodium.
- Diabetic ketoacidosis also needs to be ruled out and measurement of serum beta-hydroxybutyric acid or urine ketones may be done.
- Management includes administration of 2–4 mL/kg of 3% hypertonic saline over 20 minutes.
- In asymptomatic patients, where autocorrection is already suspected to set in, by increased water diuresis correction may be withheld.
- Autocorrection can occur if the inciting cause of hyponatremia has been reversed (e.g., drugs), the urine is dilute [specific gravity < 1.005, osmolality < 200 mOsmol/kg and increased volume, or urine cation concentration (the sum of the urine sodium and potassium concentrations) is less than one-half the serum sodium].

Ans. 246

- The aim of hyponatremia correction is to increase the serum sodium by 5 mmol/L during the initial 1 hour and up to two boluses of 2–4 mL/kg of 3% saline may be administered.
- However, if symptoms persist despite two boluses per an increase in serum sodium by 5 mmol/L, other causes of altered sensorium need to be evaluated by investigations including imaging. Attempts may be made to increase the serum sodium cautiously by 1 mmol/L with continuous infusion of 3% saline up to 10 mmol/L over 24-hours.
- Sodium should be measured at the end of first hour, 6-hour, and 12-hour with an aim not to increase correction >10 mmol/L/day.

Ans. 247

- The patient has presented with a high anion gap metabolic acidosis, dyselectrolytemia, and hypoalbuminemia. Of all the differential diagnosis, the likely diagnosis is starvation ketoacidosis, although a toxicology screen is also needed. This patient is at high risk for developing refeeding syndrome once alimentation is started.

- Refeeding syndrome is characterized by marked dyselectrolytemia due to a change in hormonal milieu from glucagon to insulin, after introduction of dextrose or glucose. The characteristic abnormalities include hypophosphatemia, hypokalemia, hypomagnesemia along with other abnormalities such as drowsiness, rhabdomyolysis, congestive heart failure, seizures, and hemolysis.
- Refeeding syndrome can be prevented by avoiding rapid increases in the caloric intake and closely monitoring the patient clinically and biochemically.
- Frequent monitoring of electrolytes and proactive corrections for the same may be needed. Early administration of vitamins and micronutrients including thiamine also may help in preventing complications of refeeding syndrome.

Ans. 248

- The patient has presented with superior vena cava (SVC) syndrome due to mediastinal mass—probably lymphoma. The wheeze heard may have been due to airway compression rather than the wheeze of a hyperdynamic airway. Thus steroid administration in this case was probably not required and harmful.
- Currently, the patient is in tumor lysis syndrome (TLS) with hyperkalemia and concurrent ECG changes.
- Urgent management includes—maintaining airway breathing and circulation, along with urgent management of hyperkalemia.
- Management of hyperkalemia include:
  - Membrane stabilizing agents—calcium gluconate.
  - Agents that cause transient hypokalemia—glucose—insulin drip, salbutamol nebulization, hydration, and diuresis.
  - Currently sodium bicarbonate is not preferred unless there is concomitant severe metabolic acidosis.
  - In massive TLS, RRT may also be required.

Ans. 249

- The patient needs emergent management of hyperkalemia, including hydration, glucose insulin drip, salbutamol nebulization, and consideration of RRT. Apart from these, hydration should be maintained providing at least 3 L/m^2 body surface area (BSA) IV fluids with urine output monitoring.
- The calcium phosphate ratio is more than 60, suggesting that RRT may be indicated.
- Rasburicase—a recombinant urate oxidase inhibitor that converts uric acid (UA) to allantoin and may be administered parenterally for acute reduction of UA.

Ans. 250

The laboratory report shows resolution of hyperkalemia, although hyperphosphatemia is persisting. The UA has reduced to low levels. However, caution may be exercised for interpreting this report as sudden disappearance of UA may be due to ex vivo effect of rasburicase (a type of preanalytical laboratory error), measures to reduce serum UA should be continued. This can be unmasked by repeating a serum sample sent to the laboratory on ice.

Ans. 251

Common causes of postpartum seizure:

Obstetric
- Eclampsia, cerebral venous sinus thrombosis
- Idiopathic epilepsy

Regional anesthesia
- Dural puncture
- Meningoencephalitis, intracranial hemorrhage, cerebral, infarction or pneumoencephalus
- Treatments used for PDPH such as caffeine, sumatriptan synacthen and epidural blood patch

Other
- Metabolic disturbances, trauma, intracranial tumor, drug, and alcohol withdrawal

(PDPH: postdural puncture headache)

- In this patient as bran imaging is normal and blood pressure remains normal eclampsia is unlikely.
- The constellation of symptoms of seizure, anemia, thrombocytopenia, suggests a microangiopathic hemolytic anemia (MAHA) like eclampsia thrombocytopenic purpura (TTP) and hemolytic uremic syndrome (HUS) management includes confirmation of diagnosis by evaluation for hemolysis and ruling out other causes. Here the peripheral smear is showing evidence of hemolysis.
- Management includes securing airway, assessing breathing and circulation and assessing the need for antiepileptics. In cases of TP, plasma exchange may be required.

Ans. 252
- Aluminum phosphide poisoning.
- *Management*: Airway, breathing, circulation (ABC).
- Vasopressors.
- Venoarterial-extracorporeal membrane oxygenation (VA-ECMO).

Ans. 253
- *Differential diagnosis*: Hypercalcemia secondary to multiple myeloma versus hyperparathyroidism versus bone secondaries.
- *Clue for multiple myeloma*: Protein albumin difference, ABG showing low anion gap metabolic acidosis, hypercalcemia, backache, renal dysfunction.
- *Management*: Hydration/RRT.
- *Workup for multiple myeloma*: Serum electrophoresis, light-chain assay.

MISCELLANEOUS

Ans. 254

Class I

Sodium (Na^+)-channel blockade inhibits action potential prolongation by blocking active and refractory sodium channels in a use-dependent fashion.

IA: Procainamide

- Prolong the atrioventricular (AV) conduction and prolong the action potential.
- Increase both QRS duration and the QT-interval.

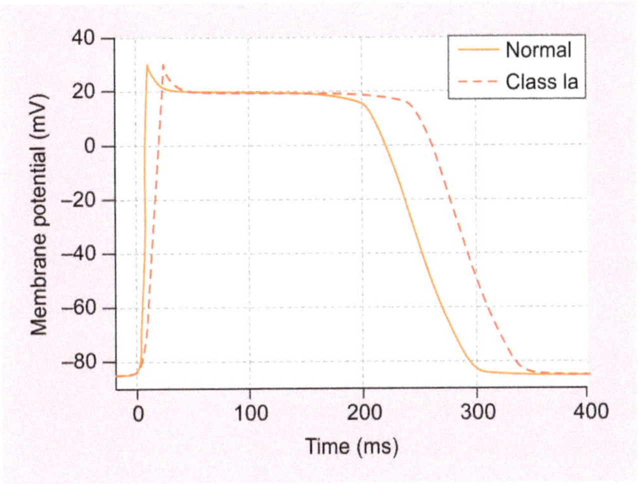

IB: Phenytoin and lignocaine

- Class IB drugs bind to open sodium channel, and will associate and dissociate from a sodium channel in the course of a normal beat.

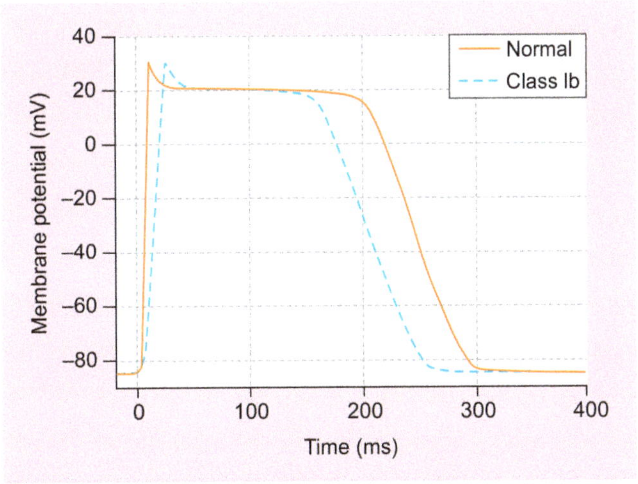

IC: Flecainide

- Associate and dissociate slowly creating a steady-state level of block.
- This causes indiscriminate blockade and general reduction in excitability.
- Suppress unidirectional or intermittent conduction pathways.
- As they markedly slow conduction velocity they increase QRS duration.

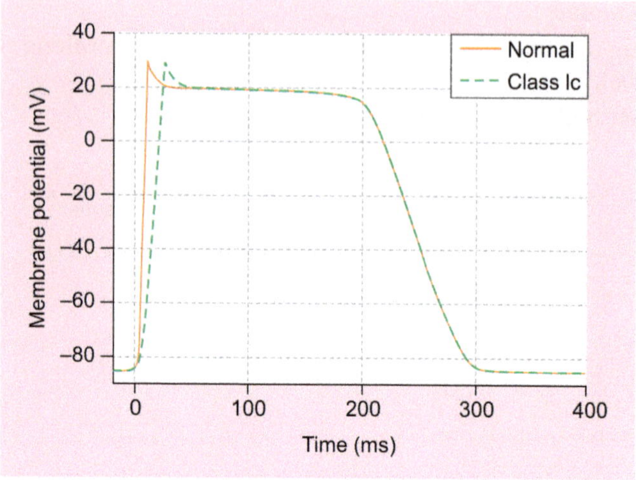

Class II

- Increased pacemaker potential current.
- Increased slow-inward Ca^{2+} current.
- Increased repolarizing K^+ and Cl^- currents.
- Increased Ca^{2+} stored in the sarcoplasmic reticulum, which may be spontaneously released causing a delayed-after-depolarizations.
- Reduced serum [K^+]*.

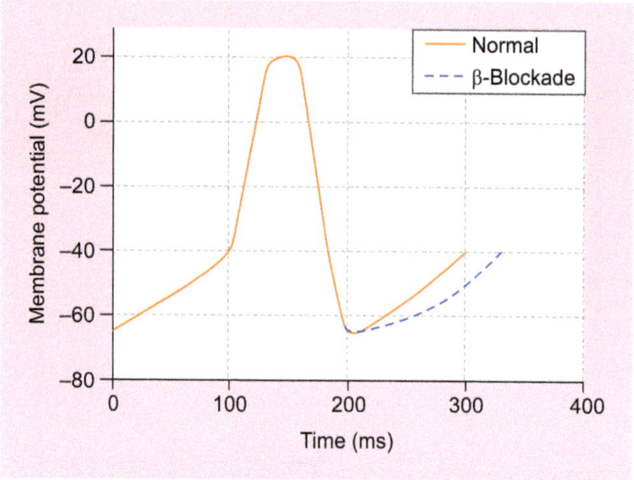

Class III

- Blocking of outward K^+ channels slows cardiac repolarization, which increases the cardiac refractory period. This has a number of beneficial effects:
  - Decreased automaticity
  - Decreased ectopy
  - Reduced defibrillation energy requirement

- Increased inotropy
- Due to the prolonged repolarization, they will also cause a *long QT*.

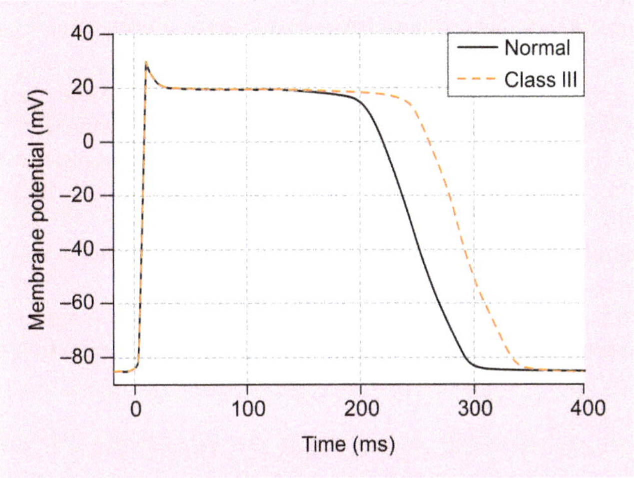

Class IV

- *Inhibit L-type Ca^{2+} channels*, inhibiting the slow-inward calcium current, which:
  - Slows sinoatrial (SA) and AV nodal conduction, AV blockade slows transmission of supraventricular arrhythmias.
  - Reduces inotropy
  - Prevents after-depolarizations. This suppresses ectopy by reducing calcium leak from sarcoplasmic reticulum.

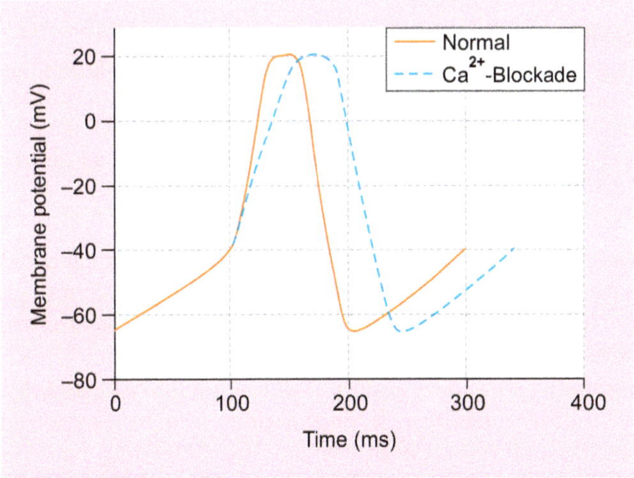

Ans. 255

- Image A shows the representation of a zero-order elimination where the elimination is not proportional to drug concentration. The rate of elimination is constant and is independent of the total drug concentration in the plasma.

- Image B shows elimination via first-order kinetics where elimination is proportional to dug concentration (higher the concentration, faster the elimination).
- *Examples of zero-order kinetics*: Phenytoin, ethanol, salicylates, theophylline, warfarin.
- Phenytoin demonstrates nonlinear (or zero order) pharmacokinetics even within the therapeutic range. The enzyme system involved in phenytoin metabolism enhances its own elimination through enzyme induction and rate of metabolism is close to the maximum capacity of the enzymes involved.
- It gradually becomes saturated, resulting in a decrease in the rate of elimination of phenytoin as the dose is increased.
- For drugs with saturable elimination, an increase in dosage can lead to a disproportionate increase in plasma drug concentration when the rate of elimination tends to reach its maximum capacity.

Further Reading

Borowy CS, Ashurst JV. Physiology, Zero and First Order Kinetics. Treasure Island (FL): StatPearls Publishing; 2020.

Ans. 256

This patient is expected to have a thrombocytopenia related to the extracorporeal circuit, volume replacement, etc., and cannot be considered as heparin-induced thrombocytopenia and thrombosis (HITT).

- The 4T score will reveal that the timing of thrombocytopenia is less than 4 days, without a history of exposure to heparin, there is no sequalae of new onset thrombosis and other causes for thrombocytopenia can exist.
- Based on the 4T score, a value of 1.45 on ELISA in low probability patients successfully rules out HIT.

Further Reading

Raschke RA, Curry SC, Warkentin TE, Gerkin RD. Improving clinical interpretation of the antiplatelet factor 4/heparin enzyme-linked immunosorbent assay for the diagnosis of heparin-induced thrombocytopenia through the use of receiver operating characteristic analysis, stratum-specific likelihood ratios, and Bayes theorem. Chest. 2013;144(4):1269-75.

Ans. 257

- This patient is at risk for refeeding syndrome—a clinical condition that occurs due to a change in endocrine homeostasis—shift from glucagon to insulin—which is associated with transcellular shift of electrolytes, sodium, and water retention.
- This possibility should be kept in mind in a high-risk patient presenting with triad of hypokalemia, hypophosphatemia, and hypomagnesemia after starting enteral or parenteral feeding. Refeeding syndrome can be prevented by prophylactic supplementation of electrolytes and by initiating a guarded calorie supplementation till phosphorous replacement is not required for three consecutive days.
- These patients require aggressive correction of dyselectrolytemia including intravenous correction, supplementation of thiamine, and reduce the calorie intake.

- Phosphorous should be given slowly as rapid administration can precipitate hypocalcemia.
- For severe hypophosphatemia (<1.25 mg/dL), a dose of 0.25–0.50 mmol/kg up to a maximum of 80 mmol should be administered over 8-12 hours.
- For milder hypophosphatemia (S PO_4 >1.25 mg/dL), a dose of 0.08–0.24 mmol/kg up to a maximum of 30 mmol is given over 6–8 hours.

Further Reading

Friedli N, Stanga Z, Culkin A, Crook M, Laviano A, Sobotka L, et al. Management and prevention of refeeding syndrome in medical inpatients: An evidence-based and consensus-supported algorithm. Nutrition. 2018;47:13-20.

Ans. 258

- In patients with acute hypocalcemia, symptoms may appear despite a calcium levels being only marginally low and is common after head and neck surgeries.
- Symptoms include mild paresthesia, laryngospasm, carpopedal spasm, tetany, and seizures.
- Common clinical signs will be positive Chvostek or Trousseau signs, bradycardia, QT-interval prolongation on echocardiogram (ECG).
- *Management*: Rule out other causes of stridor—including compression by a developing hematoma.
- In symptomatic acute hypocalcemia, 1 or 2 g of calcium gluconate can be administered slowly in 50 mL of 5% dextrose over 10-20 minutes. This is followed by an infusion of calcium gluconate. Oral supplementation of calcitriol and calcium 3-4 g/day needs to be started simultaneously.

Ans. 259

- Drug A represents a group of time-dependent antibiotics where the efficacy depends upon the percentage of time that the antibiotic concentration remains above minimum inhibitory concentration (MIC).
- Ideally the concentration should be maintained 2–4 fold above the MIC of the pathogen throughout the dosing interval. This can be attained by increasing the dose of antibiotic administered or the frequency of administration or by using continuous extended infusions.
- For example, beta-lactam.
- Drug B represents a group of concentration-dependent antibiotics where the efficacy depends upon the peak serum concentration (C_{max}).
- The peak drug concentration depends on the administered dose and is inversely related to volume of drug distribution. In critically ill patients with high volume of distribution, this can be attained by administering higher dose.
- For example, aminoglycosides and fluoroquinolones.
- Drug C—group of drugs with mixed properties—that are both time and concentration dependent and the efficacy depends upon the ratio of 24-hour area under the curve (AUC24h)/MIC.
- For example, vancomycin, azithromycin, linezolid, tigecycline.
- The efficacy of these drugs can be optimized by increasing the dosing of antibiotics.

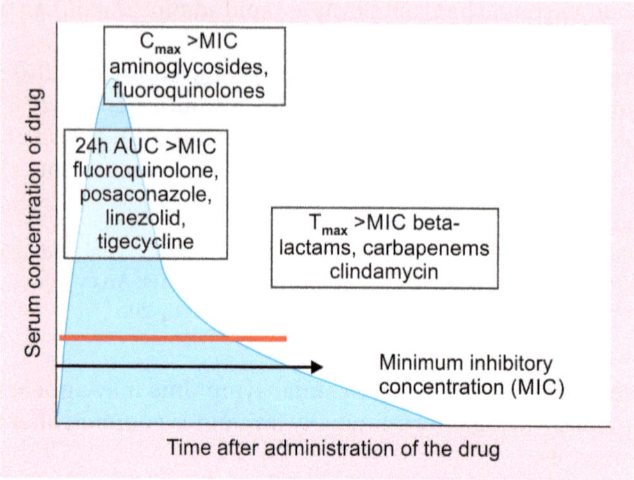

Further Reading

Al-Dorzi HM, Al Harbi SA, Arabi YM. Antibiotic therapy of pneumonia in the obese patient: Dosing and delivery. Curr Opin Infect Dis. 2014;27(2):165-73.

Ans. 260

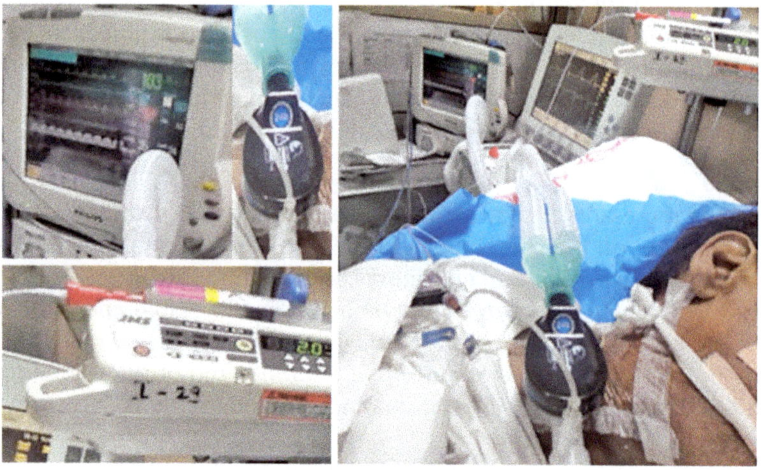

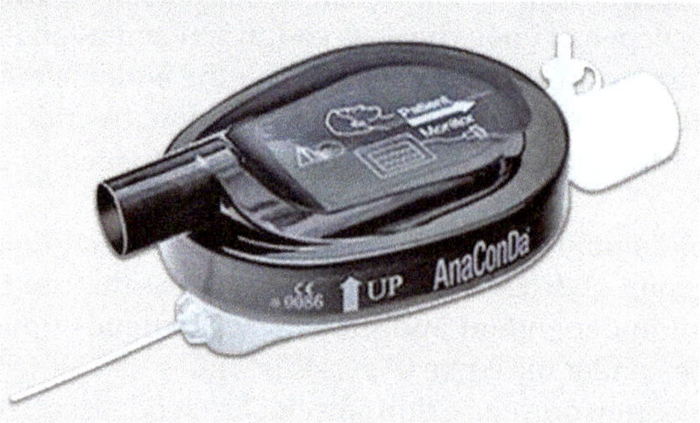

Source: Sedana Medical. [online] Available from http://www.sedanamedical.com [Last Accessed March, 2020].

The commonly used devices for inhalational sedation in ICU include AnaConDa™ and Mirus™.

This image shown is of AnaConDa (anesthesia conservation device). The activated carbon reflector adsorbs gases during expiration and delivers these gases back to the patient during next inspiration.

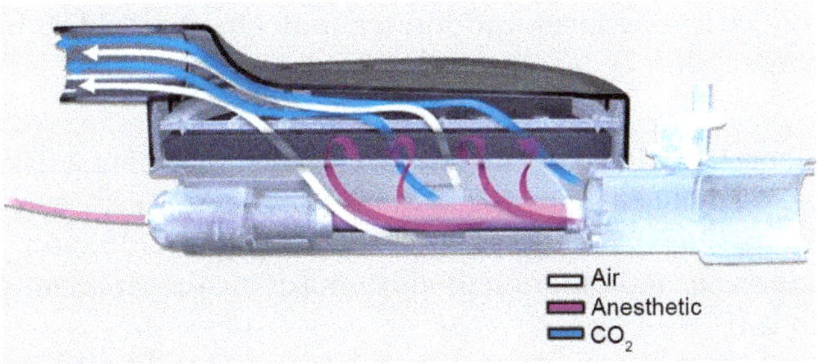

Source: Sedana Medical. [online] Available from http://www.sedanamedical.com [Last Accessed March, 2020].

Ans. 261

- Vorapaxar is a reversible antagonist of the protease-activated receptor-1 (PAR-1) on platelets. It blocks PAR-1, the primary receptor for thrombin.
- *Other drugs of the same class*:
- *Indications*: For prevention of myocardial infarction (MI), ischemic stroke recurrence, and peripheral arterial disease with aspirin and statins.

Further Reading

Morrow DA, Braunwald E, Bonaca MP, Ameriso SF, Dalby AJ, Fish MP, et al. Vorapaxar in the secondary prevention of atherothrombotic events. N Engl J Med. 2012;366(15):1404-13.

Ans. 262

- NPi-200 Pupillometer and NeuroLight Portable Pupillometer.
- Pupillary size, reactivity both can be trended over time.

Further Reading

NeurOptics. [online] Available from: https://neuroptics.com/npi-200-pupillometer/ [Last Accessed March, 2020].

Ans. 263

- Diarrhea can be classified as osmotic, secretory, exudative, and motor diarrhea.
- *Motor diarrhea*: When increased bowel motility decreases transit time for intestinal contents and intestinal absorption, large volume of stool is presented to colon. If the normal colonic absorptive capacity of 4 L (approximately) is exceeded, he can experience diarrhea.
- *Causes*: Postgastrectomy patients, postnarcotic withdrawal or use of prokinetic drugs such as metaclopramide or erythromycin.

Further Reading

Gaikwad S, Kothekar AT, Patil VP. Diarrhea in ICU. In: Freebairn RC, Kulkarni AP (Eds). Evidence Based Core Topics in Critical Care 2019, 1st edition. New Delhi: Jaypee Brothers Medical Publishers (P) Ltd; 2019.

Ans. 264

The contrast enhanced CT scan shows a hypodense filling defects in the proximal part of common hepatic artery suggestive of celiac artery thrombosis causing severe distress. Management will include a surgical opinion and interventional radiology opinion for thrombectomy. The hospital mortality for celiac artery thrombosis is around 59–93% and successful management depends on early diagnoses and interventions to re-establish blood flow management.

Ans. 265

- All patients in ICU need to be assessed for their nutritional risk. This can be done by dedicated scoring systems such as NUTRIC score and NRS (Nutritional Risk Screening) 2002 score as serum albumin, mid-arm circumference, and other methods of nutritional assessment cannot be done in ICU.
- NUTRIC score is a commonly used scoring system and incorporates points for age, APACHE score, SOFA score, number of comorbidities, duration of hospital stay, and (interleukin 6) IL-6 levels. Score of more than 6 (more than 5 if IL-6 is not measured)—at high nutritional risk. Our patient has a NUTRIC score of 1 (low risk).
- Role of immunonutrition in postoperative patients:
  - Parenteral glutamine supplementation (0.5 g/kg/d) may be considered in patients who cannot be fed adequately enterally and, therefore, require exclusive parenteral nutrition and there is no indication for oral glutamine in enterally fed patients.
  - Glutamine may reduce postoperative complication and length of stay—although the evidence is controversial.
  - Arginine—no role for supplementation.
  - Omega 3 fatty acids—only in patients who cannot be fed via enteral route adequately.

Further Reading

Heyland DK, Dhaliwal R, Jiang X, Day AG. Identifying critically ill patients who benefit the most from nutrition therapy: the development and initial validation of a novel risk assessment tool. Crit Care. 2011;15(6):R268.

Weimann A, Braga M, Carli F, Higashiguchi T, Hubner M, Klek S, et al. ESPEN guideline: Clinical nutrition in surgery. Clin Nutr. 2017;36(3):623-50.

Ans. 266

- Standardized Mortality Ratio is the ratio of the observed mortality over a period of time to the mortality predicted by scoring systems.
- Standardized Mortality Ratio is used to compare the performance among various hospitals and ICUs.
- Standardized Mortality Ratio of 1 means the mortality is as expected, <1 means a better survival, and a SMR of >1 is worse than expected.
- Causes of a high SMR:
  - False entry of data or missing data
  - Poor treatment received prior to ICU admission
  - Difference in case mix (medical vs. surgical)
  - Catering patients with higher morbidity, e.g., oncology units

- Lack of adherence to protocols
- Unforced errors due to unfamiliar staff.

Ans. 267

- *Number of VAP cases in February*: 12.
- *The total number of days that patients were on ventilators*: 36 patients × 5 days = 180 ventilator days.
- *Intensive care unit VAP rate*: The VAP rate per 1,000 ventilator days = 12/180 × 1,000 = 66.66.

Ans. 268

- The Society of Critical Care Medicine practice parameters define fever in the ICU as a temperature >38.3°C (>101 °F).
  Causes: Alcohol/drug withdrawal, postoperative fever, post-transfusion fever, drug fever, cerebral infarction/hemorrhage, adrenal insufficiency, pancreatitis, ischemic bowel, aspiration pneumonitis, subarachnoid hemorrhage, fat emboli, transplant rejection, deep venous thrombosis, pulmonary emboli, hematoma cirrhosis (without primary peritonitis), gastrointestinal (GI) bleed, phlebitis/thrombophlebitis, neoplastic fevers, decubitus ulcer.

Further Reading

Marik PE. Fever in the ICU. Chest. 2000;117(3):855-69.

O'Grady NP, Barie PS, Bartlett J, Bleck T, Garvey G, Jacobi J, et al. Practice parameters for evaluating new fever in critically ill adult patients. Crit Care Med. 1998;26(2):392-408.

Ans. 269

- This is a case of eclampsia and lab shows evidence of hemolysis, low platelet, and elevated liver enzymes.
- Differential diagnosis:
  - Incidental to the pregnant state—brain tumor, ruptured aneurysm.
  - Exacerbated by the pregnant state—thrombotic thrombocytopenic purpura (TTP), hemolytic uremic syndrome (HUS), cerebral venous thrombosis.
  - Unique to the pregnant state—eclampsia.
- Management includes:
  - Prevention of maternal hypoxia and trauma—airway, breathing, and circulation.
  - Treatment of hypertension—with intravenous (IV) labetalol or hydralazine.
  - Prevention of recurrent seizures—early administration of magnesium sulfate and monitoring.
  - Evaluation for prompt delivery as soon as feasible after discussion with gynecologist, neonatologist, and intensivist.

Ans. 270

- The peripheral smear and laboratory parameters are suggestive of hemolysis due to agglutination.

- Cold agglutination of red blood cells (RBC) is seen in cases of *M. pneumonia*, in about 60% of cases and is typically mild or subclinical and rarely requires any treatment.

Ans. 271

Of the total assessed patients, only approximately 13% were enrolled, with the remaining being excluded, and thereby introducing the possibility of selection bias in the trial results. Similarly the same results may not be applicable to the general ICU population, if such high exclusion rates are to be considered.

Ans. 272

Discrimination is the ability of the test to correctly identify the true positives and false negatives. The area under the receiver operating characteristics (ROC) curve is the percentage that a randomly drawn pair of subjects is correctly classified.

Youden index is the maximum vertical distance between the ROC curve and the chance line.

Ans. 273

- Magnetic resonance imaging shows the ventricular drain with gross hydrocephalus and periventricular ooze.
- Need to check the drain for block and proper positioning.

Ans. 274

- Figure A shows almost absent flow in pulmonary circulation while Figure B shows opened up lower lobe arteries while flow to upper lobe is still scanty.
- *Procedure done*: Catheter-directed thrombolysis for pulmonary embolism.
- A bolus of alteplase (4–6 mg) is followed by an infusion of 0.5 mg and 2 mg/h with total dose not exceeding 24 mg.
- Anticoagulation with heparin is continued at a dose of 400–600 U/ to maintain an activated partial thromboplastin time between <60 seconds.

Further Reading

Xue X, Sista AK. Catheter-directed thrombolysis for pulmonary embolism: The state of practice. Tech Vasc Interv Radiol. 2018;21(2):78-84.

Ans. 275

- The Pitt bacteremia score is used as a stratification tool in bloodstream infections due to gram-positive bacteria, gram-negative bacteria, and *Candida* species.
- A score < 4 is suggestive of a noncritically ill patient, whereas a score ≥ 4 is seen in critically ill patients and is associated with a higher mortality risk.
- It has higher discrimination than APACHE II (acute physiology and chronic health evaluation II) and the CURB-65 (confusion, uremia, respiratory rate, BP, age ≥65 years) score in ICUs.

Further Reading

Al-Hasan MN, Baddour LM. Resilience of the Pitt bacteremia score: Three decades and counting. Clin Infect Dis. 2019.

Ans. 276

- The trends show a static minute ventilation and respiratory rate.
- The compliance has progressively declined and there is a progressive increase in peak pressures.

- Differentials.
- Worsening resistance/worsening compliance.
- With background history of multiple fluid boluses in a severely ill patient, worsening pulmonary compliance should be suspected and evaluated for

Ans. 277

- Charles et al. in 2008 developed a scoring system to aid treatment decisions regarding level of care (ICU admission vs. ward admission) for patients admitted with complaints of community-acquired pneumonia. The scoring system was derived prospectively from 865 patients and later validated with various data sets.
- It consisted of 8 variables—systolic blood pressure, multilobar involvement on chest X-ray, albumin < 3.5 g/dL, RR > 25 breaths/min if aged < 50 years or > 30 breaths/min if aged > 50 years, heart rate > 125 beats/min, presence of confused mental state, P/F ratio < 333 if aged < 50 years and < 250 if aged > 50 years, and pH < 7.35.
- A score > 3 predicted a moderately high risk of needing intensive respiratory or vasopressor support.

Further Reading

Charles PG, Wolfe R, Whitby M, Fine MJ, Fuller AJ, Stirling R, et al. SMART-COP: a tool for predicting the need for intensive respiratory or vasopressor support in community-acquired pneumonia. Clin Infect Dis. 2008;47(3):375-84.

Ans. 278

- 20% w/v
- % w/v = 20 g of solute/100 mL of solution = 0.2 g/mL

Dose of intravenous NAC for paracetamol poisoning = loading of 150 mg/kg over 15 minutes, followed by 50 mg/kg over 4 hours, and then 100 mg/kg over 16 hours.

150 × 50 = 7.5 g over 15 minutes followed by 2.5 g over 4 hours and 5 g over 16 hours.

Calculation based on number of ampoules is not recommended as ampoules may vary in volume of drug contained. However, for administration, if only 5 mL vials are available, we will need 15 vials over 16 hours period.

Ans. 279

- Computed tomography shows a Foley bulb inadvertently inflated in the prostatic urethra with a full bladder.
- The Foley needs to be repositioned after deflating the bulb.
- Urinary catheter care needs to be emphasized in the unit.

Ans. 280

- This is the patient with pelvic bone fracture.
- The pelvis and femur fractures can be a major source of bleeding and even fatal hemorrhage related to direct blood loss from broken bones, ruptured major vessels, or vascular plexuses involved in pelvic trauma.
- Pelvic fracture diagnosis is based on clinical suspicion. Limb-shortening, together with abnormal movements of the pelvic bones on examination and, in many cases, visible subcutaneous hematoma suggests the clinical diagnosis. The definitive diagnosis is obtained by contrast CT scan.

- As resuscitation part control of bleeding is very important, need to activate massive transfusion protocol. Start 1:1:1 resuscitation with platelets, blood and fresh frozen plasma, prevent and treat hypothermia, acidosis, and coagulopathy.
- Early stabilization of the fracture is essential and can have an option of interventional radiology to embolize the bleeding vessel.

Ans. 281

- Patients with tibia and fibula fracture can have blood loss up to 500–1000 mL, which may collect in the calf region.
- Compartment syndrome is a painful condition that occurs when pressure within the muscles builds to dangerous levels. This pressure can decrease blood flow, which prevents nourishment and oxygen from reaching nerve and muscle cells.
- Down the line patient develops compartment syndrome, which manifests as severe pain out of proportion to clinical examination. Other manifestations include paresthesia, pulselessness, and paralysis.
- The pain is more intense than what would be expected from the injury itself. Using or stretching the involved muscles increases the pain. There may also be tingling or burning sensations (paresthesias) in the skin. The muscle may feel tight or full. Numbness or paralysis is the late sign of compartment syndrome. It usually indicates permanent tissue injury.
- The characteristic triad of complaints in rhabdomyolysis is muscle pain, weakness, and dark urine. However, more than half of patients may not report muscular symptoms; by contrast, occasional others may experience very severe pain. Patients will eventually develop acute renal failure.

Following is the way we can investigate and confirm the diagnosis:

- *Physical findings*: Muscle tenderness and swelling may be seen, but detectable muscle swelling in the extremities generally develops, when it occurs, with fluid repletion. Such swelling is much less common on hospital admission. Skin changes of ischemic tissue injury, such as discoloration or blisters, may also be seen but are present in less than 10% of patients.
- *Laboratory findings*: The hallmark of rhabdomyolysis is an elevation in creatinine kinase (CK) and other serum muscle enzymes. The other characteristic finding is the reddish-brown urine of myoglobinuria, but because this may be observed in only half of cases, its absence does not exclude the diagnosis. Routine laboratory tests, including complete blood count (CBC), erythrocyte sedimentation rate (ESR), and C-reactive protein (CRP), vary greatly depending on the underlying cause of rhabdomyolysis.
- *Creatine kinase*: Serum CK levels at presentation are usually at least five times the upper limit of normal, but range from approximately 1,500 to over 100,000 IU/L. The mean peak CK reported for each of a variety of different causes and for patients with both single and multiple causes ranged from approximately 10,000 to 25,000 in the largest series.
- The serum CK begins to rise within 2–12 hours following the onset of muscle injury and reaches its maximum within 24–72 hours. A decline is usually seen within 3–5 days of cessation of muscle injury. CK has a serum

half-life of about 1.5 days and declines at a relatively constant rate of about 40–50% of the previous day's value. In patients whose CK does not decline as expected, continued muscle injury or the development of a compartment syndrome may be present.

- *Urine findings and myoglobinuria*: Myoglobin, a heme-containing respiratory protein, is released from damaged muscle in parallel with CK. Myoglobin is a monomer that is not significantly protein-bound and is therefore rapidly excreted in the urine, often resulting in the production of red to brown urine. It appears in the urine when the plasma concentration exceeds 1.5 mg/dL. Myoglobin has a half-life of only 2–3 hours, much shorter than that of CK. Because of its rapid excretion and metabolism to bilirubin, serum levels may return to normal within 6–8 hours. Thus, it is not unusual for CK levels to remain elevated in the absence of myoglobinuria. Proteinuria may also be seen, due to the release of myoglobin and other proteins by the damaged myocytes.
- When rhabdomyolysis is suspected, regardless of the underlying etiology, one of the most important treatment goals is to avoid acute kidney injury. Because of the possible accumulation of fluids in muscular compartments and the associated hypovolemia, fluid management is imperative to prevent prerenal azotemia. Azotemia is prevented primarily by aggressive hydration at a rate of 1.5 L/h. Another option is 500 mL/h saline solution alternated every hour with 500 mL/h of 5% glucose solution with 50 mmol of sodium bicarbonate for each subsequent 2–3 L of solution. A urinary output goal of 200 mL/h, urine pH >6.5, and plasma pH <7.5 should be achieved.
- Notably, urinary alkalization with sodium bicarbonate or sodium acetate is unproven, as is the use of mannitol to promote diuresis. Drugs such as statins that are known to be a risk factor for rhabdomyolysis should also be immediately stopped. Fasciotomy may be required in compartment syndrome to limit damage to muscles and kidneys.

Further Reading

Torres PA, Helmstetter JA, Kaye AM, Kaye AD. Rhabdomyolysis: pathogenesis, diagnosis, and treatment. Ochsner J. 2015;15(1):58-69.

Ans. 282

- In the postoperative period if patient develops a triad of respiratory insufficiency, altered sensorium, and petechiae, fat embolism syndrome should be suspected. In the acute setting respiratory distress is the most clinically significant feature of fat embolism syndrome (FES). Respiratory distress from FES is indistinguishable from acute respiratory distress syndrome (ARDS) seen in polytrauma patients.
- Laboratory and imaging tests can help in the diagnosis, but are nonspecific.
- Diagnostic criteria for FES:
  - Gurd and Wilson criteria—one major + four minor.
  - One major manifestation, e.g., tachypnea, altered mentation and petachiae + four of the five minor criteria—fever, tachycardia, fall in hematocrit or thrombocytopenia, increasing ESR, retinal changes, and presence of fat globules in sputum or urine.

- Murray and Racz criteria—tachycardia, tachypnea, pyrexia, and cerebral involvement with hypoxia.
- Lindegue criteria—a sustained hypoxia of <60 mm Hg, sustained hypercarbia of >55 mm Hg, pH < 7.3, respiratory rate > 35 breaths/min despite adequate sedation and an increased work of breathing manifested as accessory muscles use, tachycardia, anxiety.
- Schonfeld score more than 5 (presence of petachiae score 5, diffuse infiltrates score 4, hypoxemia < 70 mm Hg score 3, confusion, fever, heart rate > 120 beats/min or respiratory rate > 30 breaths/min score 1 each).

Further Reading

George J, George R, Dixit R, Gupta RC, Gupta N. Fat embolism syndrome. Lung India. 2013;30(1):47-53.

Ans. 283

- Pancreatic pseudocyst.
- Pancreatitis is classified into interstitial edematous pancreatitis and necrotizing pancreatitis.
- Accordingly pancreatic fluid collections within 4 weeks are called acute peripancreatic fluid collection or acute necrotic collection depending on the initial radiological classification and collections after 4 weeks are called pseudocyst or walled-off necrosis respectively.

Modified CT severity scoring of pancreatitis

- *Presence of pancreatic inflammation is scored from 0 to 4*: 0 for a normal pancreas, 2 if there are abnormalities in pancreas with or without peripancreatic inflammation and a score of 4 if there is a pancreatic or peripancreatic fluid collection or peripancreatic fat necrosis.
- *Pancreatic necrosis is scored 0 to 4 depending upon the presence of necrosis*: 0 if there is no necrosis, 2 if the pancreatic necrosis is 30% or less, and 4 if there is >30% necrosis.
- *Extrapancreatic complications* if present (pleural effusion, ascites, vascular complication, etc.) are given a score of 2.
- *Total score*:
  - Out of 10, pancreatitis is classified as mild, moderate, and severe
  - 0–2: Mild
  - 4–6: Moderate
  - 8–10: Severe

Further Reading

Foster BR, Jensen KK, Bakis G, Shaaban AM, Coakley FV. Revised Atlanta Classification for Acute Pancreatitis: A Pictorial Essay. Radiographics. 2016;36(3):675-87.

Ans. 284

- *Diagnosis*: Emphysematous pyelonephritis.
- *Risk factors*: Diabetes, immunocompromised patients.
- *Computed tomography classification*:
  - 1: Presence of gas in the renal collecting system only.
  - 2: Presence of intrarenal gas without extension to the extrarenal space.
  - 3A: Extension of gas or abscess to the perinephric space.

- 3B: Extension of gas or abscess beyond the perinephric space, i.e., extension into adjacent tissues such as the psoas muscle.
- 4: Bilateral emphysematous pyelonephritis or emphysematous pyelonephritis in a solitary functioning kidney.

- *Management*: Urgent resuscitation with antibiotics, fluid resuscitation, percutaneous drainage of abscess, or rarely nephrectomy.

Ans. 285

- This thromboelastograph is characteristically depicting hyperfibrinolysis.
- The reaction time (R time) is normal.
- The LY30 value (lysis at 30 minutes) is prolonged to 94.5% (normal value <8%) suggestive of hyperfibrinolysis.
- Hyperfibrinolysis needs to be differentiated from clot retraction due to high platelet count by the detection of a smooth decrease of the amplitude after maximum strength (MA) in contrast to the sudden drop in amplitude in clot retraction.

Further Reading

Verma A, Hemlata. Thromboelastography as a novel viscoelastic method for hemostasis monitoring: Its methodology, applications, and constraints. Glob J Transfus Med. 2017;2(1):8-18.

Ans. 286

- Primary and secondary fibrinolysis can be differentiated from the coagulation index.
- In primary fibrinolysis, the coagulation index (CI) will be usually less than -3 while in secondary fibrinolysis where CI will be more than +3, both having increased LY30 >8%.

Further Reading

Verma A, Hemlata. Thromboelastography as a novel viscoelastic method for hemostasis monitoring: Its methodology, applications, and constraints. Glob J Transfus Med. 2017;2(1):8-18.

Ans. 287

- Prone ventilation is no longer considered a salvage therapy for refractory hypoxemia, but is used as a lung protective and recruitment strategy in moderate to severe ARDS.
- It should be started early in the course of ARDS with arterial partial pressure/fraction of inspired oxygen (PaO_2/FiO_2) ratio of <150.
- Good outcomes have been seen when used in conjunction with low tidal volumes and use of neuromuscular blockade and for prolonged durations.

Contraindications to prone ventilation:

- Facial or pelvic fractures
- Severe hemodynamic instability
- Burns or open wounds on ventral body surface
- Raised intracranial pressure.

Complications
Facial edema
Accidental extubation, removal of lines or catheters
Pressure sores
Increased need for sedation
Increased gastric residual volumes
Increased intra-abdominal pressures
Airway obstruction
Hypotension or arrhythmias

Further Reading

Scholten EL, Beitler JR, Prisk GK, Malhotra A. Treatment of ARDS with prone positioning. Chest. 2017;151(1):215-24.

Ans. 288

- In prone position, pleural pressure gradient decreases from nondependent to dependent regions, due to gravitational effects and conformational shape matching of the lung to the chest cavity.
- Improved transpulmonary pressure in the dorsal lung segments due to displacement of weight of heart/ventral lungs/abdominal viscera allows for more homogeneous lung aeration and strain distribution.
- Pulmonary blood flow is normally directed dorsally in normal and injured lungs. Due to improved ventilation in these segments in prone position, there is a reduction in the shunt and increased oxygenation.

Further Reading

Gattinoni L, Taccone P, Carlesso E, Marini JJ. Prone position in acute respiratory distress syndrome: rationale, indications, and limits. Am J Respir Crit Care Med. 2013;188(11):1286-93.

Ans. 289

- The PROSEVA trial conducted in 26 centers of France and one center in Spain, recruited almost 474 out of the 51,189 patients screened, over a period from 2008 to 2011.
- The patients were screened within 36 hours of initiation of mechanical ventilation and recruited if they had a PaO_2/FiO_2 ratio of <150 on a positive end-expiratory pressure (PEEP) of at least 5 cmH_2O and FiO_2 at least of 0.6 even after 12 hours of lung protective ventilation. Prone ventilation was offered for 16–21 hours per day.
- The stoppage rules followed in the PROSEVA trial are commonly accepted and include:
  - Maintained oxygenation, a maintained PaO_2/FiO_2 ratio of ≥150 mm Hg, with a PEEP of ≤10 cm of water and a FiO_2 of ≤0.6 for at least 4 hours.
  - A worsening in the PaO_2/FiO_2 ratio of more than 20% after proning.

- Development of complications such as accidental extubation, tube dislodgement, tube obstruction, hemoptysis, oxygen saturation (SaO_2) <85% or a PaO_2 < 55 mm Hg for more than 5 minutes with FiO_2 of 1, sudden cardiac arrest, or a periarrest situation, persistent severe hypotension, any life-threatening reason for which the clinician decided to stop the treatment.

Ans. 290

- The variable causing a breath to begin is the *trigger variable, usually patient triggered or time triggered.*
- A variable whose magnitude is constrained to some maximum value during inspiration is called a *limit variable.*
- The variable causing a breath to end is the *cycle variable.*
- During expiration, the ventilator usually maintains some level of pressure at or above atmospheric pressure (PEEP), which is referred to as the *baseline variable.*
- In the given image, the pressure time scalar is showing an ascent, peak and plateau during inspiration, followed by expiration. The flow time scalar is in square-wave pattern suggesting constant flow during inspiration—both characteristics of volume-controlled ventilation, with an end-inspiratory pause.
- In volume-controlled ventilation with inspiratory pause:
  - Trigger—time
  - Limit—volume
  - Cycling—time
  - (Here cycling takes place after the end-inspiratory pause. If the pause was not set, it would have been flow cycled)
  - Baseline—PEEP.

Ans. 291

- $P_{0.1}$ is the airway occlusion pressure in the first 100 ms of an inspiration.
- It indicates the drop in airway pressure during the first 100 ms of an occluded breath and is a measure of respiratory drive.
- Higher values are indicative of increased respiratory drive, which can lead to more stress and strain to the lung resulting in ventilator associated lung injury and diaphragm injury. $P_{0.1}$ > 3.5 cmH_2O—sensitivity of 92% and a specificity of 89% to identify excessive inspiratory effort.
- Also used to identify weaning failures, where a $P_{0.1}$/PI max >0.3 is considered as one of the indices to assess weaning failure, detection of autotriggering-> a, if the $P_{0.1}$ of zero with the measured respiratory rate is more than set.

Further Reading

Telias I, Damiani F, Brochard L. The airway occlusion pressure ($P_{0.1}$) to monitor respiratory drive during mechanical ventilation: increasing awareness of a not-so-new problem. Intensive Care Med. 2018;44(9):1532-5.

Ans. 292

Feature of HFNC	*Physiological effect*
High-flow rates	Carbon dioxide washout Reduction in anatomical dead space Provides an oxygen reservoir Reliable delivery of FiO_2 as it meets or exceeds patients' peak inspiratory flow rate Improved breathing pattern
Peak end-expiratory pressure (~5–7 cmH_2O)	Alveolar recruitment Enhanced oxygenation Decreased work of breathing
Warmed humidified gas	Reduced airway surface dehydration Improved secretion clearance Decreased atelectasis Decreased work of breathing

Ans. 293

- Time constant indicates rate of change in the volume of a lung unit that is passively inflated or deflated.
- Given by formula $V_t = V_i \times e^{-t/\zeta}$
- (V_i = starting volume of a lung unit, V_t = volume of lung unit at a given time, t = time in seconds, ζ = time constant)
- Time constant is given by the product of compliance and resistance.
- Lung units with a higher resistance or compliance empty slower, while lung units with lower resistance and compliance empty faster.
  1 time constant = 63% lung volume change, 3 time constants = 86%, 5 time constants = 99.3% change in lung volumes
- Complete emptying of alveoli occurs within 5 time constants.

Further Reading

Hess DR. Respiratory mechanics in mechanically ventilated patients. Respir Care. 2014;59(11):1773.

Ans. 294

- Static compliance = Tidal volume (V_t)/Plateau pressure (Pplat) - PEEP
- In this case 350/35 - 12 = 15.2 mL/cmH_2O
- Dynamic compliance = V_t/PIP (peak inspiratory pressure) - PEEP
- In this case 350/48 - 12 = 9.72 mL/cmH_2O
- In volume-controlled ventilation (VCV), the mechanical power can be simplistically calculated by the equation:
  Respiratory rate (RR) × Tidal volume (l) × [Peak - (Plateau - PEEP)/2] × 0.098 = 22 × 0.35 × [48 - (35 - 12)/2] × 0.098 = 27.54 J/min
- Mechanical power is defined as the amount of energy transferred per unit of time (J/min) from the mechanical ventilator to patients' lungs.
- It is a summary variable, which includes all the likely causes of ventilator-induced lung injury (VILI): tidal volume, driving pressure (i.e., the product of elastance and tidal volume), flow, respiratory rate, and PEEP.

			Mechanical power (J/MIN)					
			Power of inspiration (cmH_2O L/min)					
			Work of inspiration (cmH_2O L)					
				Pressure (cmH_2O)				
			Volume (L) ×	Elastic static component +	Elastic dynamic component +	Resistive component	× Rate (bpm)	× Conversion factor
VCV	Extended equation	Gattinoni et al	ΔV	$PEEP$	$\Delta V \cdot \frac{1}{2} ELrs$	$RR \frac{(1 + I{:}E)}{(60 \cdot I{:}E)} \cdot R_{aw}$	RR	0,098
	Simplified equation	Gattinoni et al	ΔV	$Peak\ pressure - \frac{(Plateau\ pressure - PEEP)}{2}$			RR	0,098
	Surrogate	Giosa et al	ΔV	$\frac{Peak\ pressure + PEEP + F/6}{2}$			RR	0,1
PCV	Extended equation	Van der Meijden et al	ΔV	$PEEP$	$P_{insp} \left(1 - e^{\frac{-T_{insp}}{R.C}}\right)$		RR	0,098
		Becher et al	$(PEEP + P_{insp}) \cdot \Delta V - P_{insp}^2 \cdot C \cdot 0.5 - \left(\frac{R.C}{T_{slope}}\right) + \left(\frac{R.C}{T_{slope}}\right)^2 \left(1 - e^{\frac{T_{slope}}{R.C}}\right)$				RR	0,098
	Surrogate	Becher et al	ΔV	$PEEP$	P_{insp}		RR	0,098

(PCV: Pressure-controlled ventilation)

Source: Giosa L, Busana M, Pasticci I, Bonifazi M, Maria M, Romitti F, et al. Mechanical power at a glance: a simple surrogate for volume-controlled ventilation. Intensive Care Med Exp. 2019;7:61.

- Most of the intensive care unit (ICU) patients will have a power of the range 11.7–31.2 J/min.
- Guerin et al. basis, patients studied in PROSEVA and ACURACYS trials of ARDS, showed that mechanical power above 12 J/min was associated with reduced survival.

Further Reading

Serpa Neto A, Deliberato RO, Johnson AEW, Bos LD, Amorim P, Pereira SM, et al. Mechanical power of ventilation is associated with mortality in critically ill patients: an analysis of patients in two observational cohorts. Intensive Care Med. 2018;44(11):1914-22.

Silva PL, Ball L, Rocco PRM, Pelosi P. Power to mechanical power to minimize ventilator-induced lung injury? Intensive Care Med Exp. 2019;7(Suppl 1):38.

Ans. 295

- Leak in the circuit.
- Volume is represented on the X-axis and the degree of leak can be measured by visualizing this loop.

Further Reading

Godet T, Constantin JM, Jaber S, Futier E. How to monitor a recruitment maneuver at the bedside. Curr Opin Crit Care. 2015;21(3):253-8.

Ans. 296

- This scalar shows generation of auto PEEP or intrinsic PEEP.
- This is indicated by the flow-time scalar not reaching the baseline before start of next inspiration and can be measured by using the end-expiratory hold.
- Common causes include: (a) increased flow resistance with/without expiratory flow limitation; (b) short duration of expiration; (c) increased postinspiratory muscle activity.

Further Reading

Mughal MM, Culver DA, Minai OA, Arroliga AC. Auto-positive end-expiratory pressure: mechanisms and treatment. Cleve Clin J Med. 2005;72(9):801-9.

Ans. 297

- Stress index <1.
- The stress index studies the deformations of the pressure curve which reflects alteration in the elastic properties of the lung.
- This is studied in the volume-controlled modes with constant flow.
- If the pressure-time curve had a downward concavity, it indicates an increased compliance (stress index >1), and if there is an upward concavity, there is decreasing compliance (stress index <1).

Further Reading

Hess DR. Respiratory mechanics in mechanically ventilated patients. Respir Care. 2014;59(11):1773.

Ans. 298

- Driving pressure (delta pressure) = Plateau pressure – PEEP.
- Ratio of tidal volume to respiratory system compliance.
- It indicates the tidal volume corrected for the patient's respiratory system compliance and is supposed to represent decreased functional size of the lung (baby lung).
- In this example, the driving pressure is 35 – 12 = 13 cmH_2O.
- Higher driving pressures (>14 cmH_2O) have been associated with increased mortality as compared to V_t and PEEP as per studies by Amato et al., however randomized controlled trials (RCTs) need to be done.

Further Reading

Amato MB, Meade MO, Slutsky AS, Brochard L, Costa EL, Schoenfeld DA, et al. Driving pressure and survival in the acute respiratory distress syndrome. N Engl J Med. 2015;372(8):747-55.

Ans. 299

- Equation of motion for the respiratory system of a patient on spontaneous breathing is:
- Muscle pressure + Ventilator pressure = (Elastance × Volume) + (Resistance × Flow)
- In case of a patient on mechanical ventilation, assuming they are on controlled modes, the equation is replaced by:
  Ventilator pressure = (Elastance × Volume) + (Resistance × Flow)

Further Reading

Chatburn RL. How ventilators work. Fundamentals of Mechanical Ventilation, 1st edition. Cleveland Heights: Mandu Press Ltd; 2003. pp. 17-80.

Ans. 300

Uses of end-tidal carbon dioxide ($ETCO_2$) in ICU: To confirm proper placement, patency and detect dislodgement of endotracheal tubes, track changes in alveolar ventilation following adjustment of mechanical ventilation, detect dead space ventilation such as differentiation between pulmonary edema and obstructive airway disease, judge the adequacy of resuscitative efforts during cardiopulmonary resuscitation (CPR) and detect return of spontaneous circulation (ROSC), detection of energy expenditure, estimate the changes in cardiac output to predict fluid responsiveness.

Further Reading

Nassar BS, Schmidt GA. Capnography during critical illness. Chest. 2016;149(2):576-85.

Ans. 301

- Electrical impedance tomography (EIT) is a noninvasive imaging modality that reconstructs images based on the changes in intrathoracic electrical resistivity with respiration. It is measured by passing low voltage alternating electrical currents across the thorax. The EIT image shares similar spatial orientation to that used by CT.
- Electrical impedance tomography is used to assess and quantify the changes in lung resistivity with respiration at the end of each breath, thereby detecting lung recruitment and volume losses which helps in ARDS ventilation.
- The current image shows absent ventilation in two zones and hyperinflation in one zone suggesting collapse on the left side and hyperinflation of the remaining lung.

Ans. 302

- Recruitment is a physiological process that refers to an increase in functional residual capacity due to reaeration of a previously collapsed lung, now exposed to positive pressure ventilation.
- Recruitment maneuvers are transient voluntary increase in the transpulmonary pressure, which are used to reopen the recruitable lung units.
- Application of a continuous positive pressure of 35-50 cmH_2O for duration of 20-40 s (e.g., commonly used is 40 cmH_2O over 40 s). The pressure support is usually set to 0 cmH_2O to avoid barotrauma.
- *Sigh*: Transient increase in tidal volume or PEEP, to attain a specific plateau pressure.
- *Extended sigh*: A progressive increase in PEEP, and a decrease in tidal volume for a prolonged period of time.
- Pressure-controlled ventilation during up titration or down titration of PEEP, maintaining a driving pressure of 15 cmH_2O to guarantee a tidal volume.
- *High-frequency ventilation*: Maintains significantly higher mean airway pressures, which limits cyclic alveolar closure and increases the end-expiration lung volume.
- *Prone ventilation*: Prone positioning homogenizes the transpulmonary pressure gradient, with improved ventilation-perfusion ratio causing alveolar recruitment. Although the transpulmonary pressures are not increased, there is an increase in functional residual capacity.
- *Before recruitment*: Right ventricular dysfunction should be ruled out by an echocardiography, presence of collapsed lung should be identified by ultrasound or CT scans, hypovolemia should be ruled out by clinical and echocardiography assessment.

- *During recruitment*: Monitor for improvement in oxygenation, reduction in carbon dioxide, avoidance of hypotension, and reduced cardiac output.
- *Postrecruitment*: Monitor for sustained reduction in cardiac output, complications such as barotrauma, and assessment of dead space ventilation to rule out overdistension.

Further Reading

Godet T, Constantin JM, Jaber S, Futier E. How to monitor a recruitment maneuver at the bedside. Curr Opin Crit Care. 2015;21(3):253-8.

Guerin C, Debord S, Leray V, Delannoy B, Bayle F, Bourdin G, et al. Efficacy and safety of recruitment maneuvers in acute respiratory distress syndrome. Ann Intensive Care. 2011;1(1):9.

Guérin C, Moss M, Talmor D. A glossary of ARDS for beginners. Intensive Care Med. 2016;42(5):659-62.

Ans. 303

- Ineffective trigger
- It is detected by visual inspection of the expiratory waveform.
- One can see drop in pressure below baseline with a concurrent decrease in expiratory flow.
- It ideally needs esophageal pressure (Pes) waveform or electrical activity of the diaphragm (EaDi) to detect.
- It occurs due to over-assistance from ventilator, excessive sedation, and auto-positive end expiratory pressure (auto-PEEP).
- It is rectified by checking trigger sensitivity, correcting auto-PEEP, and checking for excessive ventilator assistance (high-pressure supports, set inspiratory time, or frequency).

Further Reading

Dres M, Rittayamai N, Brochard L. Monitoring patient–ventilator asynchrony. Curr Opin Crit Care. 2016;22(3):246-53.

Subirà C, de Haro C, Magrans R, Fernández R, Blanch L. Minimizing asynchronies in mechanical ventilation: Current and future trends. Respiratory Care. 2018;63(4):464.

Ans. 304

- Reverse triggering
- Here, patient effort occurs after the initiation of a ventilator breath.
- Passive insufflation of the lungs by a ventilator breath triggers diaphragmatic muscle contractions by activation of patient's respiratory center.
- It is seen in heavily sedated patients. It is also common in those awakening from deeply sedated states.
- It can be injurious as it causes double breaths and "breath stacking."
- It can be rectified by addition of neuromuscular blockers, if patient continues to have lung injury, or decreasing sedation and attempting for spontaneous ventilation.

Further Reading

Subirà C, de Haro C, Magrans R, Fernández R, Blanch L. Minimizing asynchronies in mechanical ventilation: Current and future trends. Respir Care. 2018;63(4):464-78.

Ans. 305

An adequate flow trigger is in the range of 1-2 L/min.

A value set too low (high sensitivity) may lead to autotriggering and a value set too high (low sensitivity) means an increased work of breathing for the patient to trigger the ventilator.

In this example, at a trigger sensitivity of 10 L/min, the ventilator may fail to detect patient's respiratory efforts and will not synchronize with patient's efforts.

Further Reading

Chatburn RL. Fundamentals of Mechanical Ventilation. Ohio: Mandu Press Ltd; 2003.

CASE SCENARIOS

Ans. 306

Presently patient is on lung protective ventilation with low tidal volumes and high PEEP and continues to be hypoxemic with PaO_2/FiO_2 ratio of <50 and respiratory acidosis.

The present worsening appears due to a secondary staphylococcal bacterial infection with severe ARDS.

This patient can be given a trial of prone ventilation as a rescue maneuver. However, in view of severe hypoxemia and respiratory acidosis, ECMO would be a suitable option.

- A recruitment maneuver aims to transiently increase the transpulmonary pressure in order to reopen closed alveolar units.
- There are several methods of recruitment maneuvers which include the "40-40" methods, staircase method, sighs, etc.
- The recent Alveolar Recruitment for ARDS (ART) trial showed that recruitment maneuvers with high PEEP can increase mortality particularly in patients with moderate ARDS.
- Recruitment can be used transiently as a rescue measure for hypoxemia in severe ARDS, but should not be routinely used in all patients with ARDS. In patients with nonrecruitable lungs, harm may outweigh the benefit.

Evidence for HFOV, proning, ECMO

- In light of the OSCAR (Oscillation in ARDS) and OSCILLATE (Oscillation in ARDS Treated Early) trials published in 2013, HFOV is slowly falling out of favor, especially so with the advent of ECMO. The OSCILLATE trial showed a higher mortality in patients receiving HFOV for ARDS and was stopped prematurely, while the OSCAR showed no differences in mortality between HFOV and conventional lung protective ventilation.
- Proning is widely used as a lung protective strategy rather than just a salvage therapy in moderate to severe ARDS, particularly so after a significant mortality benefit seen in the PROSEVA study. Proning helps by improving V/Q mismatch in the dorsal lungs and thereby reducing the shunt, increases transpulmonary pressure in the dorsal regions and allows for more homogenous distribution of ventilation.
- The CESAR (Conventional Ventilatory Support vs. Extracorporeal Membrane Oxygenation for Severe Adult Respiratory Failure) trial had

shown a significant mortality benefit with patients of severe ARDS initiated on ECMO, although this trial had some limitations. Evidence for ECMO also strengthened with the Australia and New Zealand (ANZ)-ECMO case series during the H1N1 influenza pandemic. The more recent EOLIA trial done by the ANZICS group showed that early use of ECMO did not significantly improve mortality at 60 days in patients with severe ARDS, but when used as a rescue modality ECMO might help improve survival.

Role of Bicarbonate

- Although it was used in the landmark ARDSNET trial, in 2000, for cases where the pH dropped below 7.15 despite maximum permissive lung protective ventilation, the current consensus is that there is no role for bicarbonate in routine management of respiratory acidosis, as it increases the strong ion difference and can worsen the hypercapnia without a significant change in pH.
- It may be used in cases of cardiac arrest where pH is <7.

Further Reading

Combes A, Hajage D, Capellier G, Demoule A, Lavoue S, Guervilly C, et al. Extracorporeal membrane oxygenation for severe acute respiratory distress syndrome. N Engl J Med. 2018;378(21):1965-75.

Gattinoni L, Taccone P, Carlesso E. Respiratory acidosis: is the correction with bicarbonate worth? Minerva Anestesiol. 2006;72(6):551-7.

van der Zee P, Gommers D. Recruitment maneuvers and higher PEEP, the so-called open lung concept, in patients with ARDS. Crit Care. 2019;23(1):73.

Vincent JL. High-frequency oscillation in acute respiratory distress syndrome. The end of the story? Am J Respir Crit Care Med. 2017;196(6):670-1.

Ans. 307

- This patient can be initiated on venovenous ECMO primarily as he has definitive evidence of respiratory failure and no evidence of cardiogenic shock.
- The preferred route for cannulation would be insertion of the drainage cannula in the femoral vein and return cannula in the right internal jugular vein (IJV). A single dual lumen cannula inserted into the right IJV is also available.
- Extracorporeal membrane oxygenation cannulae are preferably inserted through the percutaneous route by Seldinger technique. After insertion of the guidewire, a bolus dose of 5,000 U (50-100 U/Kg) heparin is administered. The cannulae are secured and ECMO is initiated. Blood flows are kept between 2.5 L and 5 L to maintain adequate oxygenation. Anticoagulation is continued throughout and monitored. Pre- and postmembrane pressures and the transmembrane pressures are monitored.
- Resting lung ventilation should be continued for native lungs with V_t <4 mL/kg, peak inspiratory pressure (PIP) <25 cmH_2O, FiO_2 <0.5, PEEP 5–12 mm Hg.

Further Reading

Extracorporeal Life Support Organization. (2017). Guidelines for Adult Respiratory Failure. [online] Available from https://www.elso.org/Portals/0/ELSO%20Guidelines%20For%20Adult%20Respiratory%20FailuFa%201_4.pdf. [Last Accessed March, 2020].

Ans. 308

This is a picture of VA-ECMO.

- In the femorofemoral or peripheral approach to VA-ECMO, a risk of limb ischemia distal to the arterial cannula is common. A reperfusion cannula can be inserted electively to reduce the risk of limb ischemia.
- Strict monitoring of perfusion in the venous side should also be done, as a compartment syndrome can develop, if the venous drainage from the distal leg is impaired by the drainage cannula.

Ans. 309

- Adults
  - *VA-ECMO*: 50–60 cc/kg/min
  - *VV-ECMO*: 60–80 cc/kg/min

Ans. 310

Possible causes include:

- Blood flow/cardiac output <0.6
- Recirculation
- High pulmonary shunt
- Oxygenator dysfunction.

A systematic approach will be as follows:

- *Check oxygen delivery*: Flowmeter, blender, connections.
- *Check console*: Increase the rpm to increase blood flow, if desaturation occurs, consider recirculation especially if pre- and postmembrane ABGs show high PaO_2.
- In case of decreased flows, flow insufficiency maybe present and patient may be hypovolemic—look for "kicking" in the circuit.
- Optimize cardiac preload, hemoglobin.
- Check oxygenator and look for high transmembrane pressure, commonly due to clots.

Further Reading

Nunes LB, Mendes PV, Hirota AS, Barbosa EV, Maciel AT, Schettino GP, et al. Severe hypoxemia during veno-venous extracorporeal membrane oxygenation: exploring the limits of extracorporeal respiratory support. Clinics (Sao Paulo). 2014;69(3):173-8.

Ans. 311

- Carbon dioxide clearance in ECMO depends on sweep gas flow.
- The sweep gas is either 100% oxygen or carbogen (5% CO_2, 95% O_2) at a flow rate equal to the blood flow rate (1:1). Increasing the sweep flow will increase CO_2 clearance, but will not affect oxygenation.
- For selective CO_2 removal, blood flow can be as low as 1 L/min and sweep gas can be up to 15 L/min, titrated to maintain $PaCO_2$ at 40 mm Hg.
- High sweep gas flows can lead to hypocapnia, alkalosis, and decreased cerebral blood flows.

Ans. 312

- Anticoagulation is usually maintained by monitoring activated clotting time (ACT) in the first 24 hours post-ECMO. ACT should be maintained between 180 seconds and 220 seconds. Post that activated partial thromboplastin

time (PTTK) should be monitored every 6 hourly and maintained between 1.5 times and 2 times the control.
- Other methods include thromboelastography (TEG), factor Xa assays.
- Fibrinogen levels and platelet counts also need to be monitored closely during ECMO.

Further Reading

Doymaz S. Anticoagulation during ECMO: the past, present and future. J Intensive Crit Care. 2018.

Ans. 313

- The patient may be having an increased demand leading to an increase in the native cardiac output. This could be due to fever, sepsis, inadequate sedation or analgesia.
- Sepsis was thought to be a cause of high cardiac output and repeat blood cultures were sent.

Ans. 314

Changes in pharmacokinetics during ECMO are attributed to:
- Sequestration in the circuit
- Increased volume of distribution (V_d)
- Adsorption onto the membrane
- Increased clearance
- Lipophilic highly protein bound antimicrobials—large V_d—sequestered in circuit
- Hydrophilic antimicrobials with a small V_d (β-lactams, aminoglycosides, glycopeptides)—more prone to hemodilution and direct adsorption by the membrane.

Antimicrobial class	*Pharmacokinetic changes*	*Drug-dosing recommendations*
Aminoglycosides	High V_d	Increased loading doses up to 30–35 mg/kg in VA-ECMO, use therapeutic drug monitoring
Carbapenems	Meropenem—degraded and sequestered in the ECMO circuit	30% increase in loading dose with increased daily maintenance dose (2 g 8 hourly)
Piperacillin Tazobactam	Increased V_d and clearance	• Loading dose of 6.75–9 g maybe needed • Continuous infusions over 24 hours have also been recommended in cases of ventilator-associated pneumonia (VAP) to achieve desired intrapulmonary concentrations
Vancomycin	Increased V_d	Loading dose (30 mg/kg) to account for enlarged V_d. Therapeutic drug monitoring is advised

Contd...

Contd...

Colistimethate sodium	Increased V_d	Loading dose: 9 million international units (MIU) followed by 4.5 MIU three times per day (TID) has been proposed
Azoles Voriconazole	High sequestration in circuit	May need 6 mg/kg twice a day (BID) for 1st 4 days, to monitor liver function tests (LFTs) closely

Further Reading

Cheng V, Abdul-Aziz MH, Roberts JA, Shekar K. Optimising drug dosing in patients receiving extracorporeal membrane oxygenation. J Thorac Dis. 2018;10(Suppl 5):S629-41.

Honoré PM, Jacobs R, Spapen H. Antimicrobial dosing during extracorporeal membrane oxygenation. In: Vincent JL (Ed). Annual Update in Intensive Care and Emergency Medicine 2014. Cham: Springer International Publishing; 2014.

Ans. 315

- Computed tomography shows a bilateral pleural effusion with underlying collapse and consolidations of the lungs.
- In view of MSSA growing in BAL and blood, a diagnostic pleural tap maybe required to rule out an empyema.

Ans. 316

Light's criteria

Pleural effusion is likely exudative if at least one of the following exists:

- The ratio of *pleural fluid lactate dehydrogenase (LDH)* and *serum LDH* is greater than 0.6.
- Pleural fluid LDH is greater than 0.6 or 2⁄3 times the normal upper limit for serum.
- The ratio of *pleural fluid protein* and serum protein is greater than 0.5.

Bilateral thoracocentesis indications

- Empyema
- Hemothorax
- Malignancy
- Postoperative ventilation
- *Therapeutic*: Moderate to large effusions with respiratory compromise.

Investigations

Total and differential count, proteins, albumin, LDH levels, glucose, pH, Gram stain, culture and sensitivity.

Ans. 317

- Extracorporeal membrane oxygenation discontinuation can be considered when the native lung is supporting 50–80% of total gas exchange and there is improved lung compliance. Ventilator settings are adjusted as per off ECMO settings.
- The sweep gas is decreased gradually and switched off while observing patients saturation. Blood flow is kept constant, with no gas transfer. Patients are observed for few hours, during which the ventilator settings that are necessary to maintain adequate oxygenation and ventilation off

ECMO are determined. If adequate saturation is maintained and $PaCO_2$ <50 mm Hg, the cannulae are removed 30–60 minutes after stopping heparin.

- In VA-ECMO both cardiac and lung recovery should take place. Appearance of aortic pulsatility correlates with improved left ventricular ejection. Temporary clamping of both the drainage and infusion lines is done, while allowing the ECMO circuit to circulate through a bridge between the arterial and venous limbs. Anticoagulation is to be continued. If hemodynamics and oxygen delivery are optimal on minimum inotropic infusions, consider decannulation.

Further Reading

Broman LM, Malfertheiner MV, Montisci A, Pappalardo F. Weaning from veno-venous extracorporeal membrane oxygenation: how I do it. J Thorac Dis. 2018;10(Suppl 5):S692-7.

Extracorporeal Life Support Organization. (2017). Guidelines for Adult Respiratory Failure. [online] Available from https://www.elso.org/Portals/0/ELSO%20Guidelines%20For%20Adult%20Respiratory%20FailuFa%201_4.pdf. [Last Accessed March, 2020].

Ans. 318

- It is a condition seen in VA-ECMO by the femorofemoral route wherein hypoxia is noted in the upper half of the body. It is seen when cardiac recovery precedes that of the lung. Blood passing through the pulmonary circulation fails to get oxygenated due to a large shunt and leads to blood with low PaO_2 delivered to the brain and upper half of the body.
- Veno-arterial-venous (VA-V) ECMO may alleviate this problem. In this mode oxygenated blood is pumped into the contralateral femoral artery as well as the superior vena cava.

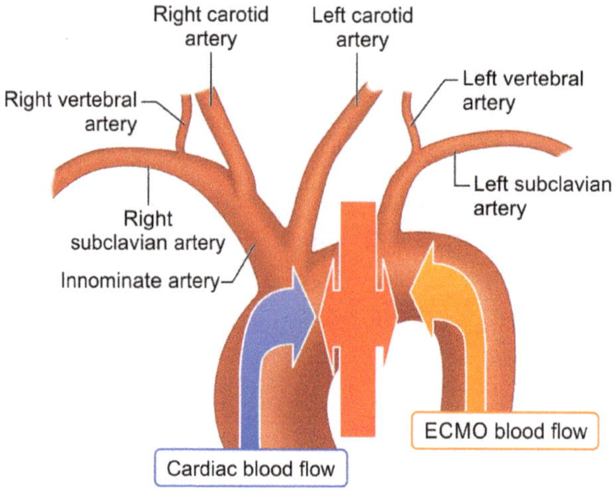

Source: Rupprecht L, Lunz D, Philipp A, Lubnow M, Schmid C. Pitfalls in percutaneous ECMO cannulation. Heart Lung Vessel. 2015;7(4):320-6.

Ans. 319

The given TEG values of R time, K Time, and angle is normal. There is no fibrinolysis as the LY 30 also is normal. Although the value of maximum amplitude (MA) is not given, the shape appears normal. Despite a normal TEG, if the patient is still bleeding, a surgical cause has to be suspected.

Ans. 320

Before placing the order, verify any religious issues that preclude blood transfusion (e.g., Jehovah Witness). Verify the type of product, quantity, and any specific requirements (e.g., irradiation) and decide on the particular sequence in which blood components are to be infused. Take appropriate history regarding any previous transfusion reactions in the past. Reconfirm that the patient's blood is again sent for grouping and cross-matching (also known as a G & S) after proper identification of the patient. Record the pretransfusion vitals and prepare for any emergency that may arise.

Once blood arrives, all blood products should be administered within 4 hours of issue. All bags should be assessed for any leak, clots, contamination, etc. Blood products are to be infused using specific tubing and no infusion or medication should be coadministered. The blood tubing needs to be changed every 4 hours or 4 units, whichever comes first. Cross check the identity by comparing patient name, ID number consent, and cross-match slip. Confirm product expiry date. Reconfirm the physician order before starting blood transfusion.

During blood transfusion, monitor vitals carefully, prior to transfusion and then frequently. Closely monitor for transfusion reaction. Once transfusion is complete, the transfusion record form may be filled and sent back to blood bank.

Further Reading

Doyle GR, McCutcheon JA. Clinical Procedures for Safer Patient Care. Victoria, BC: BCcampus; 2015.

Ans. 321

Massive transfusion is defined as "need of > 10 units of PRBCs in the initial 24 hours of admission" or "need of > 4 packet cell volumes in an hour with anticipation of ongoing need" or "the need to replace at least 50% of the estimated blood volume with blood and blood products within 3 hours of admission." Early initiation of protocolized transfusion aims at replacement of the intravascular volume, prevention of coagulopathy, reduction in the mortality, and blood requirement.

Clinical astuteness is not adequate to predict the need of massive transfusion and hence numerous score have been proposed such as the Assessment of Blood Consumption (ABC) Vandromme score, the Baker Model, Trauma-Associated Severe Haemorrhage (TASH score), the Larson Model, the Cincinnati Individual Transfusion Trigger study (CITT SCORE), the Prince of Wales Hospital (PWH) score, the Massive Transfusion Score, the Shock Index [heart rate/systolic blood pressure (HR/SBP > 0.9)], the Modified Shock Index (MSI) and the Age Shock Index (Age SI), traumatic bleeding severity score (TBSS) and the Trauma-Induced Coagulopathy Clinical Score (TICCS score).

Once the clinical need of massive transfusion is identified, the blood bank needs to be informed regarding the same and a protocolized system of transfusion needs to be called into force **(Flowchart)**. Cross-match is needed for only PRBC concentrate and granulocyte concentrate, and all other blood products such as platelets, fresh frozen plasma (FFP), cryoprecipitate, prothrombin concentrate may be given irrespective of ABO group. In case of emergency, the universal donor is O negative blood and AB plasma.

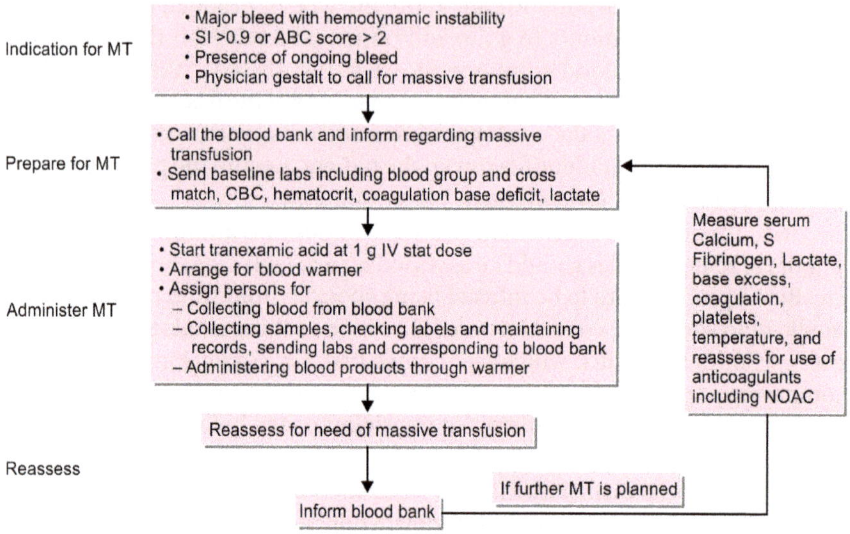

(ABC: assessment of blood consumption; CBC: complete blood count; IV: intravenous; MT: massive transfusion; NOAC: non-vitamin K antagonist oral anticoagulant; SI: shock index)

Ans. 322

Complications of massive transfusion

Transfusion-associated acute lung injury (TRALI) Acute respiratory distress syndrome (ARDS)	• Limit further transfusion. • Lung protective ventilation strategy
Transfusion-associated cardiac overload (TACO)	• Consider stopping further transfusion, respiratory support/higher PEEP • Diuretics, vasodilators
Transfusion-associated immunomodulation (TRIM)	• Use leukodepleted blood
Transmission of infections	• Management as per infection • Send culture from the bag also
Electrolyte abnormalities—hyperkalemia, hypocalcemia	• Management of hyperkalemia
Citrate toxicity	• Calcium supplementation • Watch for seizure
Acidosis	• Usually transient
Hypothermia	• Use of blood warmer for transfusion

Contd...

Contd...

Compartment syndrome	• Surgical consultation, diuretics, decompression of abdomen with Ryle's tube and flatus tube, controlled ventilation
Dilutional coagulopathy	• Use of a massive transfusion protocol or hemostatic resuscitation
Hemolytic transfusion reactions	• Immediately stop the transfusion, send a blood sample for cross-match again • Manage symptomatically with hydration, and vasopressors if needed. Inform blood bank and send the unused blood back.
Allergy reactions	• Stop transfusion and administer antihistamine and corticosteroids

Ans. 323

TRALI is classified as:

- *TRALI type I*: Patients who have no risk factors for ARDS and meet the following criteria: acute nature of onset with hypoxemia documented as a P/F ≤ 300* or SpO_2 < 90% on room air, having clear evidence of bilateral pulmonary edema on imaging (e.g., chest radiograph, chest CT, or ultrasound) with no evidence of left atrial hypertension, or, if left atrial hypertension is present, it is not the main contributor to the hypoxemia that co-occurs during or within 6 hours of transfusion, and the patient had no temporal relationship to any risk factor for ARDS.
- *TRALI type II*: Patients who have risk factors for ARDS (but who have not been diagnosed with ARDS) or who have existing mild ARDS (P/F of 200–300), but whose respiratory status deteriorates§ and is judged to be due to transfusion based on findings as described in categories a and b of TRALI type I, and stable respiratory status in the 12 hours before transfusion.
- Patients who have risk factors for ARDS, and deteriorate not due to transfusion, but as a consequence of the already present ARDS, risk factors will be continued to be labeled as ARDS, similar to those patients whose onset of ARDS was within 6 hours after transfusion but respiratory status was deteriorating in the 12 hours before transfusion or had pre-existing ARDS that further deteriorates after transfusion where the respiratory status was already deteriorating in the 12 hours before transfusion.

Further Reading

Vlaar AP, Toy P, Fung M, Looney MR, Juffermans NP, Bux J, et al. A consensus redefinition of transfusion-related acute lung injury. Transfusion. 2019;59(7):2465-76.

Ans. 324

The figure shows an elevated peak pressure, elevated plateau pressure, and increased oxygen requirement suggestive of significant reduction of intra-abdominal compliance. The differential diagnosis would include pulmonary causes such as ARDS, TRALI, TACO, etc. and extrapulmonary complications such as intra-abdominal hypertension and abdominal compartment syndrome. Given the presence of organ damage, the possibility of intra-abdominal hypertension needs to be kept in mind. Abdominal hypertension is defined as a sustained intra-abdominal pressure (IAP) ≥ 12 mm Hg and if the IAP is sustained > 20 mm Hg (irrespective of abdominal perfusion pressures) and is associated with new organ dysfunction, it is called abdominal compartment syndrome.

Normal IAP is 5–7 mm Hg in critically ill adults.

Intra-abdominal hypertension is further graded as:

- Grade I, IAP 12–15 mm Hg
- Grade II, IAP 16–20 mm Hg
- Grade III, IAP 21–25 mm Hg
- Grade IV, IAP > 25 mm Hg

Inadequate renal perfusion pressure and a reduced renal filtration gradient are the causative factors in the development of renal failure due to abdominal compartment syndrome. The renal filtration gradient across the glomerulus is the difference between the glomerular filtration pressure (GFP) and the pressure in the proximal tubules. In cases of intra-abdominal hypertension, the pressure inside the tubules parallels the IAP.

As the GFP is estimated as MAP minus IAP, the filtration gradient is calculated as = GFP – PTP = (MAP – IAP) – IAP = MAP – 2 × IAP. Thus, it can be seen that the renal filtration gradient is dependent on both MAP and IAP.

Ans. 325

Intra-abdominal pressure is measured in mm Hg at the end of expiration, keeping the patient completely supine. All abdominal muscle activities are to be ruled out. Twenty-five milliliters of saline is instilled into the bladder and the transducer should be zeroed in the midaxillary line at the level of the iliac crest.

It was decided to open up the sutures and release the tension. Abdominal wall was opened up and vacuum system applied. Patient was shifted back to ICU for further stabilization.

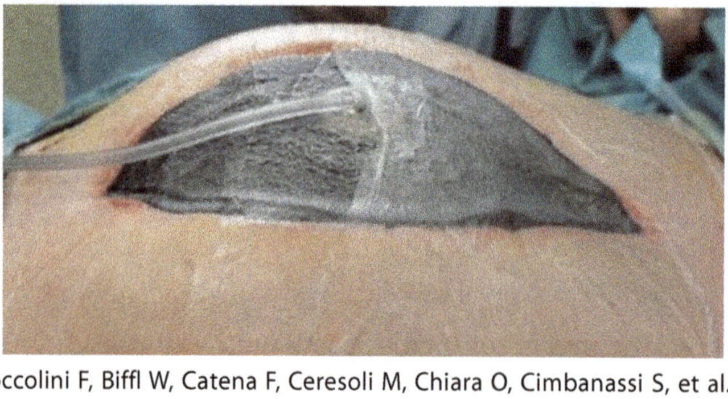

Source: Coccolini F, Biffl W, Catena F, Ceresoli M, Chiara O, Cimbanassi S, et al. The open abdomen, indications, management and definitive closure. World J Emerg Surg. 2015;10:32.

Further Reading

Malbrain ML, Cheatham ML, Kirkpatrick A, Sugrue M, Parr M, De Waele J, et al. Results from the International Conference of Experts on Intra-abdominal Hypertension and Abdominal Compartment Syndrome. I. Definitions. Intensive Care Med. 2006;32(11):1722-32.

Ans. 326

- In nerve studies, with demyelination, the motor conduction velocity reduces and distal motor latency is prolonged. The sensory neurons are usually spared. The compound muscle action potentials amplitude is usually reduced in cases of axonopathies such as diabetes, traumatic nerve injury, and in critical illness polyneuromyopathy but can be reduced in demyelination also due to conduction blocks. The F wave denotes changes in roots, are prolonged, or absent in cases of demyelination.
- The above report suggests features of early demyelinating axonopathy of the median ulnar and tibial nerve roots with normal sensory pattern. In the clinical background, the diagnosis is probably acute motor axonal neuropathy (AMAN) variant of Guillain-Barré syndrome (GBS).

Further Reading

Mallik A, Weir AI. Nerve conduction studies: essentials and pitfalls in practice. J Neurol Neurosurg Psychiatr. 2005;76:ii23-ii31.

Ans. 327

Dose of plasmapheresis is usually calculated as:

One to one-and-a half times the plasma volume is replaced per schedule, and the whole procedure is repeated four to six treatments over 7–10 days. The estimated plasma volume (in liters) = 0.07 × bodyweight (kg) × (1 - hematocrit). In acute GBS, it may be necessary to perform plasma exchange once or twice a week till clinical improvement.

TABLE 1: ASFA category I indications for therapeutic plasma exchange.

Specialty	*Condition*
Neurology	Acute Guillain-Barré syndrome
	Chronic inflammatory demyelinating polyneuropathy
	Myasthenia gravis
	Polyneuropathy associated with paraproteinemias
	Pediatric autoimmune neuropsychiatric disorder (PANDAS)*
Hematology	Thrombotic thrombocytopenic purpura
	Atypical hemolytic uremic syndrome (autoantibody to factor H)
	Hyperviscosity syndromes (paraproteinemias)
	Severe/symptomatic cryoglobulinemia
Renal	Good pasture's syndrome (antiglomerular basement membrane antibodies)
	Antineutrophil cytoplasmic antibody (ANCA)-associated rapidly progressive glomerulonephritis
	Recurrent focal segmental glomerular sclerosis
	Antibody-mediated renal transplant rejection
Metabolic	Familial hypercholesterolemia (homozygous)
	Fulminant Wilson's disease

(ASFA: American Society for Apheresis)

*Pediatric autoimmune neuropsychiatric disorders associated with streptococcal infection.

TABLE 2: ASFA category II indications for therapeutic plasma exchange (established second-line therapy).

Specialty	*Condition*
Neurology	Lambert-Eaton myasthenic syndrome
	Acute exacerbation of multiple sclerosis
	Chronic focal encephalitis
	Neuromyelitis optica
Hematology	ABO-incompatible hemopoietic stem-cell transplantation
	Pure red cell aplasia
	Life-threatening cold agglutinin disease
	Atypical hemolytic uremic syndrome (complement factor gene mutations)
	Myeloma with cast nephropathy
	Red cell alloimmunization in pregnancy
Immunological	Catastrophic antiphospholipid syndrome
	Cerebral systemic lupus erythematosus (SLE)
Metabolic	Refsum's disease

(ASFA: American Society for Apheresis)
Source: Norfolk D. Handbook of Transfusion Medicine, 5th edition. 2013.

Ans. 328

- The Kidney Disease Improving Global Outcomes (KDIGO) definition and staging system is the most recent and preferred definition.
- The KDIGO guidelines define AKI as follows:
  - Increase in serum creatinine by ≥0.3 mg/dL (≥26.5 µmol/L) within 48 hours, or
  - Increase in serum creatinine to ≥1.5 times baseline, which is known or presumed to have occurred within the prior seven days, or
  - Urine volume <0.5 mL/kg/hour for six hours
- Before diagnosing and classifying AKI, one should assess and optimize volume status and exclude obstruction.
- Classification of AKI:
  - *Stage 1:* Increase in serum creatinine to 1.5 to 1.9 times baseline, or increase in serum creatinine by ≥0.3 mg/dL (≥26.5 µmol/L), or reduction in urine output to <0.5 mL/kg/hour for 6 to 12 hours.
  - *Stage 2:* Increase in serum creatinine to 2.0 to 2.9 times baseline, or reduction in urine output to <0.5 mL/kg/hour for ≥12 hours.
  - *Stage 3:* Increase in serum creatinine to 3.0 times baseline, or increase in serum creatinine to ≥4.0 mg/dL (≥353.6 µmol/L), or reduction in urine output to <0.3 mL/kg/hour for ≥24 hours, or anuria for ≥12 hours, or the initiation of renal replacement therapy, or, in patients <18 years, decrease in estimated glomerular filtration rate (eGFR) to <35 mL/min/1.73 m^2.

Ans. 329

As per the definition:

- There is no mention of increasing PEEP and FiO2 requirement after a period of stable oxygenation
- Although WBC is elevated and temperature spikes are present, there is no mention of change in antibiotics
- As per definition, enterococci, Candida, and coagulase negative Staphylococcus aureus in BAL is not considered as VAP, unless isolated from lung tissue or pleural fluid.

Further Reading

CDC. Pneumonia (Ventilator-associated [VAP] and non-ventilator-associated Pneumonia [PNEU]) Event. [online] Available from https://www.cdc.gov/nhsn/pdfs/pscmanual/6pscvapcurrent.pdf [Last accessed February, 2020].

Ans. 330

It is CODMAN MICROSENSOR® Ventricular Catheter Kit. It measures the intracranial pressure (ICP) via a strain gauge microchip located at the tip of the catheter. Pressure is reflected as an electrical voltage that is transmitted to the proximal end of the catheter through nylon encapsulated copper wires. The catheter is connected to the Codman ExpressTM monitor, which displays the ICP.

EU GSPR Authorised Reprsentative
Logos Europe, 9 rue Nicolas Poussin
1700, La Rochelle, France
Phone: +33 (0) 6 67 93 73 78
E-mail: contact@logoseurope.eu

www.ingramcontent.com/pod-product-compliance
Ingram Content Group UK Ltd.
Pitfield, Milton Keynes, MK11 3LW, UK
UKHW050427150426
5217IPUK00019B/1271
9789390020492